P9-AFZ-460

Advances in
Neurochemistry

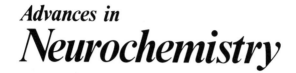

Volume 4

Advances in Neurochemistry

ADVISORY EDITORS

J. Axelrod	E. M. Gál	F. Margolis	J. S. O'Brien
F. Fonnum	H. R. Mahler	P. Morell	E. Roberts

A Continuation Order Plan is available for this series. A continuation order will bring delivery of each new volume immediately upon publication. Volumes are billed only upon actual shipment. For further information please contact the publisher.

Advances in
Neurochemistry

Volume 4

Edited by

B. W. Agranoff
Mental Health Research Institute and
Department of Biological Chemistry
University of Michigan
Ann Arbor, Michigan

and

M. H. Aprison
Institute of Psychiatric Research and
Department of Psychiatry and Biochemistry
Indiana University School of Medicine
Indianapolis, Indiana

PLENUM PRESS • NEW YORK AND LONDON

The Library of Congress cataloged the first volume of this series as follows:

Advances in neurochemistry/edited by B.W. Agranoff and M.H. Aprison.
–New York: Plenum Press, [1975-
v.   : ill.; 24 cm.
Includes bibliographies and index.
ISBN 0-306-39221-6 (v. 1)

1. Neurochemistry. I. Agranoff, Bernard W., 1926-   II. Aprison, M. H.,
1923-
[DNLM: 1. Neurochemistry — Period. W1 AD684E]
QP356.3.A37   612'.822   75-8710

LIBRARY

MAY 1 8 1982

UNIVERSITY OF THE PACIFIC

393405
Science

ISBN 0-306-40678-0

© 1982 Plenum Press, New York
A Division of Plenum Publishing Corporation
233 Spring Street, New York, N.Y. 10013

All rights reserved

No part of this book may be reproduced, stored in a retrieval system, or transmitted,
in any form or by any means, electronic, mechanical, photocopying, microfilming,
recording, or otherwise, without permission from the Publisher

Printed in the United States of America

CONTRIBUTORS

E. MARTIN GÁL ● *Neurochemical Research Laboratories, Department of Psychiatry, University of Iowa, Iowa City, Iowa*

LOUIS SOKOLOFF ● *Laboratory of Cerebral Metabolism, National Institute of Mental Health, U.S. Public Health Service, Department of Health and Human Services, Bethesda, Maryland*

HERBERT WIEGANDT ● *Physiologisch Chemisches Institut, Philipps Universität Marburg, Marburg, German Federal Republic*

PREFACE

This series has been directed at providing scientists possessing considerable biochemical background with specialized reviews of neurobiological interest. Some have dealt with completed bodies of research, while others consist of extensive reports of research in progress, judged to be of current interest to the active researcher. We have selected recognized scientists and allowed them freedom to reflect and speculate in the field in which they have achieved prominence. We note with sadness the passing of Dr. Jordi Folch-Pi, who served as an advisory editor when the series was initiated. He played a central role in the development of neurochemistry, as well as the creation of professional societies and journals. He will be remembered fondly by all those whose lives he touched.

The editors acknowledge the cooperation of the Upjohn Company in the preparation of the color plate included in this volume. We also acknowledge the skillful editorial assistance of Dr. Kenneth C. Leskawa. We are pleased to honor the retirement of Dr. E. Martin Gál, a former advisory editor of *Advances*, with the inclusion of a chapter by him in this volume.

B. W. Agranoff
M. H. Aprison

CONTENTS

CHAPTER 2

**BIOSYNTHESIS AND FUNCTION OF UNCONJUGATED
PTERINS IN MAMMALIAN TISSUES**

E. MARTIN GÁL

CHAPTER 3
THE GANGLIOSIDES
HERBERT WIEGANDT

THE RADIOACTIVE DEOXYGLUCOSE METHOD

THEORY, PROCEDURE, AND APPLICATIONS FOR THE MEASUREMENT OF LOCAL GLUCOSE UTILIZATION IN THE CENTRAL NERVOUS SYSTEM

LOUIS SOKOLOFF

Laboratory of Cerebral Metabolism
National Institute of Mental Health
U.S. Public Health Service
Department of Health and Human Services
Bethesda, Maryland

1. INTRODUCTION

The brain is a complex, heterogeneous organ composed of many anatomical and functional components with markedly different levels of functional activity that vary independently with time and function. Other tissues are generally far more homogeneous with most of their cells functioning similarly and synchro-

Abbreviations used in this chapter: DG, 2-deoxyglucose; DG-6-P, 2-deoxyglucose-6-phosphate; G-6-P, glucose-6-phosphate

nously in response to a common stimulus or regulatory influence. The central nervous system, however, consists of innumerable subunits each integrated into its own set of functional pathways and networks and subserving only one or a few of the many activities in which the nervous system participates. Understanding how the nervous system functions requires knowledge not only of the mechanisms of excitation and inhibition but even more so of their precise localization in the nervous system and the relationships of neural subunits to specific functions.

Historically, studies of the central nervous system have concentrated heavily on localization of function and mapping of pathways related to specific functions. These have been carried out neuroanatomically and histologically with staining and degeneration techniques, behaviorally with ablation and stimulation techniques, electrophysiologically with electrical recording and evoked electrical responses, and histochemically with a variety of techniques, including fluorescent and immunofluorescent methods and autoradiography of orthograde and retrograde axoplasmic flow. Many of these conventional methods suffer from a sampling problem. They generally permit examination of only one potential pathway at a time, and only positive results are interpretable. Furthermore, the demonstration of a pathway reveals only a potential for function; it does not reveal its significance in normal function.

Tissues that do physical and/or chemical work, such as heart, kidney, and skeletal muscle, exhibit a close relationship between energy metabolism and functional activity. From the measurement of energy metabolism it is possible to estimate the level of functional activity. The existence of a similar relationship in the tissues of the central nervous system has been more difficult to prove, partly because of uncertainty about the nature of the work associated with nervous functional activity, but mainly because of the difficulty in assessing the levels of functional and metabolic activities in the same functional component of the brain at the same time. Much of our present knowledge of cerebral energy metabolism *in vivo* has been obtained by means of the nitrous oxide technique of Kety and Schmidt (1948*a*) and its modifications (Scheinberg and Stead, 1949; Lassen and Munck, 1955; Eklöf *et al.*, 1973; Gjedde *et al.*, 1975), which measure the average rates of energy metabolism in the brain as a whole. These methods have demonstrated changes in cerebral metabolic rate in association with gross or diffuse alterations of cerebral function and/or structure, such as, for example, those that occur during postnatal development, aging, senility, anesthesia, disorders of consciousness, and convulsive states (Kety, 1950, 1957; Lassen, 1959; Sokoloff, 1960, 1976). However, these methods have not detected changes in cerebral metabolic rate in a number of conditions with, perhaps, more subtle alterations in cerebral functional activity, e.g., deep slow-wave sleep, performance of mental arithmetic, sedation and tranquilization, schizophrenia, and LSD-induced psychosis (Kety, 1950; Lassen, 1959; Sokoloff, 1969). It is possible that there are no changes in cerebral energy metabolism in these conditions. The apparent lack of change could also be explained by either a redistribution of local levels of functional and metabolic activity, without significant change in the average of the brain as a whole, or the restriction of altered metabolic activity to regions too small to be detected in measurements of the brain as a whole. What has clearly been needed is a method that measures the rates of energy metabolism in specific discrete regions of the brain in normal and altered states of functional activity.

Kety and associates (Landau *et al.*, 1955; Freygang and Sokoloff, 1958; Kety, 1960; Reivich *et al.*, 1969) developed a quantitative autoradiographic technique to measure the local tissue concentrations of chemically inert, diffusible, radioactive tracers, which they used to determine the rates of blood flow simultaneously in all the structural components visible and identifiable in autoradiographs of serial sections of the brain. The application of this quantitative autoradiographic technique to the determination of local cerebral metabolic rate has proved to be more difficult because of the inherently greater complexity of the problem and the unsuitability of the labeled species of the normal substrates of cerebral energy metabolism, oxygen and glucose. The radioisotopes of oxygen have too short a physical half-life. Both oxygen and glucose are too rapidly converted to carbon dioxide (CO_2), which is then cleared from the cerebral tissues too rapidly. Sacks (1957), for example, has found in man significant losses of $^{14}CO_2$ from the brain within 2 min after the onset of an intravenous infusion of [^{14}C]glucose, labeled either uniformly or in the C-1, C-2, or C-6 position. These limitations of [^{14}C]glucose have been avoided by the use of 2-deoxy-D-[^{14}C]glucose, a labeled analogue of glucose with special properties that make it particularly appropriate for this application (Sokoloff *et al.*, 1977). It is metabolized through part of the pathway of glucose metabolism at a definable rate relative to that of glucose. Unlike glucose, however, its product, [^{14}C]deoxyglucose-6-phosphate, is essentially trapped in the tissues, thus allowing the application of the quantitative autoradiographic technique. The use of radioactive 2-deoxyglucose to trace glucose utilization and the autoradiographic technique to achieve regional localization has recently led to the development of a method that measures the rates of glucose utilization simultaneously in all components of the central nervous system in the normal conscious state and during experimental physiological, pharmacological, and pathological conditions (Sokoloff *et al.*, 1977). Because the procedure is so designed that the concentrations of radioactivity in the tissues during autoradiography are more or less proportional to the rates of glucose utilization, the autoradiographs provide pictorial representations of the relative rates of glucose utilization in all the cerebral structures visualized. Numerous studies with this method have established that there is a close relationship between functional activity and energy metabolism in the central nervous system (Sokoloff,

1977; Plum *et al.*, 1976). The method has become a potent new tool for mapping functional neural pathways on the basis of evoked metabolic responses.

2. THEORETICAL BASIS OF THE RADIOACTIVE 2-DEOXYGLUCOSE METHOD

2.1. Biochemical Properties of 2-Deoxyglucose in Brain

2-Deoxy-D-glucose differs from glucose only in the replacement of the hydroxyl group on the second carbon atom by a hydrogen atom. The remainder of the molecule is indistinguishable from that of glucose. It is metabolized qualitatively exactly like glucose until a point in the glycolytic pathway is reached where its anomalous structure prevents its further metabolism. Thus, deoxyglucose is transported between blood and brain tissues by the same saturable carrier that transports glucose (Bidder, 1968; Bachelard, 1971; Oldendorf, 1971; Horton *et al.*, 1973). In the tissues it competes with glucose for hexokinase, which phosphorylates both substrates to their respective hexose-6-phosphates (Sols and Crane, 1954). It is at this point in the biochemical pathway that the further metabolism of the two compounds diverges.

Glucose-6-phosphate is converted to fructose-6-phosphate by phosphohexoseisomerase and metabolized further via the glycolytic pathway and tricarboxylic acid cycle. 2-Deoxyglucose-6-phosphate cannot be isomerized to fructose-6-phosphate because of the lack of a hydroxyl group on its second carbon atom; therefore, its metabolism ceases at this point in the pathway (Sols and Crane, 1954; Wick *et al.*, 1957; Tower, 1958; Bachelard *et al.*, 1971; Horton *et al.*, 1973). Although not a substrate for further metabolism, deoxyglucose-6-phosphate does have an affinity for the phosphohexoseisomerase and, when present in sufficiently high concentrations, can competitively inhibit glucose-6-phosphate metabolism at this point (Wick *et al.*, 1957; Tower, 1958; Horton *et al.*, 1973). Indeed, it is probably mainly by this competitive inhibition at the phosphohexoseisomerase step that pharmacological doses of deoxyglucose lead to an inhibition of glycolysis and produce a clinical syndrome like that of hypoglycemic coma (Tower, 1958; Landau and Lubs, 1958; Horton *et al.*, 1973; Meldrum and Horton, 1973); inhibition at the hexokinase step, either competitively by deoxyglucose or by depletion of adenosine triphosphate (ATP), may also be contributory (Tower, 1958; Horton *et al.*, 1973).

There are alternative pathways of glucose-6-phosphate metabolism, but these do not appear to have significant influence on the fate of deoxyglucose-6-

phosphate in brain. Glucose-6-phosphate can be oxidized by glucose-6-phosphate dehydrogenase, the first step in the hexosemonophosphate shunt, but deoxyglucose-6-phosphate does not appear to be a substrate for this enzyme (Sols and Crane, 1954; Tower, 1958; Horton *et al.*, 1973). Glucose-6-phosphate can also be hydrolyzed back to free glucose by glucose-6-phosphatase. The activity of this enzyme has been reported to be very low in mammalian brain (Hers and DeDuve, 1950; Hers, 1957; Raggi *et al.*, 1960; Prasannan and Subrahmanyam, 1968), but its possible influence in the deoxyglucose technique will be considered in greater detail in Section 4.3.

2.2. Description of Theoretical Model

The theoretical basis of the [^{14}C]deoxyglucose technique is derived from the analysis of a model of the biochemical behavior of deoxyglucose in brain. This model is diagrammatically illustrated in Figure 1. According to the model, [^{14}C]deoxyglucose and glucose in the plasma share and compete for a common carrier in the blood–brain barrier for transport from plasma to brain. [^{14}C]Deoxyglucose and glucose, transported into a homogeneous tissue, enter a common precursor pool in which they compete either for the carrier for trans-

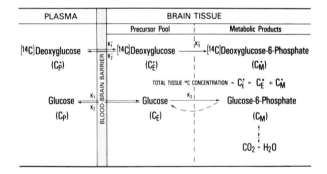

FIGURE 1. Diagrammatic representation of the theoretical model. C_i^* represents the total ^{14}C concentration in a single homogeneous tissue of the brain. C_P^* and C_P represent the concentrations of [^{14}C]-DG and glucose in the arterial plasma, respectively; C_E^* and C_E represent their respective concentrations in the tissue pools that serve as substrates for hexokinase. C_M^* represents the concentration of [^{14}C]-DG-6-P in the tissue. The constants k_1^*, k_2^*, and k_3^* represent the rate constants for carrier-mediated transport of [^{14}C]-DG from plasma to tissue and back from tissue to plasma, and for phosphorylation by hexokinase, respectively. The constants k_1, k_2, and k_3 are the equivalent rate constants for glucose. [^{14}C]-DG and glucose share and compete for the carrier, which transports both between plasma and tissue, and for hexokinase, which phosphorylates them to their respective hexose-6-phosphates. The dashed arrow represents the possibility of G-6-P hydrolysis by glucose-6-phosphatase activity. (From Sokoloff *et al.*, 1977.)

port back from brain to plasma or for the enzyme, hexokinase, which phosphorylates them to [^{14}C]deoxyglucose-6-phosphate ([^{14}C]-DG-6-P) and glucose-6-phosphate (G-6-P), respectively. The hexokinase reaction is essentially irreversible, and inasmuch as [^{14}C]-DG-6-P is not a suitable substrate for any other enzymes known to be present in significant amounts, it is trapped and accumulates as it is formed. On the other hand, G-6-P does not accumulate but is eventually metabolized further to CO_2 and water. The model allows for the possibility that a fraction of the G-6-P is hydrolyzed back to free glucose by glucose-6-phosphatase activity (broken arrow in Figure 1).

The essential features of the model are founded on these experimentally established biochemical properties of deoxyglucose (DG) in cerebral metabolism. The application of this model to the quantification of local cerebral glucose utilization is dependent, however, on the validity of some additional assumptions and/or conditions:

1. The model is applicable only to a localized region of tissue that is homogeneous with respect to the following: rate of blood flow; rates of transport of [^{14}C]-DG and glucose between plasma and tissue; concentrations of [^{14}C]-DG, glucose, [^{14}C]-DG-6-P, and G-6-P; and rate of glucose utilization.

2. The [^{14}C]-DG and [^{14}C]-DG-6-P are present in tracer amounts, i.e., their molecular concentrations in blood and/or tissues are quantitatively negligible and pharmacologically inactive.

3. To facilitate mathematical analysis of the model it is assumed that all of the free [^{14}C]-DG and glucose in each homogeneous element of tissue is present in a single compartment in which their concentrations are those of the precursor pools for the hexokinase reaction and the carrier-mediated transport from tissue to plasma. Inasmuch as there are extracellular and intracellular spaces and multiple cell types in each such element of tissue, this assumption is not fully valid. It will be seen (Section 2.3), after the operational equation is derived and the finally adopted procedure is described, that the design of the procedure serves to minimize, if not eliminate, possible errors arising from invalidity of this assumption.

4. Carbohydrate metabolism in the brain is in a steady state. The plasma glucose concentration, the rate of local cerebral glucose utilization, and the concentrations of the intermediates of the glycolytic pathway remain constant throughout the period of measurement.

5. The capillary plasma concentrations of [^{14}C]-DG and glucose are approximately equal to or bear a constant relationship to their arterial plasma concentrations. Experiments in this laboratory have demonstrated that the cerebral extraction ratio of [^{14}C]-DG is normally very low, approximately 5%; the mean capillary plasma concentration can-

not differ, therefore, by more than 5% from the arterial plasma level. In the case of glucose a constant relationship between arterial and capillary concentrations is implicit in the assumption of steady state conditions for glucose delivery and metabolism.

2.3. Mathematical Analysis of Model

At any time following the introduction of [^{14}C]-DG into the blood, C_i^*, the total content of ^{14}C per unit mass of any tissue, i, is equal to the sum of the concentrations of the free [^{14}C]-DG in the precursor pool in the tissue, C_E^*, and its product, [^{14}C]-DG-6-P, C_M^*, in that tissue (Figure 1). Therefore,

$$C_i^* = C_E^* + C_M^* \tag{1}$$

and the derivative of equation (1) with respect to time, t, is

$$dC_i^*/dt = dC_E^*/dt + dC_M^*/dt \tag{2}$$

The rate of change of the free [^{14}C]-DG concentration in the tissue, dC_E^*/dt, is equal to the difference between the rates of its transport into the tissue from the plasma and its loss from the tissue by transport back to the plasma or by hexokinase-catalyzed phosphorylation to [^{14}C]-DG-6-P. This relationship can be described by the equation

$$dC_E^*/dt = k_1^* C_P^* - k_2^* C_E^* - k_3^* C_E^* \tag{3}$$

where C_P^* equals the concentration of [^{14}C]-DG in the arterial plasma, and k_1^*, k_2^*, and k_3^* are the rate constants for the transport of [^{14}C]-DG from plasma to brain tissue, for the transport of free [^{14}C]-DG back from tissue to plasma, and for the phosphorylation of [^{14}C]-DG in the tissue, respectively. The term in which each rate constant appears represents the rate of the process to which it applies.

It should be noted that C_P^* actually represents mean capillary rather than arterial plasma concentration. Capillary concentration, however, is not readily measured. Inasmuch as the difference between arterial and cerebral venous [^{14}C]-DG concentrations is generally less than 5% of the arterial level, the mean capillary plasma concentration can reasonably closely be approximated by the arterial plasma concentration. Furthermore, as will be seen in this section, any potential error associated with this approximation is partially counteracted by a corresponding approximation made for the plasma glucose concentration.

The assumption of first-order rate constants, k_1^*, k_2^*, and k_3^*, in the mathematical description of saturable processes, such as carrier-mediated transport and enzyme-catalyzed reactions, might appear to be questionable. With saturable processes first-order kinetics apply to only a narrow range of the lowest substrate concentrations. The basic requirements and assumptions of the model presented above provide conditions, however, in which k_1^*, k_2^*, and k_3^* behave as true first-order rate constants. For example, [^{14}C]-DG and glucose compete for the same carrier for transport from plasma into brain. The rate of inward transport of [^{14}C]-DG can, therefore, be described by the classical Michaelis–Menten equation, modified for the influence of the presence of the competitive substrate, glucose (Dixon and Webb, 1964). Thus,

$$v_i^* = \frac{V_M^* C_P^*}{K_M^*(1 + C_P/K_M) + C_P^*} \tag{4}$$

where v_i^* represents the rate of inward transport of [^{14}C]-DG, V_M^* represents the maximal velocity of [^{14}C]-DG transport, K_M^* and K_M are the apparent Michaelis–Menten constants of the carrier for [^{14}C]-DG and glucose, respectively, and C_P^* and C_P are the plasma concentrations of [^{14}C]-DG and glucose, respectively.

The model, however, requires that the [^{14}C]-DG be administered in tracer amounts and that tracer theory apply. C_P^* can therefore be considered to be negligible compared to $K_M^* (1 + C_P/K_M)$ and thus

$$v_i^* = \left[\frac{V_M^*}{K_M^*(1 + C_P/K_M)} \right] C_P^* \tag{5}$$

In equation (3) it is assumed that

$$v_i^* = k_1^* C_P^* \tag{6}$$

Equating equations (5) and (6),

$$k_1^* = \frac{V_M^*}{K_M^*(1 + C_P/K_M)} \tag{7}$$

The model also requires a steady state of cerebral glucose utilization and a constant arterial plasma glucose concentration, i.e., a constant C_P. It is apparent then that within the constraints imposed by the model k_1^* is a constant independent of the plasma [^{14}C]-DG concentration and, therefore, a true first-order rate constant.

By comparable analyses k_2^* and k_3^* can be similarly defined and shown to be true rate constants as used in equation (3). Equation (3) can therefore be integrated and solved for C_E^* as a function of time as follows:

$$C_E^*(T) = k_1^* e^{-(k_2^*+k_3^*)} T \int_0^T C_P^* e^{(k_2^*+k_3^*)t} dt \tag{8}$$

where T is any given time elapsed following the introduction of the $[^{14}C]$-DG into the circulation.

The tissue concentration of $[^{14}C]$-DG-6-P as a function of time can also be mathematically described. dC_M^*/dt equals the rate of formation and accumulation of $[^{14}C]$-DG-6-P per unit mass of tissue. Thus

$$dC_M^*/dt = k_3^* C_E^* \tag{9}$$

Substituting for C_E^* its equivalent function defined in equation (8) and integrating and solving for C_M^*,

$$C_M^*(\tau) = k_1^* k_3^* \int_0^\tau \left[e^{-(k_2^*+k_3^*)T} \int_0^T C_P^* e^{(k_2^*+k_3^*)t} dt \right] dT \tag{10}$$

where τ is any given time elapsed following the introduction of the $[^{14}C]$-DG into the circulation.

The functions for C_E^* and C_M^* defined in equations (8) and (10), respectively, can now be substituted for these variables in equation (1) to obtain the following equation:

$$C_i^*(\tau) = k_1^* e^{-(k_2^*+k_3^*)\tau} \int_0^\tau C_P^* e^{(k_2^*+k_3^*)t} dt \tag{11}$$

$$+ k_1^* k_3^* \int_0^\tau \left[e^{(k_2^*+k_3^*)T} \int_0^T C_P^* e^{(k_2^*+k_3^*)t} dt \right] dT$$

Equation (11) defines the total tissue concentration of ^{14}C as a function of time in terms of the history of the plasma concentration from zero time to any given time, τ, and the rate constants k_1^*, k_2^*, and k_3^*. The application of this equation to the determination of the rate constants will be described.

The behavior of glucose is similar to that of $[^{14}C]$-DG, but its mathematical description is simpler because of the assumptions of a constant arterial plasma glucose concentration and a steady state of glucose uptake and metabolism in brain. Thus,

$$dC_E/dt = k_1 C_P - k_2 C_E - k_3 C_E \tag{12}$$

where C_P and C_E represent the free glucose concentrations in arterial plasma and brain tissue, respectively, and k_1, k_2, and k_3 represent the rate constants for transport of glucose from plasma to tissue, for transport back from tissue to plasma, and for the phosphorylation of free glucose in the tissue to G-6-P by hexokinase, respectively.

Again, as in the case of $[^{14}C]$-DG, C_P should represent mean capillary plasma glucose concentration but can be approximated by the arterial plasma concentration because of the generally low net extraction of glucose from cerebral blood. Furthermore, as can be seen in the operational equation (Section 2.3.1) on which the method is based, it is the ratio of plasma $[^{14}C]$-DG and glucose concentrations that is most critical. The application of the same approximation to both substances therefore tends to cancel the effects of the approximations.

The constants, k_1, k_2, and k_3, also behave as first-order rate constants. With saturable processes such as carrier-mediated transport and enzyme-catalyzed reactions, they are obviously influenced by the plasma and tissue concentrations of glucose. However, the model requires steady state conditions, e.g., constant plasma and tissue concentrations of glucose, throughout the duration of the procedure. Under those circumstances k_1, k_2, and k_3 become constants of proportionality between the constant rates of the process and the constant glucose concentrations in the pools to which they apply. They are, however, affected by the glucose concentration; the higher the glucose concentration, the lower the value of the rate constant.

The assumption of a steady state also means that dC_E/dt in equation (12) equals zero. Equation (12) can then be solved as follows:

$$C_E = [k_1/(k_2 + k_3)] C_P \qquad (13)$$

The combination of constants, $k_1/(k_2 + k_3)$, is therefore equal to the distribution ratio of glucose between the tissue and plasma in the steady state. It is equivalent to the tissue–plasma partition coefficient or, more appropriately, the distribution volume for glucose per unit mass of tissue.

2.3.1. Derivation of Operational Equation

The mathematical analysis of the model has been extended to derive an operational equation that defines the variables to be measured and the procedures to be followed to determine local cerebral glucose utilization.

When $[^{14}C]$-DG is introduced into the circulation, the ^{14}C is taken up by the tissues of the brain. Because the ^{14}C can be present in only two chemical species, $[^{14}C]$-DG and $[^{14}C]$-DG-6-P, then the rate of change of the total concentration of ^{14}C in any tissue, C_i^*, must be equal to the sum of the rates of change of the concentrations of $[^{14}C]$-DG and $[^{14}C]$-DG-6-P in that tissue. Thus

$$dC_i^*/dt = dC_E^*/dt + dC_M^*/dt \qquad (14)$$

dC_M^*/dt is the rate of change of the $[^{14}C]$-DG-6-P concentration in the tissue. Inasmuch as it is assumed that the $[^{14}C]$-DG-6-P is trapped as it is formed, the rate of change in its concentration must be equal to its rate of formation. Therefore,

$$dC_M^*/dt = v^* \qquad (15)$$

where v^* equals the velocity of the hexokinase-catalyzed phosphorylation of $[^{14}C]$-DG per unit mass of the tissue.

Combining equations (14) and (15):

$$dC_i^*/dt = dC_E^*/dt + v^* \qquad (16)$$

Because glucose metabolism in the tissue is assumed to be in a steady state, the rate of glucose uptake by the tissue from the blood is equal to the rate of glucose utilization, R_i. When a metabolic pathway is in a steady state, there is no change in concentration of any of the intermediates of that pathway; therefore, the net rate through any step in that pathway is equal to the overall rate of the pathway as a whole. It follows that with glucose metabolism in a steady state, the net rate of G-6-P formation is equal to the rate of glucose utilization. The net rate of G-6-P formation equals the difference between its rate of synthesis by hexokinase-catalyzed phosphorylation of glucose and its rate of dephosphorylation by phosphatase activity, if any. Therefore,

$$R_i = v - r \qquad (17)$$

where v represents the rate of phosphorylation of glucose, and r represents the rate of G-6-P hydrolysis, indicated by the dashed arrow in Figure 1. Factoring out v in Equation (17),

$$R_i = (1 - r/v)v = \Phi v \qquad (18)$$

where $\Phi = 1 - r/v$.

In a steady state v and r are constants. Therefore, Φ is also a constant, between zero and one, that represents the fraction of glucose which, once phosphorylated, is metabolized further, and Φv equals the rate of glucose utilization. Inasmuch as there is little glucose-6-phosphatase in brain, Φ can be expected to be very close to one.

Dividing equation (16) by R_i or its equivalent Φv,

$$\frac{dC_i^*/dt}{R_i} = \frac{dC_E^*/dt}{R_i} + \frac{v^*}{\Phi v} \tag{19}$$

[^{14}C]-DG and glucose are competitive substrates for hexokinase, and v^* and v represent their rates of phosphorylation, respectively, under these conditions of mutual competitive inhibition. Solution of the rate equations for two substrates competing for the same enzyme leads to the classical Michaelis–Menten relationship, which is modified to take into account the influence of the competitive substrate (Dixon and Webb, 1964). Thus

$$v^*/v = \frac{C_E^* V_m^*/[K_m^*(1 + C_E/K_m) + C_E^*]}{C_E V_m/[K_m(1 + C_E^*/K_m^*) + C_E]} \tag{20}$$

where V_m^* and V_m are the maximal velocities, K_m^* and K_m are the apparent Michaelis–Menten constants, and C_E^* and C_E are the substrate concentrations for [^{14}C]-DG and glucose respectively, in the hexokinase reactions.

With tracer amounts of [^{14}C]-DG, however, C_E^* is negligible. Therefore,

$$K_m^*(1 + C_E/K_m) + C_E^* \approx K_m^*(1 + C_E/K_m) \tag{21}$$

and

$$K_m(1 + C_E^*/K_m^*) + C_E \approx K_m + C_E = K_m(1 + C_E/K_m) \tag{22}$$

Equation (20) reduces to

$$v^*/v = \frac{C_E^* V_m^*/[K_m^*(1 + C_E/K_m)]}{C_E V_m/[K_m(1 + C_E/K_m)]} \tag{23}$$

and after cancellation and rearrangement

$$v^*/v = (C_E^*/C_E)(V_m^* K_m/V_m K_m^*) \tag{24}$$

Substituting for v^*/v in equation (19) and rearranging,

$$\frac{(dC_i^*/dt - dC_E^*/dt)}{R_i} = (C_E^*/C_E)(V_m^* K_m/\Phi V_m K_m^*) \tag{25}$$

C_E^* and C_E are defined in equations (8) and (13) respectively. After dividing equation (8) by equation (13),

$$C_E^*/C_E = \frac{k_1^* e^{-(k_2^*+k_3^*)T} \int_0^T C_P^* e^{(k_2^*+k_3^*)t}\, dt}{[k_1/(k_2+k_3)]C_P} \tag{26}$$

After multiplying the numerator by $(k_2^* + k_3^*)/(k_2^* + k_3^*)$ and dividing through by C_P, which is a constant and can therefore be incorporated under the integral, it follows that

$$C_E^*/C_E = \lambda(k_2^* + k_3^*)e^{-(k_2^*+k_3^*)T} \int_0^T (C_P^*/C_P)e^{(k_2^*+k_3^*)t}\, dt \tag{27}$$

where λ is the constant $[k_1^*/(k_2^* + k_3^*)]\big/[k_1/(k_2 + k_3)]$, which is equal to the ratio of the distribution volumes for $[^{14}C]$-DG to glucose in the tissue.

Substituting for C_E^*/C_E in equation (25), rearranging, and integrating from zero time to the final time, τ,

$$C_i^*(\tau) - C_E^*(\tau) = R_i \int_0^\tau \left[\lambda(k_2^* + k_3^*)e^{-(k_2^*+k_3^*)T} \right. \tag{28}$$
$$\left. \int_0^T (C_P^*/C_P)e^{(k_2^*+k_3^*)t}\, dt \right] dt\, (V_m^*K_m/\Phi V_m K_m^*)$$

Substituting for C_E^* its equivalent function defined in equation (8), and solving for R_i,

$$R_i = \frac{C_i^*(\tau) - k_1^* e^{-(k_2^*+k_3^*)\tau} \int_0^\tau C_P^* e^{(k_2^*+k_3^*)t}\, dt}{\left(\dfrac{\lambda V_m^* K_m}{\Phi V_m K_m^*}\right) \int_0^\tau \left[(k_2^* + k_3^*)e^{-(k_2^*+k_3^*)T} \int_0^T (C_P^*/C_P)e^{(k_2^*+k_3^*)t}\, dt \right] dT} \tag{29}$$

The denominator of equation (29) can be integrated by parts to yield the following simpler and more useful form of the equation:

$$R_i = \frac{C_i^*(\tau) - k_1^* e^{-(k_2^*+k_3^*)\tau} \int_0^\tau C_P^* e^{(k_2^*+k_3^*)t}\, dt}{(\lambda V_m^* K_m/\Phi V_m K_m^*)\int_0^\tau (C_P^*/C_P)\, dt - e^{-(k_2^*+k_3^*)\tau} \int_0^\tau (C_P^*/C_P)e^{(k_2^*+k_3^*)t}\, dt} \tag{30}$$

Equation (30) is the operational equation of the method. It states that if [^{14}C]-DG is introduced into the blood and allowed to circulate for time τ, then the rate of glucose consumption, R, in any cerebral tissue, i, can be calculated, provided that the total concentration of ^{14}C in that tissue, C_i^*, is measured at time, τ; the entire histories of the arterial plasma concentrations of [^{14}C]-DG and glucose from zero time to τ are determined; and the rate constants, k_1^*, k_2^*, and k_3^*, and the single lumped constant (a combination of six other constants) are known. The conditions necessary for equation (30) to apply are that the [^{14}C]-DG be present in tracer amounts, that the arterial plasma glucose concentration remain constant, and that the glucose metabolism of the tissue be in a steady state during the period of measurement.

Despite its complex appearance, the operational equation is essentially nothing more than a general statement of the standard relationship by which rates of enzymatic reactions are routinely determined from measurements made with radioactive tracers (Figure 2). The rate of the enzymatic reaction is equal to the amount of radioactive product formed in a given period of time divided by the integrated specific activity of the precursor during that interval of time. If the radioactive precursor exhibits an isotope effect, i.e., kinetic differences from the natural, unlabeled precursor, then a correction factor for the isotope effect must be included. When the assay is carried out in the test tube, all the necessary variables to calculate the rate can be measured directly and/or controlled by the selection of the appropriate reaction mixture. The complexity of the operational equation derives from the fact that in this application the assay is carried out not in a test tube but in all the structural components of the brain in living, conscious animals. The necessary variables cannot be measured or controlled directly in the tissues and must be determined indirectly from measurements in the arterial plasma. The functional anatomy of the operational equation is described in Figure 2. The numerator of the equation represents the amount of radioactive product formed in the interval of time 0 to T; it is equal to C_i^*, the combined concentrations of [^{14}C]-DG and [^{14}C]-DG-6-P in the tissue at time T, measured by the quantitative autoradiographic technique, less a term that represents the free unmetabolized [^{14}C]-DG still remaining in the tissue.

Because it is impractical if not impossible to measure the free [^{14}C]-DG concentration directly in all the cerebral structures visualized in the autoradiographs, the free [^{14}C]-DG concentration is computed from the time course of the [^{14}C]-DG concentration in the arterial plasma and the appropriate rate constants. The denominator represents the integrated specific activity of the precursor pool times the lumped constant. The term with the exponential factor in the denominator takes into account the lag in the equilibration of the tissue precursor pool with the plasma in which the specific activity is directly measured. The lumped constant corrects for the differences in the kinetic behavior

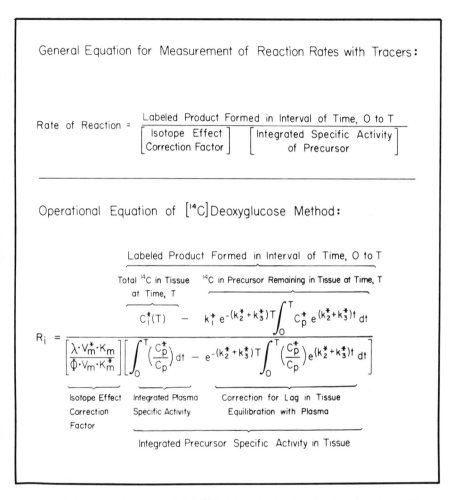

FIGURE 2. Operational equation of the [14C]-DG method and its functional anatomy. *T* represents the time at the termination of the experimental period; λ equals the ratio of the distribution space of DG in the tissue to that of glucose; Φ equals the fraction of glucose that, once phosphorylated, continues down the glycolytic pathway; and K_m^* and V_m^* and K_m and V_m represent the familiar Michaelis–Menten kinetic constants of hexokinase for DG and glucose, respectively. The other symbols are the same as those defined in Figure 1. (From Sokoloff, 1978.)

of DG and glucose with hexokinase. Although the kinetic differences are not as a result of the isotopic label but rather to the slight structural difference, the lumped constant is kinetically equivalent to the correction factor for an isotope effect.

2.3.2. Determination of the Rate Constants

Equation (11) provides the theoretical basis for the determination of the rate constants, k_1^*, k_2^*, and k_3^*. It describes the time course of the total concentration of ^{14}C in a tissue as a function of time, the history of the plasma $[^{14}C]$-DG concentration, and the three rate constants. If the time courses of the tissue and plasma concentrations are known, then the three rate constants can be estimated by computerized nonlinear, least-squares fitting routines. These rate constants have been fully determined in the conscious albino rat (Sokoloff *et al.*, 1977). Because only a single measurement of the ^{14}C concentration in the cerebral tissues was possible in any one animal, the studies were carried out in a group of 15 rats matched for age and weight. Each animal was infused intravenously at a constant rate with a total dose of 20–50 μCi of $[^{14}C]$-DG for 5, 10, 20, 30, or 45 min and decapitated at the end of that time. Three animals were studied for each period. Timed arterial blood samples were drawn during the infusion and assayed for the history of plasma $[^{14}C]$-DG concentration prior to the time of killing. The local cerebral ^{14}C concentrations at the time of decapitation were determined by the quantitative autoradiographic technique. Equation (11) was then fitted to the cerebral tissue ^{14}C concentrations and the time courses of the plasma $[^{14}C]$-DG concentration obtained from all the rats. The values for k_1^*, k_2^*, and k_3^* providing the least-squares best-fit of the equation to the experimental data were obtained on a PDP-10 computer by means of a nonlinear iterative process employing the MLAB program (Knott and Shrager, 1972; Knott and Reece, 1972).

The values of the rate constants obtained by this method in a number of gray and white structures in the brain of the conscious rat are presented in Table 1. The values for each of the rate constants are higher in gray matter than in white matter, but within each class of structures there is relatively little variation. It is possible, therefore, to use only the mean values of the rate constants for gray matter and for white matter in order to simplify calculations.

The constants, k_2^* and k_3^*, always appear as their sum in equation (30), the operational equation for the determination of local cerebral glucose utilization. The term $(k_2^* + k_3^*)$ is the exponential constant in all the exponential terms that appear in these equations. From the model and equation (3) it can also be seen that $(k_2^* + k_3^*)$ is equal to the rate constant for the turnover of the $[^{14}C]$-DG precursor pool in the tissue and can be used to calculate the half-lives of these pools. The half-lives are uniformly and significantly greater in

TABLE 1. Values of Rate Constants in the Normal Conscious Albino Rat[a]

| Structure | Rate constants (min^{-1}) | | | Distribution volume (ml/g) $k_1^*/(k_2^* + k_3^*)$ | Half-life of precursor pool (min) $\log_e 2/(k_2^* + k_3^*)$ |
	k_1^*	k_2^*	k_3^*		
		Gray matter			
Visual cortex	0.189 ± 0.048	0.279 ± 0.176	0.063 ± 0.040	0.553	2.03
Auditory cortex	0.226 ± 0.068	0.241 ± 0.198	0.067 ± 0.057	0.734	2.25
Parietal cortex	0.194 ± 0.051	0.257 ± 0.175	0.062 ± 0.045	0.608	2.17
Sensorimotor cortex	0.193 ± 0.037	0.208 ± 0.112	0.049 ± 0.035	0.751	2.70
Thalamus	0.188 ± 0.045	0.218 ± 0.144	0.053 ± 0.043	0.694	2.56
Medial geniculate body	0.219 ± 0.055	0.259 ± 0.164	0.055 ± 0.040	0.697	2.21
Lateral geniculate body	0.172 ± 0.038	0.220 ± 0.134	0.055 ± 0.040	0.625	2.52
Hypothalamus	0.158 ± 0.032	0.226 ± 0.119	0.043 ± 0.032	0.587	2.58
Hippocampus	0.169 ± 0.043	0.260 ± 0.166	0.056 ± 0.040	0.535	2.19
Amygdala	0.149 ± 0.028	0.235 ± 0.109	0.032 ± 0.026	0.558	2.60
Caudate–putamen	0.176 ± 0.041	0.200 ± 0.140	0.061 ± 0.050	0.674	2.66
Superior colliculus	0.198 ± 0.054	0.240 ± 0.166	0.046 ± 0.042	0.692	2.42
Pontine gray matter	0.170 ± 0.040	0.246 ± 0.142	0.037 ± 0.033	0.601	2.45
Cerebellar cortex	0.225 ± 0.066	0.392 ± 0.229	0.059 ± 0.031	0.499	1.54
Cerebellar nucleus	0.207 ± 0.042	0.194 ± 0.111	0.038 ± 0.035	0.892	2.99
Mean ± S.E.M.	0.189 ± 0.012	0.245 ± 0.040	0.052 ± 0.010	0.647 ± 0.073	2.39 ± 0.40
		White matter			
Corpus callosum	0.085 ± 0.015	0.135 ± 0.075	0.019 ± 0.033	0.552	4.50
Genu of corpus callosum	0.076 ± 0.013	0.131 ± 0.075	0.019 ± 0.034	0.507	4.62
Internal capsule	0.077 ± 0.015	0.134 ± 0.085	0.023 ± 0.039	0.490	4.41
Mean ± S.E.M.	0.079 ± 0.008	0.133 ± 0.046	0.020 ± 0.020	0.516 ± 0.171	4.51 ± 0.90

[a] From Sokoloff et al. (1977).

white matter than in gray matter (Table 1). The average half-life of the precursor pool is approximately 2.4 min in gray matter and 4.5 min in white matter.

The distribution ratios for $[^{14}C]$-DG between the plasma and the various cerebral tissues, determined from $k_1^*/(k_2^* + k_3^*)$, appear to be greater in gray matter than in white matter (Table 1), but in each group they are rather uniform. These distribution ratios, calculated on the basis of the rate constants, agree quite well with the value, 0.575 (S.D. = ±0.019), that R. Fishman (personal communication) has found experimentally to be the average distribution ratio in rat brain as a whole. This agreement provides some evidence for the reliability of the computed values for the rate constants in Table 1.

The values of the rate constants have thus far been determined fully only in normal conscious rats. Partial determinations indicate that they are similar in the monkey and cat, but they probably vary with the condition of the animal. For example, k_3^* is the rate constant for the phosphorylation of $[^{14}C]$-DG by hexokinase and is likely to be altered by changes in metabolic rate. The values for the rate constants for the transport of $[^{14}C]$-DG between blood and tissue, k_1^* and k_2^*, are influenced not only by the properties of the transport system but also by the steady state levels of glucose in the plasma and tissue and, to a smaller extent, by the blood flow to the tissue. For greatest accuracy, therefore, it is advisable to determine the rate constants for the condition and species of the animal desired to be studied. For studies in the normal animal, however, and particularly in gray matter, the quantitative nature of the rate constants combined with the design of the experimental procedure (Section 3) serve to permit a considerable latitude in the values of the constants around those in Table 1 without any major influence on the calculated values for local cerebral glucose utilization.

2.3.3. Determination of the Lumped Constant

The lumped constant combines six constants into one. However, to determine even that one constant separately in each of the structural components of the brain would represent a formidable undertaking. Fortunately, the composition of the lumped constant is such that it can reasonably be assumed to be relatively uniform throughout the brain. For example, the lumped constant $[\lambda V_m^* K_m / \Phi V_m K_m^*]$ is really the product of the four factors $1/\Phi$, λ, V_m^*/V_m, and K_m/K_m^*. The first factor is the reciprocal of Φ, a constant between zero and one that reflects the amount of glucose-6-phosphatase activity; in view of the almost negligible activity of this enzyme in mammalian brain (Hers, 1957) Φ is likely to be equal or close to one throughout the brain. The second factor, λ, represents the ratio of distribution volumes for $[^{14}C]$-DG and glucose in the tissue.

Although the distribution volume for $[^{14}C]$-DG varies in the different tissues of the brain (Table 1), the distribution volume for glucose probably varies proportionately so that the ratio, λ, can be expected to remain constant throughout the brain. V_m^*/V_m is the ratio of the maximal velocities of phosphorylation of $[^{14}C]$-DG and glucose by hexokinase. Maximal velocity reflects total amount of enzyme, which certainly varies from tissue to tissue, but then the two maximal velocities would vary in proportion so that V_m^*/V_m remains constant. Similarly, the ratio of the Michaelis–Menten constants, K_m/K_m^*, which represent kinetic properties of the enzyme, can be expected to be uniform throughout the brain. It is therefore likely that a lumped constant determined for the brain as a whole would be representative of the lumped constants in its component parts.

Further analysis of the theoretical model and appropriate manipulation of the equations developed in Section 2.3.1 leads to a mathematical definition of the lumped constant for the whole brain in terms of measurable physiological variables.

When $[^{14}C]$-DG is introduced into the circulation, the rate of change in concentration of ^{14}C in the brain tissue is equal to the difference between the rate of its delivery to the tissue by the arterial blood and its removal by the venous blood. Thus

$$F(C_A^* - C_V^*) = dC_i^*/dt \tag{31}$$

where F is the rate of blood flow per unit mass of tissue, C_A^* is the concentration of $[^{14}C]$-DG in the arterial blood, and C_V^* equals the concentration of $[^{14}C]$-DG in the representative cerebral venous blood.

Cerebral glucose metabolism is assumed to be in a steady state, and the concentration of glucose in the tissue does not change. Its net uptake is therefore equivalent to its rate of utilization and is equal to the difference between the rates of its delivery by the arterial blood and removal by the venous blood. Thus

$$F(C_A - C_V) = R_i \tag{32}$$

where C_A and C_V equal the concentrations of glucose in arterial and cerebral venous blood, respectively.

Substituting $F(C_A^* - C_V^*)$ and $F(C_A - C_V)$ for dC_i^*/dt and R_i, respectively, in equation (19),

$$\frac{F(C_A^* - C_V^*)}{F(C_A - C_V)} = \frac{dC_E^*/dt}{R_i} + \frac{V^*}{\Phi v} \tag{33}$$

Cancelling out F and factoring out C_A^* and C_A leads to

$$\left(\frac{C_A^*}{C_A}\right)\left(\frac{E^*}{E}\right) = \frac{dC_E^*/dT}{R_i} + \frac{v^*}{\Phi v} \tag{34}$$

where E^* and E equal $(C_A^* - C_V^*)/C_A^*$ and $(C_A - C_V)/C_A$, the cerebral extraction ratios for $[^{14}C]$-DG and glucose, respectively. Substituting for v^*/v its equivalent function defined in equation (24),

$$\left(\frac{C_A^*}{C_A}\right)\left(\frac{E^*}{E}\right) = \frac{dC_E^*/dT}{R_i} + \frac{C_E^*}{C_E}\left(\frac{V_m^*K_m}{\Phi V_m K_m^*}\right) \tag{35}$$

and substituting for C_E^*/C_E according to equation (27),

$$\left(\frac{C_A^*}{C_A}\right)\left(\frac{E^*}{E}\right) = \frac{dC_E^*/dT}{R_i}$$
$$+ (k_2^* + k_3^*)e^{-(k_2^*+k_3^*)T}\int_0^T (C_P^*/C_P)e^{(k_2^*+k_3^*)t}dt\left(\frac{\lambda V_m^*K_m}{\Phi V_m K_m^*}\right) \tag{36}$$

C_P, the arterial plasma glucose concentration, is already assumed to be constant, and if C_P^* can also be maintained constant from zero time to time T, then the integration in equation (36) can be performed explicitly to yield

$$\left(\frac{C_A^*}{C_A}\right)\left(\frac{E^*}{E}\right) = \frac{dC_E^*/dT}{R_i} + \frac{C_P^*}{C_P}(1 - e^{-(k_2^*+k_3^*)T})\left(\frac{\lambda V_m^*K_m}{\phi V_m K_m^*}\right) \tag{37}$$

If C_P^* is a constant, then integration of equation (3) yields

$$C_E^* = [k_1^*/(k_2^* + k_3^*)]C_P^*(1 - e^{-(k_2^*+k_3^*)T}) \tag{38}$$

which when differentiated leads to the following:

$$dC_E^*/dT = k_1^*C_P^*e^{-(k_2^*+k_3^*)T} \tag{39}$$

Substituting for dC_E^*/dT in equation (35),

$$\left(\frac{C_A^*}{C_A}\right)\left(\frac{E^*}{E}\right) = \frac{k_1^*C_P^*e^{-(k_2^*+k_3^*)T}}{R_i} + \frac{C_P^*}{C_P}(1 - e^{-(k_2^*+k_3^*)T})\left(\frac{\lambda V_m^*K_m}{\Phi V_m K_m^*}\right) \tag{40}$$

As T approaches infinity, all the terms containing the exponential factor approach zero, and at $T = \infty$,

$$\left(\frac{C_A^*}{C_A}\right)\left(\frac{E^*}{E}\right)(\infty) = \frac{C_P^*}{C_P}\left(\frac{\lambda V_m^* K_m}{\Phi V_m K_m^*}\right) \tag{41}$$

and

$$\left(\frac{\lambda V_m^* K_m}{\Phi V_m K_m^*}\right) = \left(\frac{E^*}{E}\right)\left(\frac{C_A^*}{C_A}\right)\Big/\left(\frac{C_P^*}{C_P}\right)(\infty) \tag{42}$$

Equations (40) and (42) prescribe the procedure to determine the lumped constant. They state that if [^{14}C]-DG is so administered to the animal that C_P^* is maintained constant long enough for the exponential factor $e^{-(k_2^*+k_3^*)T}$ to approach zero, then the ratio of the fractional extractions of [^{14}C]-DG and glucose by the brain multiplied by the ratio of the specific activities (i.e., ratio of [^{14}C]-DG to glucose concentrations) in arterial blood and plasma declines exponentially with a rate constant equal to $(k_2^* + k_3^*)$ until it reaches an asymptotic value equal to the lumped constant. The factor $(C_A^*/C_A)/(C_P^*/C_P)$ merely takes into account the possibility that [^{14}C]-DG and glucose may distribute disproportionately between plasma and red cells.

The derivation of the definition of the lumped constant in terms of variables measurable in blood assumes a single homogeneous tissue with a common rate of glucose utilization and single values for $(k_2^* + k_3^*)$ and the lumped constant. Inasmuch as representative cerebral venous blood can be sampled only from the entire brain, in practice more than one tissue is represented. Equation (40) can readily be modified to take into account multiple tissues. The equation becomes more complex with additional exponential terms, one each for every value of $(k_2^* + k_3^*)$. The principles and conclusions remain the same except that the left side of the equation then declines multiexponentially, one exponential compartment for each value of $(k_2^* + k_3^*)$. If, as expected for the reasons given above, the lumped constant is uniform throughout the brain, then the asymptotic value equals that lumped constant. If, on the other hand, the lumped constant varies among the tissues, then the value so obtained is equal to the weighted average of the lumped constant for the brain as a whole.

The design of the procedures used to determine the lumped constant, $\lambda V_m^* K_m/\Phi V_m K_m^*$, is based on equations (40) and (42). These equations state that if the [^{14}C]-DG is administered in such a way that its concentration in arterial plasma achieves and maintains a constant level for a sufficiently long time, the concentrations of free [^{14}C]-DG and its rates of phosphorylation in the tissues will reach a steady state like that already existing for glucose. When steady states exist for both [^{14}C]-DG and glucose, then the ratio of the cerebral extraction ratio of [^{14}C]-DG to that of glucose, corrected by the ratio of the specific activities (i.e., ratio of [^{14}C]-DG to glucose concentrations) in arterial blood and plasma, becomes equal to the lumped constant [equation (42)]. In other words, the lumped constant is really the constant of proportionality between the steady state rates of [^{14}C]-DG and glucose phosphorylation by the brain when it is exposed to equal arterial plasma concentrations of both.

In order to determine the lumped constant, it is first necessary to design an intravenous infusion schedule that produces and maintains a constant concentration of [^{14}C]-DG in the arterial plasma. To achieve this animals are administered intravenous pulses of [^{14}C]-DG and timed arterial blood samples are drawn for at least 45 min for the measurement of the plasma [^{14}C]-DG concentrations. The plasma disappearance curve is then fitted by an iterative, nonlinear least-squares routine to the sum of three or four exponential terms. From a Laplace transform of the relationship between the impulse input and the multiexponential output, it is possible to compute the input function (e.g., the infusion schedule) necessary to achieve a constant arterial plasma level. The details of the mathematical procedures have been published elsewhere (Patlak and Pettigrew, 1976). The infusion schedule consists of an intravenous pulse of [^{14}C]-DG followed by a continuous infusion with specified changes in rate every minute. The controlled infusion can be achieved by means of a calibrated peristaltic pump with a speed control that is changed manually every minute. If available, a microprocessor-controlled infusion pump would be far more convenient.

The lumped constants have been determined by this method for the following animals: the albino rat, both conscious and anesthetized (Sokoloff *et al.*, 1977); the conscious Rhesus monkey (Kennedy *et al.*, 1978); the anesthetized cat (J. Magnes, C. Kennedy, M. Miyaoka, M. Shinohara, and L. Sokoloff, unpublished data); the beagle puppy (Duffy *et al.*, 1979). The data and their use to determine the lumped constant in a representative experiment performed on a monkey are illustrated in Figure 3. The values for the lumped constants in the various species of animals are summarized in Table 2. The lumped constant clearly varies with the species, but significant variation within a species under different conditions has not yet been observed, except under conditions of severe hypoglycemia (S. Suda, C. Kennedy, and L. Sokoloff, unpublished observations), and hyperglycemia (F. Schuier, F. Orzi, and L. Sokoloff, unpublished observations). For example, in the albino rat the lumped constant does not change significantly between the conscious and anesthetized states or while breathing high concentrations of carbon dioxide (Table 2).

3. EXPERIMENTAL PROCEDURE FOR MEASUREMENT OF LOCAL CEREBRAL GLUCOSE UTILIZATION

3.1. Theoretical Considerations in the Design of the Procedure

Equation (30) is the operational equation of the method. It specifies the variables to be measured in order to determine R_i, the local rate of glucose consumption in the brain. The following variables are measured in each experiment: (1) the entire history of the arterial plasma $[^{14}C]$-DG concentration, C_P^*, from zero time to the time of killing, τ; (2) the steady state arterial plasma glucose level, C_P, over the same interval; and (3) the local concentration of ^{14}C in the tissue at the time of killing, $C_i^*(\tau)$. The rate constants k_1^*, k_2^*, and k_3^* and the lumped constant $\lambda V_m^* K_m / \Phi V_m K_m^*$ are not measured in each experiment; the values for these constants that are used are those determined separately in other groups of animals as described above and presented in Tables 1 and 2.

Equation (30) is generally applicable with all types of arterial plasma $[^{14}C]$-DG concentration curves. Its configuration, however, suggests that a declining curve approaching zero by τ is the choice to minimize certain potential errors. The quantitative autoradiographic technique measures only total ^{14}C concentration in the tissue and does not distinguish between $[^{14}C]$-DG-6-P and $[^{14}C]$-DG. It is, however, the $[^{14}C]$-DG-6-P concentration that must be known to determine glucose consumption. The $[^{14}C]$-DG-6-P concentration is calculated in the numerator of equation (30), which equals the total tissue ^{14}C content, $C_i^*(\tau)$, minus the $[^{14}C]$-DG concentration present in the tissue estimated by the term containing the exponential factors and rate constants. In the denominator of equation (30) there is also a term containing exponential factors and rate constants. Both these terms have the useful property of approaching zero with increasing time if C_P^* is also allowed to approach zero. The rate constants, k_1^*, k_2^*, and k_3^*, are not measured in the same animals in which local glucose consumption is being measured. It is conceivable that the rate constants in Table 1 are not equally applicable in all physiological, pharmacological, and pathological states. One possible solution is to determine the rate constants for each condition to be studied. An alternative solution (that chosen) is to administer the $[^{14}C]$-DG as a single intravenous pulse at zero time and to allow sufficient time for (1) the clearance of $[^{14}C]$-DG from the plasma and (2) the terms containing the rate constants to fall to levels too low to influence the final result. To wait until these terms reach zero is impractical because of the long time required and the risk of effects of the small but finite rate of loss of $[^{14}C]$-DG-6-P from the tissues. A reasonable time interval is 45 min; by this time the plasma level has fallen very low and, on the basis of the values of

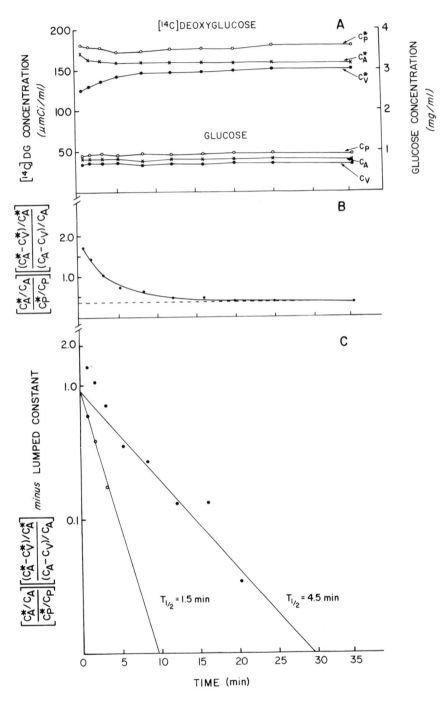

TABLE 2. Values of the Lumped Constant in the Albino Rat,
Rhesus Monkey, Cat, and Dog[a]

Animal	No. of animals	Mean ± S.D.	S.E.M.
Albino rat			
Conscious	15	0.464 ± 0.099[b]	± 0.026
Anesthetized	9	0.512 ± 0.118[b]	± 0.039
Conscious (5% CO_2)	2	0.463 ± 0.122[b]	± 0.086
Combined	26	0.481 ± 0.119	± 0.023
Rhesus monkey			
Conscious	7	0.344 ± 0.095	± 0.036
Cat			
Anesthetized	6	0.411 ± 0.013	± 0.005
Dog (beagle puppy)			
Conscious	7	0.558 ± 0.082	± 0.031

[a] The values were obtained as follows: rat, Sokoloff et al. (1977); monkey, Kennedy et al. (1978); cat, (M. Miyaoka, J. Magnes, C. Kennedy, M. Shinohara, and L. Sokoloff, unpublished data); dog, Duffy et al. (1979) (From Sokoloff, 1979).
[b] No statistically significant difference between normal conscious and anesthetized rats ($0.3 < p < 0.4$) and conscious rats breathing 5% CO_2 ($p > 0.9$).

($k_2^* + k_3^*$) in Table 1, the exponential factors have declined through at least ten half-lives.
The time courses of the concentrations of [^{14}C]-DG and [^{14}C]-DG-6-P in arterial plasma and/or representative gray and white matter following an intravenous pulse of [^{14}C]-DG are illustrated in Figure 4. As the plasma concentration falls from its peak following the pulse, the tissue concentrations of

←

FIGURE 3. Data obtained and their use in determination of the lumped constant and the combination of rate constants, ($k_2^* + k_3^*$), in a representative experiment. (A) Time courses of arterial blood and plasma concentrations of [^{14}C]-DG and glucose and cerebral venous blood concentrations of [^{14}C]-DG and glucose during programmed intravenous infusion of [^{14}C]-DG. (B) Arithemetic plot of the function derived from the variables in (A) and combined as indicated in the formula on the ordinate against time. This function declines exponentially, with a rate constant equal to ($k_2^* + k_3^*$), until it reaches an asymptotic value equal to the lumped constant (0.35) in this experiment (dashed line). (C) Semilogarithmic plot of the curve in (B) less the lumped constant, i.e., its asymptotic value. Solid circles represent actual values. This curve is analyzed into two components by a standard curve-peeling technique to yield the two straight lines representing the separate components. Open circles are points for the fast component, obtained by subtracting the values for the slow component from the solid circles. The rate constants for these two components represent the values of ($k_2^* + k_3^*$) for two compartments; the fast and slow compartments are assumed to represent gray and white matter, respectively. In this experiment the values for ($k_2^* + k_3^*$) were found to equal 0.462 ($T_{1/2}$ = 1.5 min) and 0.154 ($T_{1/2}$ = 4.5 min) in gray and white matter, respectively. (From Kennedy et al., 1978.)

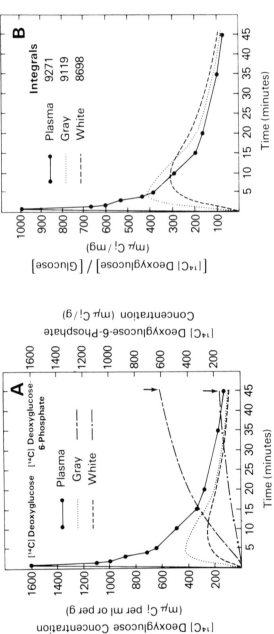

FIGURE 4. Graphical representation of the significant variables in equation (30) used to calculate local cerebral glucose utilization. (A) Time courses of [^{14}C]-DG concentrations in arterial plasma and in average gray and white matter and [^{14}C]-DG-6-P concentrations in average gray and white matter following an intravenous pulse of 50 μCi of [^{14}C]-DG. The plasma curve is derived from measurements of plasma [^{14}C]-DG concentration. The tissue concentrations were calculated from the plasma curve and the mean values of k_1^*, k_2^*, and k_3^* for gray and white matter in Table 1 according to equation (8), which is equivalent to the second term in the numerator of equation (30). The [^{14}C]-DG-6-P concentrations in the tissues were calculated from the same variables and constants according to equation (10). The arrows point to the concentrations of [^{14}C]-DG and [^{14}C]-DG-6-P in the tissues at the time of killing; the autoradiographic technique measures the total ^{14}C content (i.e., the sum of these concentrations) at that time, which is equal to $C_i^*(\tau)$, the first term in the numerator of equation (30). Note that at the time of killing, the total ^{14}C content represents mainly the [^{14}C]-DG-6-P concentration, especially in gray matter. (B) Time courses of ratios of the [^{14}C]-DG to glucose concentrations (i.e., specific activities) in plasma and average gray and white matter. The curve for plasma was determined by division of the plasma curve in (A) by the plasma glucose concentrations. The curves for the tissues were calculated by the function in brackets in the denominator of equation (29). The integrals in (B) are the integrals of the specific activities with respect to time and represent the areas under the curves. The integrals under the tissue curves are equivalent to all of the denominator of equation (30), except for the lumped constant. Note that by the time of killing, the integrals of the tissue curves approach equality with each other and with that

[^{14}C]-DG rise until the tissues and plasma reach equilibrium. As the plasma concentration continues to fall below its equilibrium levels, there is a net loss of [^{14}C]-DG from the tissues back to the plasma, as well as continued conversion of tissue [^{14}C]-DG to [^{14}C]-DG-6-P, and the concentrations of free [^{14}C]-DG in the tissues then decline (Figure 4A). The higher the blood flow in the tissue, the more rapidly it initially takes up [^{14}C]-DG, however, it reaches equilibrium with plasma sooner and loses [^{14}C]-DG more rapidly after the point of equilibrium. These opposing effects of blood flow before and after equilibrium tend to cancel out the effects of blood flow. After 45 min the tissue and plasma levels of free [^{14}C]-DG have reached very low levels. On the other hand, the [^{14}C]-DG-6-P concentrations in the tissues rise continuously and by 45 min are responsible for most of the ^{14}C in the tissues, particularly in gray matter (Figure 4A). The numerator of equation (30) represents the final total tissue ^{14}C concentration, measured autoradiographically, minus the final point on the tissue [^{14}C]-DG curve; it is equal, therefore, to the final [^{14}C]-DG-6-P concentration in the tissue (Figure 4A).

The physical significance of the denominator of equation (30) is illustrated in Figure 4B. The curves in Figure 4B are derived from the curves for [^{14}C]-DG concentration in plasma and average gray and white matter (Figure 4A) by dividing them by the glucose concentrations in those tissues. In effect they represent the time courses of the specific activities in those tissues. The integrals in Figure 4B are the integrated specific activities, i.e., the areas under each of the curves between zero and 45 min. The denominator of equation (30) is equal to the product of the lumped constant and the integral appropriate to the tissue. It should be noted that the integrals for gray and white matter are almost equal to the integral for plasma (Figure 4B). As can be seen from equation (30), this phenomenon merely reflects the diminished contributions of the terms containing the exponential factors at 45 min after the pulse of [^{14}C]-DG; at infinite time all the integrals would be equal to the integral of the plasma curve. It may be recalled that the model assumes only a single compartment for free [^{14}C]-DG in each tissue. It can be shown that at infinite time following a pulse the integrals of the specific activities of all compartments (either in series or parallel) which derive their [^{14}C]-DG ultimately from the plasma compartment, become equal to each other and to the integral of the plasma specific activity (C. Patlak, unpublished). It would then be immaterial if there were, indeed, more than one compartment, and 45 min is sufficiently close to infinity (i.e., at least 10 half-lives) to minimize possible errors due to that assumption.

3.2. Experimental Protocol

The animals are prepared for the experiment by the insertion of polyethylene catheters in an artery and a vein. Any convenient artery or vein can be used. In the rat the femoral or the tail arteries and veins have been found satisfactory. In the monkey and cat the femoral vessels are probably most convenient. The catheters are inserted under anesthesia, and anesthetic agents without long-lasting aftereffects should be used. Light halothane anesthesia with or without supplementation with nitrous oxide has been found to be quite satisfactory. At least 2 hr are allowed for recovery from the surgery and anesthesia before initiation of the experiment.

The design of the experimental procedure for the measurement of local cerebral glucose utilization was based on the theoretical considerations discussed in Section 3.1. At zero time a pulse of no more than 125 μCi of [^{14}C]-DG per kg of body weight is administered to the animal via the venous catheter. Arterial sampling is initiated with the onset of the pulse, and timed 50- to 100-μl samples of arterial blood are collected consecutively as rapidly as possible during the early period so as not to miss the peak of the arterial curve. Arterial samping is continued at less frequent intervals later in the experimental period but at sufficient frequency to define fully the arterial curve. The arterial blood samples are immediately centrifuged to separate the plasma, which is stored on ice until assayed for [^{14}C]-DG by liquid scintillation counting and glucose concentrations by standard enzymatic methods. After approximately 45 min the animal is decapitated, and the brain is removed and frozen in Freon XII or isopentane maintained between -50 and $-75\,^\circ$C with liquid nitrogen. When fully frozen, the brain is stored at $-70\,^\circ$C until sectioned and autoradiographed. The experimental period may be limited to 30 min. This is theoretically permissible and may sometimes be necessary for reasons of experimental expediency, but greater errors owing to possible inaccuracies in the rate constants may result.

3.3. Autoradiographic Measurement of Tissue ^{14}C Concentration

The ^{14}C concentrations in localized regions of the brain are measured by a modification of the quantitative autoradiographic technique previously described (Reivich *et al.*, 1969). The frozen brain is coated with chilled embedding medium (Lipshaw Manufacturing Company, Detroit, Michigan) and fixed to object holders appropriate to the microtome to be used.

Brain sections, precisely 20 μm in thickness, are prepared in a cryostat maintained at -21 to $-22\,^\circ$C. The brain sections are picked up on glass coverslips, dried on a hot plate at 60 $^\circ$C for at least 5 min, and placed sequentially in an X-ray cassette. A set of [^{14}C]methylmethacrylate standards (Amersham Corporation, Arlington Heights, Illinois), which include a blank and a series of progressively increasing ^{14}C concentrations, are also placed in the cassette. These standards must previously have been calibrated for their autoradiographic equivalence to the ^{14}C concentrations in brain sections (20 μm in thickness) prepared as described above. The method of calibration has been described previously (Reivich et al., 1969). Autoradiographs are prepared from these sections directly in the X-ray cassette with Kodak single-coated, blue-sensitive Medical X-ray Film, Type SB-5 (Eastman Kodak Company, Rochester, New York). The exposure time is generally 5–6 days with the doses used as described above, and the exposed films are developed according to the instructions supplied with the film. The SB-5 X-ray film is rapid but coarse grained. For finer grained autoradiographs and, therefore, better defined images with higher resolution, it is possible to use mammographic films such as DuPont LoDose or Kodak MR-1 films, or fine grain panchromatic film such as Kodak Plus-X, but the exposure times are 2–3 times longer. The autoradiographs provide a pictorial representation of the relative ^{14}C concentrations in the various cerebral structures and the plastic standards. A calibration curve of the relationship between optical density and tissue ^{14}C concentration for each film is obtained by densitometric measurements of the portions of the film representing the various standards. The local tissue concentrations are then determined from the calibration curve and the optical densities of the film in the regions representing the cerebral structures of interest. Local cerebral glucose utilization is calculated from the local tissue concentrations of ^{14}C and the plasma $[^{14}C]$-DG and glucose concentrations according to equation (30).

4. THEORETICAL AND PRACTICAL CONSIDERATIONS AND LIMITATIONS

Equation (30), the operational equation of the method, defines the variables to be measured to determine local cerebral glucose utilization. This equation is generally applicable, but it contains several constants, i.e., the rate constants k_1^*, k_2^*, and k_3^*, and the lumped constant, which are not determined uniquely in each animal at the time of the experiment but are evaluated in separate groups of animals of the same species under conditions often different from those of the experiment. There is no assurance, of course, that these constants are universal and apply to all individual animals of a species under all conditions. Also, equation (30) is derived on the basis of the assumption that $[^{14}C]$-DG-6-P, once formed, remains trapped for the duration of the experiment. $[^{14}C]$-DG-6-P cannot leave the tissue directly. It must first be hydrolyzed to free $[^{14}C]$-DG by phosphatase, and glucose-6-phosphatase activity is very low in brain (Hers and DeDuve, 1950; Hers, 1957). Although low, however, glucose-6-phosphatase activity is not entirely absent and some finite rate of hydrolysis of $[^{14}C]$-DG-6-P is to be expected. All these factors are potential sources of error, and special considerations are necessary to define their effects and the limitations that they impose, as well as to design measures to minimize their influence.

4.1. The Rate Constants

The operational equation contains terms that incorporate the rate constants k_1^* and $(k_2^* + k_3^*)$. The combination $(k_2^* + k_3^*)$ is equal to the rate constant for the turnover of the free $[^{14}C]$-DG pool in the tissue; it is related to the half-life of this pool by the relationship

$$T_{1/2} = \frac{0.693}{(k_2^* + k_3^*)}$$

Obviously, the half-life of the $[^{14}C]$-DG pool in the tissue will vary with the blood flow, blood–brain barrier transport, plasma glucose concentration, and the rate of metabolism; k_1^* varies with the blood flow, blood–brain barrier transport, and plasma glucose level. These are all functions that may vary from structure to structure within the brain, from animal to animal, and from condition to condition. The single set of rate constants in Table 1 was determined in normal conscious rats and cannot possibly be accurate for all conditions.

The influence of inaccuracies in the rate constants is minimized, however, by the design of the procedure adopted for the measurement of local cerebral glucose utilization, namely, the use of an intravenous pulse of $[^{14}C]$-DG at zero time followed by a long interval of time before killing. The configuration of the operational equation is such that if the $[^{14}C]$-DG is so administered that the plasma $[^{14}C]$-DG concentration approaches zero with increasing time, then the terms containing the rate constants also approach zero while the terms from which they are subtracted are increasing with time. At infinite time the terms containing the rate constants reach zero, and then the values of the rate constants have absolutely no influence on the final calculated value for local cerebral glucose utilization. The influence of the rate constants is predominant early after the pulse but diminishes with increasing time until it is almost insignificant at 45 min. The terms with the rate constants are then between 5 and 10% of the terms from which they are subtracted in the gray matter of normal conscious rats. Considerable errors in the rate constants can then be tolerated with negligible error in the final results. Figure 5 illustrates the influence of different values for the rate constant $(k_2^* + k_3^*)$ on the denominator of the equation as a function of time. The family of curves in Figure 5 was computed from a typical curve for plasma $[^{14}C]$-DG concentration following a pulse at zero time and five different values for $(k_2^* + k_3^*)$ between infinity and 0.139 per min; this corresponds to tissue $[^{14}C]$-DG half-lives from 0 to 5 min. It can

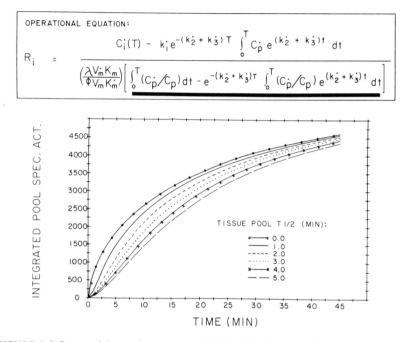

OPERATIONAL EQUATION:

$$R_i = \frac{C_i^*(T) - k_i^* e^{-(k_2^* + k_3^*)T} \int_0^T C_p^* e^{(k_2^* + k_3^*)t} \, dt}{\left(\frac{\lambda V_m^* K_m}{\phi V_m K_m^*}\right)\left[\int_0^T (C_p^*/C_p) \, dt - e^{-(k_2^* + k_3^*)T} \int_0^T (C_p^*/C_p) e^{(k_2^* + k_3^*)t} \, dt\right]}$$

TISSUE POOL T 1/2 (MIN):

- •——• 0.0
- —— 1.0
- ----- 2.0
- ········ 3.0
- ×——× 4.0
- —— 5.0

INTEGRATED POOL SPEC. ACT.

TIME (MIN)

FIGURE 5. Influence of time and rate constant ($k_2^* + k_3^*$) on integrated precursor pool specific activity. The portion of the equation underlined, corresponding to integrated pool specific activity, was computed as a function of time with different values of ($k_2^* + k_3^*$), as indicated by their equivalent half-lives and calculated according to $T_{1/2} = 0.693/(k_2^* + k_3^*)$. (From Sokoloff, 1979.)

be seen that enormous errors of several hundred percent can be encountered with erroneous values of the rate constants early following the pulse, but the curves all rise and converge within a narrow range by 45 min, despite the wide span of rate constants used. It is obvious that there is then little difference in the final result, regardless of the rate constants used.

The variety of rate constants used in Figure 5 adequately covers the range to be expected in reasonably normal physiological states. There are, however, extreme conditions in which the rate constants might be expected to fall below this range (i.e., increased half-life of the [^{14}C]-DG pool above 5 min). For example, blood flow influences k_1^* and k_2^*. Extreme reductions in blood flow may, therefore, cause these rate constants to fall severely, and the half-life of the pool may then markedly exceed 5 min. Increased plasma glucose concentration lowers all the rate constants. Studies in this laboratory have demonstrated no detectable influence on the measured rate of local cerebral glucose utilization over a plasma glucose concentration range of 85–300 mg%, but above this range there are progressively falling values for calculated local cerebral glucose utilization with increasing plasma glucose concentration. Presumably, the normal rate constants determined in normal animals (Table 1), which are used in these calculations, are adequate to cover the range from 85 to 300 mg% but are too far above the true values of the rate constants, which are certainly much lower in severe hyperglycemia. It is recommended, therefore, that the rate constants be redetermined for studies in conditions in which the rate constants may be markedly reduced.

4.2. The Lumped Constant

The lumped constant is composed of six separate constants. One of these, Φ, is influenced by hydrolysis of G-6-P to free glucose and phosphate. Because there is little phosphohydrolase activity in normal brain tissue, Φ is normally approximately equal to unity. The other components are arranged in three ratios: λ, which is the ratio of distribution spaces in the tissue for DG and glucose; V_m^*/V_m; and K_m/K_m^*. Although each individual constant may vary from structure to structure and condition to condition, it is likely that the ratios remain the same. For reasons described in detail above, it is assumed that the lumped constant is the same throughout the brain and is characteristic of the species of animal, but only under normal conditions. Although reasonable, this assumption is not certain, and theoretically it may not be so; however, empirical experience thus far indicates that it is. The greatest experience is with the albino rat. In this species the lumped constant for the brain as a whole has been determined under a variety of conditions. In the normal conscious rat local cerebral glucose utilization, determined by the [^{14}C]-DG method with the single value of the lumped constant for the brain as a whole, correlates almost perfectly ($r = 0.96$) with local cerebral blood flow measured by the [^{14}C]iodoantipyrine method, an entirely independent method. It is generally recognized that local blood flow is adjusted to local metabolic rate, but if the single value of the lumped constant did not apply to the individual structures studied, then errors in local glucose utilization would occur that might be expected to obscure the correlation. Also, the lumped constant has been directly determined in the albino rat in the normal conscious state, under barbiturate anesthesia, and during the inhalation of 5% CO_2; no significant differences were observed (Table 2).

The lumped constant does vary with the species of animal. It has now also been determined in the Rhesus monkey, cat, and Beagle puppy; each species has a different value (Table 2). The values for local rates of glucose utilization determined with these lumped constants in these species are very close to what might be expected from measurement of energy metabolism in the brain as a whole by other methods.

Although there is yet no definitive experimental evidence to indicate that the lumped constants determined in animals with normal brain tissues do not apply to pathological states, such a possibility must be seriously considered. Tissue damage may disrupt the normal cellular compartmentation. There is no assurance that λ, the ratio of the distribution spaces for [^{14}C]-DG and glucose, is the same in damaged tissue as in normal tissue. Also in pathological states there may be release of lysosomal acid hydrolases that may hydrolyze G-6-P and thus alter the value of Φ.

Current studies in our laboratory suggest that even with anatomically normal brain tissue, extreme changes in the plasma glucose level may alter the lumped constant. Theoretical analysis of the relationship between λ, the component of the lumped constant that represents the ratio of the tissue distribution spaces for DG and glucose, and the plasma glucose concentration indicates that this quantity rises with decreasing plasma glucose level. This means that changes in plasma glucose level may alter the values for the DG and glucose spaces in the tissue and that these alterations are disproportionate. Over the normal range of plasma glucose concentrations, 85–300 mg%, λ changes very gradually, less than 5% over the entire range. The changes in λ are more pronounced in severe hypoglycemia and hyperglycemia. Because of this change in λ, the lumped constant can be expected to be higher in hypoglycemia and lower in hyperglycemia than the values determined in normoglycemic animals. We have, indeed, obtained higher than expected values for cerebral glucose utilization in rats with plasma glucose concentrations at 50 mg% or less, and lower than normal values in rats with plasma glucose concentrations in the range of 330–600 mg% when the rates of glucose utilization were calculated with the values of the lumped constant and rate constants determined in normoglycemic rats. The inappropriateness of the rate constants may explain part but not all of the errors; it is likely that the problem lies mainly with the lumped constant. Indeed, initial experiments indicate that the lumped constant may be significantly higher in severely hypoglycemic and lower in severe hyperglycemic than in normal rats. Studies are currently in progress to determine the lumped and rate constants in rats with different ranges of plasma glucose concentrations, including severe hypoglycemia and hyperglycemia.

4.3.   Role of Glucose-6-Phosphatase

An essential premise of the model on which the operational equation is based is that once [^{14}C]-DG-6-P is formed, the radioactive tag remains trapped in the tissue for the duration of the period of measurement. The label need not remain in [^{14}C]-DG-6-P. All that is required is that it be in either [^{14}C]-DG-6-P or any derivative of it that retains the ^{14}C within the tissue. The label could even be in free [^{14}C]-DG, provided that the [^{14}C]-DG is derived from [^{14}C]-DG-6-P and is in a compartment that does not lose label to the blood. It is highly unlikely that [^{14}C]-DG-6-P could be lost from the tissue directly because it could not cross the blood–brain barrier; it probably does not even leave the cell. Evidence in the literature (Section 2.1) indicates that DG-6-P is a poor substrate for enzymes known to exist in brain in significant amounts, and activities of enzymes for which it might be a good substrate appear to be very low in brain. The validity of this premise could, therefore, be reasonably assumed, but because of its critical importance, experiments have been carried out to test it directly.

The possibility was considered that [^{14}C]-DG-6-P might be cleared directly from the tissues by the circulation without prior hydrolysis. This possibility was examined in cats. A pulse of [^{14}C]-DG was administered intravenously, and timed arterial and cerebral venous blood samples were then drawn. The blood samples were centrifuged, and their plasma fractions were assayed for ^{14}C concentrations in a liquid scintillation counter. Despite the rapidly falling arterial and cerebral venous concentrations, there was initially a positive cerebral arteriovenous difference, indicating net uptake of ^{14}C by the brain. This difference diminished gradually until at approximately 7 min the arterial and cerebral venous curves intersected and a negative arteriovenous difference appeared that persisted for at least 25 min. The plasma samples taken during the period of the negative cerebral arteriovenous difference were analyzed by ion-exchange column chromatography, paper chromatography, and thin layer chromatography for their [^{14}C]-DG and [^{14}C]-DG-6-P contents. There was no trace of [^{14}C]-DG-6-P in any of the samples. Despite the fact that there was clearly a net loss of ^{14}C from the brain to the blood during this period, all of the loss could be accounted for as [^{14}C]-DG. These results not only confirmed that there is bidirectional transport of free [^{14}C]-DG between blood and brain but also demonstrated that there is no direct loss of [^{14}C]-DG-6-P from the cerebral tissues to the blood.

It was possible that some of the [^{14}C]-DG lost from the brain tissues to the blood was derived from the hydrolysis of [^{14}C]-DG-6-P. The activity of glucose-6-phosphatase, an enzyme that might be expected to hydrolyze [^{14}C]-DG-6-P, is generally believed to be very low in mammalian brain. For example, Hers (1957) found a maximal rate of G-6-P hydrolysis of only 0.06 μmol/g per min in rat brain homogenates assayed at 37 °C, at an optimal pH of 6.5, and with saturating concentrations of substrate. Even this maximal rate, which might be expected to be considerably greater than the rate under more physiological conditions of pH and substrate concentration *in vivo,* is only approximately 5% of the glycolytic flux *in vivo* in the brain of the conscious rat (see Table 3). To test the possibility that DG-6-P hydrolysis might be more rapid we carried out similar experiments at a pH of 7.4 and with saturating concentrations of [^{14}C]-DG-6-P as the substrate. The maximal rate of hydrolysis was even lower, 0.03 μmol/g per min, indicating that deoxyglucose-6-phosphatase activity did not present a serious problem.

Although the results of assays of brain homogenates *in vitro* indicated very little deoxyglucose-6-phosphatase activity, there remained a possibility that *in vivo* there might be, in some cerebral tissues, significant hydrolysis of [^{14}C]-DG-6-P and subsequent clearance of the released [^{14}C]-DG from the tissue by the circulation. Experiments were therefore carried out to estimate the rates of disappearance of [^{14}C]-DG-6-P from the various structural components of the brain.

A group of rats, matched for age and weight, were administered equal intravenous pulses of [^{14}C]-DG. The arterial plasma [^{14}C]-DG concentration of each animal was monitored by liquid scintillation counting and found to reach very low levels by 6 hr after the pulse. Animals were killed by decapitation at 6, 17, and 24 hr after the pulse; their brains were removed and frozen in Freon XII chilled to $-75\,°$C in liquid nitrogen, and the local cerebral tissue concentrations of ^{14}C were determined by the quantitative autoradiographic procedure described in Section 3.3. By 17 hr the plasma concentrations had reached and remained at negligible levels long enough for any free [^{14}C]-DG in the cerebral tissues to have been cleared by the circulation or metabolized to [^{14}C]-DG-6-P. Any loss of ^{14}C from the tissues thereafter could reasonably be assumed to represent the loss of [^{14}C]-DG-6-P and/or its labeled products. The ^{14}C concentrations in a variety of gray and white cerebral structures at 17 hr and 24 hr after the pulse were plotted semilogarithmically and their half-lives estimated. The mean half-lives in gray and white matter were 7.7 hr (S.D. $= \pm 1.6$) and 9.7 hr (S.D. $= \pm 2.6$), respectively. The shortest half-life, which was found in the inferior colliculus, was 6.1 hr. These results indicate that the loss of ^{14}C from [^{14}C]-DG-6-P in cerebral tissues is sufficiently slow that it could be considered to be essentially trapped if the experimental procedure were limited to less than 1 hr.

The trapping of [^{14}C]-DG-6-P has recently been questioned by Hawkins and Miller (1978), who presented what they considered to be evidence of significant loss of [^{14}C]-DG-6-P under the conditions specified by the [^{14}C]-DG method. First, they cited a number of references in the literature that have reported higher levels of glucose-6-phosphatase activity than were observed by Hers and DeDuve (1950) and Hers (1957). It should be noted, however, that Hers (1957) and Hers and DeDuve (1950) assayed the activity of the native enzyme in broken cell homogenates of whole brain whereas in most of the studies cited by Hawkins and Miller (1978) the enzyme activity was estimated from assays carried out with isolated microsomes at pH 5.5–6.5 in the presence of deoxycholate, which activates this normally enzyme-bound enzyme.

Futhermore, the assay of glucose-6-phosphatase *in vitro* under optimized conditions neglects a number of other factors which might restrict the enzyme's activity *in vivo*. Glucose-6-phosphatase is a multifunctional enzyme that catalyzes a number of other reactions in addition to its glucose phosphohydrolase activity (Nordlie, 1971, 1974), and a number of the enzyme molecules can be expected to be committed to some of these other reactions. Also, the enzyme is inhibited by many compounds normally present intracellularly in brain, e.g., citrate, glucose, inorganic phosphate, and bicarbonate (Nordlie, 1974). Finally, one must consider intracellular compartmentation, which is disrupted in *in vitro* assays with subcellular components but which has a critical influence *in vivo*. Glucose-6-phosphatase is compartmentalized on the inner surfaces of the cisterns of the endoplasmic reticulum (Ballas and Arion, 1977). The hexose phosphates are formed in the cytosol and must be transported through the membranes of the endoplasmic reticulum before they can be hydrolyzed (Ballas and Arion, 1977). There is evidence that the transport of DG-6-P may be slower than that of G-6-P and may in fact be rate limiting in its hydrolysis by glucose-6-phosphatase (M. Karnovsky, personal communication).

The only phosphohydrolase activity of relevance to the [^{14}C]-DG method is the [^{14}C]deoxyglucose-6-phosphatase activity that occurs *in vivo*. Hawkins and Miller (1978) attempted to evaluate this activity as well. They applied the [^{14}C]-DG method to a series of rats but killed them at various times after the intravenous pulse of [^{14}C]-DG and measured the [^{14}C]-DG-6-P concentrations in brain as a function of time by direct chemical analyses. They also measured the time courses of the arterial plasma [^{14}C]-DG and glucose concentrations up to the time of killing, and with these data they used a transposed version of the operational equation (Figure 2) to calculate the time course of tissue [^{14}C]-DG-6-P concentration (i.e., the numerator of the operational equation) predicted by the equation, which assumes no loss of [^{14}C]-DG-6-P owing to phosphatase activity. Their computed curve was 2- to 3-fold higher than their measured concentrations (Figure 6), and they interpreted their results as proof that there was significant loss of [^{14}C]-DG-6-P during the experimental period. To make the computation with the transposed equation, however, it was necessary for them to assume values for R_i, the rate of cerebral glucose utilization, and the lumped constant. They assumed a value of 0.8 μmol/g per min for R_i—a reasonable value for the average rate of glucose utilization in the conscious rat brain. For the lumped constant, however, they assumed a value of 1.1. The lumped constant has, however, been directly determined in the rat and found to be 0.48 (Sokoloff *et al.,* 1977). If their computed curve is corrected for the error in the lumped constant that they used, then the theoretical curve obtained fits their experimental data remarkably well through all of the 45-min experimental period (Figure 6). Quite contrary to their conclusions, the experimental data of Hawkins and Miller (1978) offer the most convincing evidence that there is no significant loss of [^{14}C]-DG-6-P from brain owing to glucose-6-phosphatase activity or any other cause during the first 45 min after the pulse of [^{14}C]-DG.

It should be noted, however, that although it is low, the rate of loss of DG-6-P from brain tissue is not zero. DG-6-P formed in brain is not retained indef-

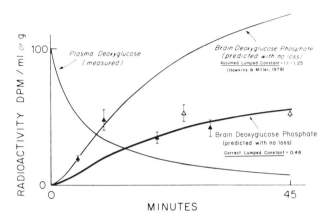

MINUTES

FIGURE 6. Comparison of time courses of [¹⁴C]-DG-6-P concentration in rat brain measured experimentally (triangles) and computed (continuous lines) by transposed version of equation (30), which assumes no loss owing to glucose-6-phosphatase activity. ▲, Mean ± S.E.M. of 4–12 rats; △, mean ± range of 2 animals. (Modified from Figure 1 in report of Hawkins and Miller, 1978.)

initely; it is lost with a half-life of several hours (Sokoloff *et al.*, 1977), presumably because of glucose-6-phosphatase activity. If the experimental period between the intravenous pulse of [¹⁴C]-DG and the time of killing is kept within 45 min, then the rate of loss can be ignored, and the standard operational equation of the method [equation (30)] can be used with negligible error. There may be occasions, however, when for special reasons longer experimental periods must be used. One example is the [¹⁸F]fluorodeoxyglucose adaptation of the [¹⁴C]-DG method for human use in which the local tissue concentrations of radioactivity are measured not by autoradiography but by positron emission tomography (Reivich *et al.*, 1979; Phelps *et al.*, 1979). [¹⁸F]Fluorodeoxyglucose-6-phosphate has been found to have a half-life in human brain of approximately 3 hr (Phelps *et al.*, 1979), but because of the slowness of presently available positron emission scanners, the period of measurement must be extended to 1–2 hr. Loss of product due to phosphatase activity cannot then be ignored. To make the method applicable in such situations the original model represented in Figure 1 has been modified by the addition of a k_4^*, representing the rate constant of hydrolysis and loss of the labeled phosphorylated product owing to phosphatase activity. The revised model has been mathematically analyzed and a modified operational equation has been derived that includes k_4^* and takes loss of labeled product into account. If k_4^* is assumed to be equal to zero, as is done in the original model, then the revised equation reduces to the original operational equation. The newly derived equation [equation (43)] therefore represents a more general case that is applicable to all conditions. The revised generalized equation to take phosphatase activity into account is as follows:

$$
R_i = \frac{C_i^*(\tau) - C_E^*(\tau) + k_4^* \int_0^\tau C_M^* dt}{\left(\frac{\lambda V_m^* K_m}{\Phi V_m K_m^*}\right)\left\{\int_0^\tau\left[(k_2^* + k_3^*)e^{-AT}\int_0^T (C_P^*/C_P)e^{At}dt\right]dT + \int_0^\tau\left[\left(\frac{k_4^*}{k_1^*}\right)(k_2^* + k_3^*)e^{-AT}\int_0^T (C_P^*/C_P)e^{+At}dt\right]dT\right\}} \tag{43}
$$

where $A = k_2^* + k_3^* + k_4^*$

$$
C_E^* = k_1^* e^{-AT}\int_0^T C_P^* e^{At}dt + k_4^* e^{-AT}\int_0^T C_i^* e^{At}dt
$$

$$
k_4^* \int_0^\tau C_M^* dt =
$$

$$
k_4^* \int_0^T \left\{ k_3^* e^{-k_4^* \tau}\int_0^\tau \left[k_1^* e^{-(k_2^*+k_3^*)T}\int_0^T C_P^* e^{At}\,dt + k_4^* e^{-(k_2^*+k_3^*)T}\int_0^T C_i^* e^{At}\,dt\right]\right\}dt
$$

The availability of the generalized equation has made it possible to test the limits of the validity of the assumption of no loss of product owing to phosphatase activity made in the derivation of the original operational equation. If the original operational equation is used under conditions in which there is significant phosphatase activity, then the rate of glucose utilization will be underestimated, and the degree of underestimation increases with increasing interval between the pulse of [14C]-DG and the time of killing and also with increasing phosphatase activity (i.e., the value of k_4^*). If the value of k_4^* is known, the magnitude of underestimation can be determined by comparison of the results obtained with the original operational equation and the generalized equation. A large group of normal conscious rats of approximately equal weight and age was studied by means of the DG method, but were killed at various times from 20 to 120 min following a pulse of [14C]-DG. The rates of glucose utilization were calculated by both equations. The three broken lines in Figure 7 represent the values for average glucose utilization in gray matter that should have been obtained with the standard operational equation in the presence of phosphatase activities equivalent to k_4^* values of 0.002, 0.005, and 0.01 per min; these lines also illustrate the magnitudes of the underestimations that would have occurred. The solid line in Figure 7 represents, however, the actual values calculated with the standard operational equation. It can be seen that up to 45 min there is no significant change with time in the

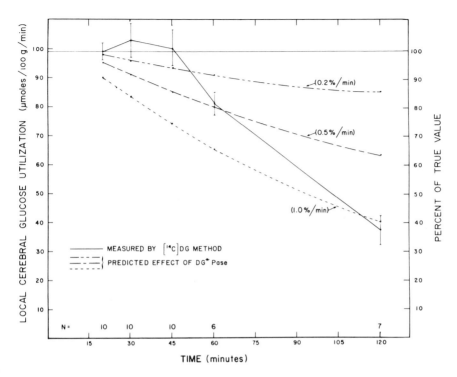

FIGURE 7. Effect of duration of experimental period on average (arithmetic) gray matter glucose utilization calculated by the standard operational equation (equation (30)), which assumes
no deoxyglucose-6-phosphatase (DG*Pase) activity (solid line). The points and bars at 20, 30,
45, 60, and 120 min represent the means and standard errors of the number of animals indicated
as *N*. Note that there is no significant change in the calculated value for glucose utilization
between 20 and 45 min. This indicates no influence of phosphatase activity during this period.
The broken lines represent the theoretical values for glucose utilization that should have been
obtained with the standard operational equation if there were loss of ^{14}C from the tissue owing
to DG*Pase activity or any other cause at rates equal to those indicated. Note the appearance
of loss of ^{14}C at later times.

calculated value of glucose utilization and no underestimation. This result con-
firms that there is no significant influence of phosphatase activity (i.e., k_4^*
equals zero) up to 45 min. However, at 60 min there is an underestimation of
approximately 18% (i.e., equivalent to a k_4^* of 0.005 per min) and at 120 min
the underestimation is approximately 60% (i.e., equivalent to a k_4^* of 0.01 per
min). These results demonstrate that there is no significant influence of phosphatase activity and the standard operational equation is valid for the first 45
min after the pulse. Thereafter, the generalized equation must be used to take
progressively increasing phosphatase activity into account.

The results also demonstrate another phenomenon. The influence of phosphatase activity is initially absent, becomes evident after a long lag, and then increases in magnitude with increasing time. This type of kinetics is consistent with a model based on compartmentation in which transport of the substitute into the compartment containing the enzyme is rate-limiting. It would appear then that the rate of hydrolysis and loss of label from $[^{14}C]$-DG-6-P is limited not by the level of glucose-6-phosphatase activity but by the accessibility of the substrate to the enzyme.

4.4. Influence of Varying Plasma Glucose Concentration

In the derivation of the operational equation of the method [equation (30)], the assumption was made that the arterial plasma glucose concentration, C_P, remains constant throughout the duration of the experimental period. This assumption is explicitly stated in the mathematical analysis of the model at the point where equation (27) is derived from equation (26). The reason for the assumption was that it simplified the mathematical analysis. Once made, this assumption established a necessary condition for the operational equation to be valid, and the method was then applicable only to experiments in which the plasma glucose concentration remained constant during the procedure. This restraint has proved cumbersome. A new operational equation has, therefore, been derived which allows for a varying C_P. The equation is as follows:

$$R_i = \frac{C_i^*(\tau) - k_1^* e^{-(k_2^*+k_3^*)\tau} \int_0^\tau C_p^* e^{(k_2^*+k_3^*)t}\, dt}{\left(\dfrac{\lambda V_m^* K_m}{\Phi V_m K_m^*}\right) \displaystyle\int_0^\tau \left[\dfrac{(k_2^*+k_3^*)e^{-(k_2^*+k_3^*)T}\int_0^T C_p^* e^{(k_2^*+k_3^*)k}\, dt}{C_P(0)e^{(k_2+k_3)T} + (k_2+k_3)e^{-(k_2+k_3)T}\int_0^T C_p e^{(k_2+k_3)t}\, dt}\right] dT} \tag{44}$$

where $(k_2 + k_3)$ equals the turnover rate constant of the free glucose pool in the brain; $C_P(0)$ equals the arterial plasma glucose concentration at zero time; τ equals the time of killing; and all other symbols are as in equation (30).

Equation (44) requires an estimate of the turnover rate constant or half-life of the free glucose pool in the tissue. The rate constant equals 0.693 divided by the half-life of the pool. A method has been developed to measure the half-life of the free glucose pool in brain tissue *in vivo*. This half-life has been found to equal 1.2 and 1.8 min in normal conscious and anesthetized rats, respectively, and to vary with the plasma glucose concentration (Savaki *et al.,* 1980). The equation is relatively insensitive to the value of the half-life of the glucose pool in the range in which it usually falls, and, therefore, only an approximation of this value is sufficient without any serious impairment to the accuracy of the final result. It should be noted that equation (44) is only an approximation of the actual situation which is immensely more complex. Specifically, equation (44) assumes that $(k_2 + k_3)$ remains constant with changing plasma glucose concentration. It has been found, however, that $(k_2 + k_3)$ does change with the plasma glucose concentration (Savaki et al., 1980). The slope, however, is quite shallow, and a change of 200 mg% in plasma glucose concentration changes the value of $(k_2 + k_3)$ by approximately 25%. Simulation analyses of equation (44) have demonstrated that changes in the value of $(k_2 + k_3)$ by 25% from its value normally existing at plasma glucose concentrations between 100 and 200 mg% have negligible effects on the final results. Also, recent studies in our laboratory have revealed that hypoglycemia, i.e., plasma glucose concentrations below 70 mg% (S. Suda, M. Miyaoka, C. Kennedy, L. Sokoloff, unpublished observations) and hyperglycemia, i.e., plasma glucose concentrations above 300 mg% (F. Schuier, F. Orzi, and L. Sokoloff, unpublished observations) alter the lumped constant from its value in normoglycemic conditions. Therefore the DG method should not be used at present with plasma glucose levels outside these limits. Within these limits equation (44), though an approximation, is fully satisfactory with conditions of changing plasma glucose concentration.

4.5.   [^{14}C] Deoxyglucose vs. [^{14}C] Glucose

The DG method has the unique feature that it utilizes a labeled analogue which serves as a competitive substrate to measure the rate of metabolism of a natural substrate, in this case glucose. It is reasonable to ask why the analogue is used when labeled preparations of the natural substrate are readily available. The reason is that the use of DG makes it possible to bypass certain extremely difficult, if not insurmountable, problems associated with the use of glucose. The problem with [^{14}C]glucose is that labeled CO_2 is rapidly lost from the brain (within 2 min after its introduction into the circulation) regardless of which carbon is labeled (Sacks, 1957). The same probably applies to water if [^{3}H]glucose is used. It is impossible to obtain an accurate estimate of the amount of product formed if the product is continuously being lost and at a rate that varies with time. To derive a correction for the loss of product is an extraordinarily complex and probably impossible goal because the loss of labeled CO_2 is dependent not only on the rate of glucose utilization but also on the fluxes of glucose carbon, turnover rate constants, and pool sizes for every single intermediate in the entire metabolic pathway between glucose and the points at which CO_2 is released. Furthermore, these determinant factors are likely to be different for each structure of the brain.

To minimize the problem of loss of $^{14}CO_2$, it is necessary to keep the experimental period very short before there has been significant formation and loss of $^{14}CO_2$. This, however, introduces another equally complex problem. The rate of formation of labeled product depends not only on the rate of the chemical reaction but also on the specific activity of the precursor pool. In the intact animal it is impossible to measure the time courses of the specific activity of the glucose pool in all the structures of the brain. It is necessary to measure the time course of the specific activity in the arterial plasma and then to calculate the specific activities in the tissues from the plasma specific activities and the separately determined kinetic constants governing the equilibration of tissue and plasma specific activities (see Figure 2). The rate constants are used to correct for the lag in the equilibration of the precursor pool specific activity of the tissue with that of plasma. The shorter the interval of time the more critical the rate constants become. Figure 5 applies to the use of labeled glucose as well as labeled DG. The half-life of the glucose pool in normal conscious rat brain is approximately 1.5 min (Savaki *et al.,* 1980), which falls well within the range of those included in the family of curves in Figure 5. It can be seen that at early times relatively small errors in the values of the rate constants used can produce enormous errors in the final value of the integrated specific activity of the precursor pool in the tissue. Inasmuch as the rate constants cannot be measured in the same animal at the same time that glucose utilization is being measured, it is almost certain that the values of the rate constants used are not very accurate for that particular animal. Furthermore, with the short experimental periods required for the use of labeled glucose, the rate constants become so critical that it is necessary to have accurate values of the rate constants for each individual cerebral structure, not average values for gray matter, white matter, or the brain as a whole. On the other hand, if the experimental period is prolonged, then the rate constants become uncritical, and large errors in the values of the rate constants lead to only slight errors in the final result.

There is, therefore, a major dilemma associated with the use of [^{14}C]glucose. If the experimental period is kept short to avoid loss of $^{14}CO_2$, then large errors occur due to inaccurate estimation of the precursor pool specific activities. If the experimental period is lengthened to minimize these errors, the equally serious errors due to loss of $^{14}CO_2$ ensue. Hawkins *et al.* (1974) ignored this dilemma when they described their method for the measurement of cerebral glucose utilization based on the use of [2-^{14}C]glucose. They assumed that the glucose pool in the tissue was in instantaneous and continuous equilibrium with that of the plasma (i.e., tissue glucose pool half-life equals zero) so they used the plasma glucose specific activity as the value for the tissue glucose specific activity. This assumption is obviously invalid; the half-life of the glucose pool in the tissue is finite and significant and cannot be ignored.

It is precisely to avoid this dilemma associated with the use of

[^{14}C]glucose that [^{14}C]-DG is used. Because of the relative stability and retention of the product [^{14}C]-DG-6-P, it becomes possible to extend the experimental interval to a period long enough to minimize errors in the estimation of the tissue precursor specific activity while at the same time avoiding errors due to loss of product. The price that must be paid for this advantage is the appearance of a lumped constant not equal to unity. Because of differences in the kinetic constants of hexokinase for DG and glucose, the lumped constant is less than one, whereas with labeled glucose the kinetic constants are the same and the lumped constant equals unity. The lumped constant, however, has been rigorously defined, can be reasonably accurately determined, and presents far less serious problems than those associated with the use of [^{14}C]glucose.

5. RATES OF LOCAL CEREBRAL GLUCOSE UTILIZATION IN THE NORMAL CONSCIOUS STATE

Thus far quantitative measurements of local cerebral glucose utilization have been reported only for the albino rat (Sokoloff *et al.,* 1977) and monkey (Kennedy *et al.,* 1978). These values are presented in Table 3. The rates of local cerebral glucose utilization in the normal conscious rat vary widely throughout the brain. The values in white structures tend to group together and are always considerably below those of gray structures. The average value in gray matter is approximately 50–200 μmol of glucose/100 g per min. The highest values are in the structures involved in auditory functions, with the inferior colliculus clearly the most metabolically active structure in the brain.

The rates of local cerebral glucose utilization in the conscious monkey exhibit similar heterogeneity, but they are generally one-third to one-half of the values in corresponding structures of the rat brain (Table 3). The differences in rates in the rat and monkey brain are consistent with the different cellular packing densities in the brains of these two species.

6. EFFECTS OF GENERAL ANESTHESIA

General anesthesia produced by thiopental reduces the rates of glucose utilization in all structures of the rat brain (Table 4) (Sokoloff *et al.,* 1977). The effects are not uniform. The greatest reductions occur in the gray structures, particularly those of the primary sensory pathways. The effects in white matter, though definitely present, are relatively small compared to those of gray matter. These results are in agreement with those of previous studies in which anesthesia has been found to decrease the cerebral metabolic rate of the brain as a whole (Kety, 1950; Lassen, 1959; Sokoloff, 1976).

TABLE 3. Representative Values for Local Cerebral Glucose Utilization in the Normal Conscious Albino Rat and Monkey (μmoles/100 g per min)[a]

Structure	Albino rat[b] (10)	Monkey[c] (7)
Gray matter		
Visual cortex	107 ± 6	59 ± 2
Auditory cortex	162 ± 5	79 ± 4
Parietal cortex	112 ± 5	47 ± 4
Sensorimotor cortex	120 ± 5	44 ± 3
Thalamus		
Lateral nucleus	116 ± 5	54 ± 2
Ventral nucleus	109 ± 5	43 ± 2
Medial geniculate body	131 ± 5	65 ± 3
Lateral geniculate body	96 ± 5	39 ± 1
Hypothalamus	54 ± 2	25 ± 1
Mamillary body	121 ± 5	57 ± 3
Hippocampus	79 ± 3	39 ± 2
Amygdala	52 ± 2	25 ± 2
Caudate–putamen	110 ± 4	52 ± 3
Nucleus accumbens	82 ± 3	36 ± 2
Globus pallidus	58 ± 2	26 ± 2
Substantia nigra	58 ± 3	29 ± 2
Vestibular nucleus	128 ± 5	66 ± 3
Cochlear nucleus	113 ± 7	51 ± 3
Superior olivary nucleus	133 ± 7	63 ± 4
Inferior colliculus	197 ± 10	103 ± 6
Superior colliculus	95 ± 5	55 ± 4
Pontine gray matter	62 ± 3	28 ± 1
Cerebellar cortex	57 ± 2	31 ± 2
Cerebellar nuclei	100 ± 4	45 ± 2
White matter		
Corpus callosum	40 ± 2	11 ± 1
Internal capsule	33 ± 2	13 ± 1
Cerebellar white matter	37 ± 2	12 ± 1

[a] The values are the means ± standard errors from measurements made in the number of animals indicated in parentheses.
[b] From Sokoloff *et al.* (1977).
[c] From Kennedy *et al.* (1978).

TABLE 4. Effects of Thiopental Anesthesia on Local Cerebral Glucose Utilization in the rat[a,b]

Structure	Local cerebral glucose utilization (μmoles/100 g per min)		% Effect
	Control[c] (6)	Anesthetized[c] (8)	
Gray matter			
Visual cortex	111 ± 5	64 ± 3	−42
Auditory cortex	157 ± 5	81 ± 3	−48
Parietal cortex	107 ± 3	65 ± 2	−39
Sensorimotor cortex	118 ± 3	67 ± 2	−43
Lateral geniculate body	92 ± 2	53 ± 3	−42
Medial geniculate body	126 ± 6	63 ± 3	−50
Thalamus			
Lateral nucleus	108 ± 3	58 ± 2	−46
Ventral nucleus	98 ± 3	55 ± 1	−44
Hypothalamus	63 ± 3	43 ± 2	−32
Caudate–putamen	111 ± 4	72 ± 3	−35
Hippocampus: Ammon's Horn	79 ± 1	56 ± 1	−29
Amygdala	56 ± 4	41 ± 2	−27
Cochlear nucleus	124 ± 7	79 ± 5	−36
Lateral lemniscus	114 ± 7	75 ± 4	−34
Inferior colliculus	198 ± 7	131 ± 8	−34
Superior olivary nucleus	141 ± 5	104 ± 7	−26
Superior colliculus	99 ± 3	59 ± 3	−40
Vestibular nucleus	133 ± 4	81 ± 4	−39
Pontine gray matter	69 ± 3	46 ± 3	−33
Cerebellar cortex	66 ± 2	44 ± 2	−33
Cerebellar nucleus	106 ± 4	75 ± 4	−29
White matter			
Corpus callosum	42 ± 2	30 ± 2	−29
Genu of corpus callosum	35 ± 5	30 ± 2	−14
Internal capsule	35 ± 2	29 ± 2	−17
Cerebellar white matter	38 ± 2	29 ± 2	−24

[a] From Sokoloff *et al.* (1977).
[b] Determined at 30 min following pulse of [^{14}C]-DG.
[c] The values are the means ± standard errors obtained in the number of animals indicated in parentheses. All the differences are statistically significant at the $p < 0.05$ level.

Preliminary studies indicate that thiopental anesthesia has effects in the Rhesus monkey like those in the rat (Shapiro *et al.,* 1975). The effects of halothane anesthesia in the monkey are similar, except that it appears to leave the basal ganglia unaffected (Shapiro *et al.,* 1975). In contrast, phencyclidine, which is often used as an anesthetic agent but is probably a convulsant, causes 10–50% increases in glucose consumption in all gray structures, except the inferior colliculus, pontine nuclei, and cerebellar cortex where significant decreases are observed (Shapiro *et al.,* 1975).

7. RELATION BETWEEN LOCAL FUNCTIONAL ACTIVITY AND ENERGY METABOLISM

The results of a variety of applications of the method demonstrate a clear relationship between local cerebral functional activity and glucose consumption. The most striking demonstrations of the close coupling between function and energy metabolism are seen with experimentally induced local alterations in functional activity that are restricted to a few specific areas in the brain. The effects on local glucose consumption are then so pronounced that they not only are observed in the quantitative results but also can be visualized directly on the autoradiographs, which are really pictorial representations of the relative rates of glucose utilization in the various structural components of the brain.

7.1. Effects of Increased Functional Activity

7.1.1. Effects of Sciatic Nerve Stimulation

Electrical stimulation of one sciatic nerve in the rat under barbiturate anesthesia causes pronounced increases in glucose consumption (i.e., increased optical density in the autoradiographs) in the ipsilateral dorsal horn of the lumbar spinal cord (Figure 8) (Kennedy *et al.,* 1975).

7.1.2. Effects of Olfactory Stimulation

The [^{14}C]-DG method has been used to map the olfactory system of the rat (Sharp *et al.,* 1975). Olfactory stimulation with amyl acetate has been found to produce increased labeling in localized regions of the olfactory bulb. Preliminary results obtained with other odors, such as camphor and cheese, suggest different spatial patterns of increased metabolic activity with different odors.

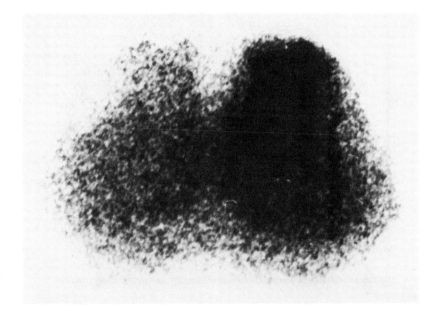

FIGURE 8. Effects of unilateral electrical stimulation of the sciatic nerve on local utilization of glucose in the lumbar spinal cord of the anesthetized rat. The illustration is an autoradiograph of a section of the lumbar spinal cord, which provides a pictorial representation of the relative rates of local glucose utilization in the tissues. The greater the optical density, the greater the rate of glucose utilization. Note the asymmetrical increased density in the region of the dorsal horn on the side ipsilateral to the stimulated nerve. (From Kennedy *et al.*, 1975.)

7.1.3. Effects of Experimental Focal Seizures

The local injection of penicillin into the hand–face area of the motor cortex of the Rhesus monkey has been shown to induce electrical discharges in the adjacent cortex and to result in recurrent focal seizures involving the face, arm, and hand on the contralateral side (Caveness, 1969). Such seizure activity causes selective increases in glucose consumption in areas of motor cortex adjacent to the penicillin locus and in small discrete regions of the putamen, globus pallidus, caudate nucleus, thalamus, and substantia nigra of the same side (Figure 9) (Kennedy *et al.*, 1975). Similar studies in the rat have led to comparable results and provided evidence on the basis of an evoked metabolic response of a "mirror" focus in the motor cortex contralateral to the penicillin-induced epileptogenic focus (Collins *et al.*, 1976).

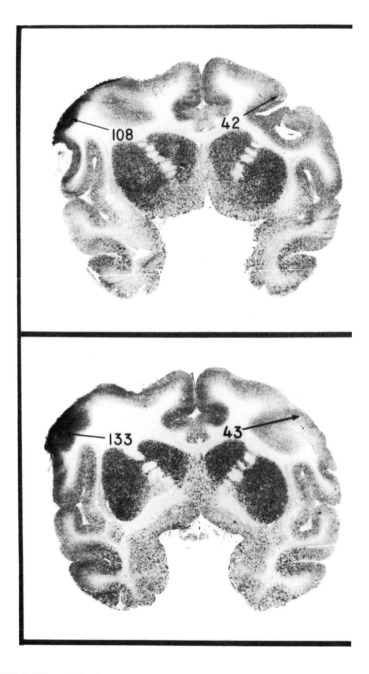

FIGURE 9. Effects of focal seizures produced by local application of penicillin to motor cortex on local cerebral glucose utilization in the Rhesus monkey. The penicillin was applied to the hand and face area of the left motor cortex. The left side of the brain is on the left in each of the autoradiographs in the figure. The numbers are the rates of local cerebral glucose utilization in μmol/100 g tissue per min. Note the following: Upper left, Motor cortex in region of penicillin

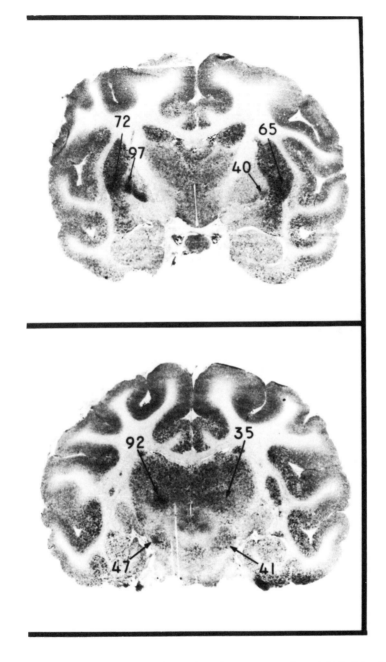

application and corresponding region of contralateral motor cortex; lower left, ipsilateral and contralateral motor cortical regions remote from area of penicillin applications; upper right, ipsilateral and contralateral putamen and globus pallidus; lower right, ipsilateral and contralateral thalamic nuclei and substantia nigra. (From Sokoloff, 1977.)

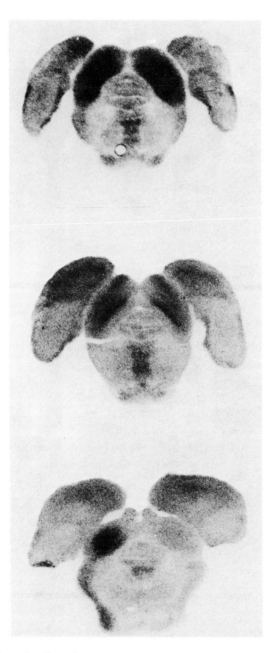

FIGURE 10. Effects of auditory deprivation on cerebral glucose utilization of some components of the auditory system of the albino rat. Upper, Autoradiograph of section of brain from normal conscious rat with intact bilateral hearing in ambient noise of laboratory. The autoradiograph

7.2. Effects of Decreased Functional Activity

Decrements in functional activity result in reduced rates of glucose utilization. These effects are particularly striking in the auditory and visual systems of the rat and the visual system of the monkey.

7.2.1. Effects of Auditory Deprivation

In the albino rat some of the highest rates of local cerebral glucose utilization are found in components of the auditory system, i.e., auditory cortex, medial geniculate ganglion, inferior colliculus, lateral lemniscus, superior olive, and cochlear nucleus (Table 3). The high metabolic activities of some of these structures (e.g., inferior colliculus, nuclei of lateral lemniscus, and superior olive) are clearly visible in the autoradiographs (Figure 10). Bilateral auditory deprivation by occlusion of both external auditory canals with wax markedly depresses the metabolic activity in all of these areas (Figure 10) (M. H. Des Rosiers, C. Kennedy, and L. Sokoloff, unpublished observations). The reductions are symmetrical bilaterally and range from 35 to 60%. Unilateral auditory deprivation also depresses the glucose consumption of these structures but to a lesser degree, and some of the structures are asymmetrically affected. For example, the metabolic activity of the ipsilateral cochlear nucleus is 75% of the activity of the contralateral nucleus. The lateral lemniscus, superior olive, and medial geniculate ganglion are slightly lower on the contralateral side, while the contralateral inferior colliculus is markedly lower in metabolic activity than the ipsilateral structure (Figure 10). These results demonstrate that there is some degree of lateralization and crossing of auditory pathways in the rat.

7.2.2. Visual Deprivation in the Rat

In the rat the visual system is 80–85% crossed at the optic chiasma (Lashley, 1934; Montero and Guillery, 1968) and unilateral enucleation removes most of the visual input to the central visual structures of the contralateral side. In the conscious rat studied 2–24 hr after unilateral enucleation, there are marked decrements in glucose utilization in the contralateral superior collicu-

---

shows the inferior colliculi, the lateral lemnisci, and the superior olives, all of which exhibit bilateral symmetry of optical densities. Autoradiograph (middle) of comparable section of brain from rat with bilateral occlusion of external auditory canals with wax and kept in a soundproof room. Note the virtual disappearance of the inferior colliculi, lateral lemnisci, and superior olives. Autoradiograph (lower) of comparable section of brain from rat with one external auditory canal blocked. Note the asymmetry of the inferior colliculi and the almost symmetrical intermediate reductions of densities in the lateral lemnisci and superior olives. The ear that was blocked was contralateral to the inferior colliculus that was markedly depressed. (From Sokoloff, 1977.)

lus, lateral geniculate ganglion and visual cortex as compared to the ipsilateral side (Figure 11) (Kennedy *et al.*, 1975). In the rat with both eyes intact, no asymmetry in the autoradiographs is observed (Figure 11).

7.2.3.   Visual Deprivation in the Monkey

In animals with binocular visual systems, such as the Rhesus monkey, there is only approximately 50% crossing of the visual pathways, and the structures of the visual system on each side of the brain receive equal inputs from both retinae. Although each retina projects more or less equally to both hemispheres, their projections remain segregated and terminate in six well-defined laminae in the lateral geniculate ganglia, three each for the ipsilateral and contralateral eyes (Hubel and Wiesel, 1968, 1972; Wiesel *et al.*, 1974; Rakic, 1976). This segregation is preserved in the optic radiations, which project the monocular representations of the two eyes for any segment of the visual field to adjacent regions of Layer IV of the striate cortex (Hubel and Wiesel, 1968, 1972). The cells responding to the input of each monocular terminal zone are distributed transversely through the thickness of the striate cortex resulting in a mosaic of columns, 0.3–0.5 mm in width, alternately representing the monocular inputs of the two eyes. The nature and distribution of these ocular dominance columns have previously been characterized by electrophysiological techniques (Hubel and Wiesel, 1968), by Nauta degeneration methods (Hubel and Wiesel, 1972), and by autoradiographic visualization of axonal and transneuronal transport of [³H]proline- and [³H]fucose-labeled protein and/or glycoprotein (Wiesel *et al.*, 1974; Rakic, 1976). Bilateral or unilateral visual deprivation, either by enucleation or by the insertion of opaque plastic discs, produces consistent changes in the pattern of distribution of the rates of glucose consumption, all clearly visible in the autoradiographs, that coincide closely with the changes in functional activity expected from known physiological and anatomical properties of the binocular visual system (Kennedy *et al.*, 1976).

In animals with intact binocular vision no bilateral asymmetry is seen in the autoradiographs of the structures of the visual system (Figures 12A and 13A). The lateral geniculate ganglia and oculomotor nuclei appear to be of fairly uniform density and essentially the same on both sides (Figure 12A). The visual cortex is also the same on both sides (Figure 13A), but throughout all of Area 17 there is heterogeneous density distributed in a characteristic laminar pattern. These observations indicate that in animals with binocular visual input the rates of glucose consumption in the visual pathways are essentially equal on both sides of the brain and relatively uniform in the oculomotor nuclei and lateral geniculate ganglia, but markedly different in the various layers of the striate cortex.

Autoradiographs from animals with both eyes occluded exhibit generally decreased labeling of all components of the visual system, but the bilateral symmetry is fully retained (Figures 12B and 13B) and the density within each lateral geniculate body is for the most part fairly uniform (Figure 12B). In the striate cortex, however, the marked differences in the densities of the various layers seen in the animals with intact bilateral vision (Figure 13A) are virtually absent so that, except for a faint delineation of a band within Layer IV, the concentration of the label is essentially homogeneous throughout the striate cortex (Figure 13B).

Autoradiographs from monkeys with only monocular input because of unilateral visual occlusion exhibit markedly different patterns from those described above. Both lateral geniculate bodies exhibit exactly inverse patterns of alternating dark and light bands corresponding to the known laminae representing the regions receiving the different inputs from the retinae of the intact and occluded eyes (Figure 12C). Bilateral asymmetry is also seen in the oculomotor nuclear complex; a lower density is apparent in the nuclear complex contralateral to the occluded eye (Figure 12C). In the striate cortex the pattern of distribution of the $[^{14}C]$-DG-6-P appears to be a composite of the patterns seen in the animals with intact and bilaterally occluded visual input. The pattern found in the former regularly alternates with that of the latter in columns oriented perpendicularly to the cortical surface (Figure 13C). The dimensions, arrangement, and distribution of these columns are identical to those of the ocular dominance columns described by Hubel and Wiesel (Hubel and Wiesel, 1968, 1972; Wiesel *et al.*, 1974). These columns reflect the interdigitation of the representations of the two retinae in the visual cortex. Each element in the visual fields is represented by a pair of contiguous bands in the visual cortex, one for each of the two retinae or their portions that correspond to the given point in the visual fields. With symmetrical visual input bilaterally, the columns representing the two eyes are equally active and, therefore, not visualized in the autoradiographs (Figure 13A). When one eye is blocked, however, only those columns representing the blocked eye become metabolically less active, and the autoradiographs then display the alternate bands of normal and depressed activities corresponding to the regions of visual cortical representation of the two eyes (Figure 13C).

A pair of regions in the folded calcarine cortex can be seen in the autoradiographs (from the animals with unilateral visual deprivation) that exhibit bilateral asymmetry (Figure 13C). The ocular dominance columns are absent on both sides, but on the side contralateral to the occluded eye this region has the appearance of visual cortex from an animal with normal bilateral vision. Furthermore, on the ipsilateral side this region looks like cortex from an animal with both eyes occluded (Figure 13). These regions are the loci of the cortical representation of the blind spots of the visual fields and normally have only monocular input (Kennedy *et al.*, 1975, 1976). The area of the optic disc in

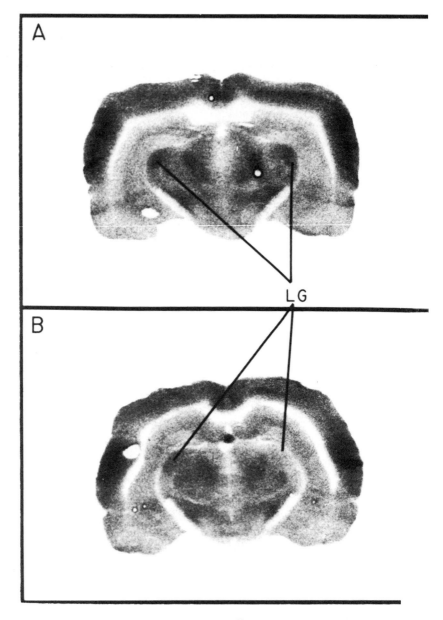

FIGURE 11. Effects of unilateral enucleation on [^{14}C]-DG uptake in components of the visual system in the rat. In the normal rat with both eyes intact the uptakes in the lateral geniculate bodies (LG), superior colliculi (SC), and striate cortex (Str C) are approximately equal on both

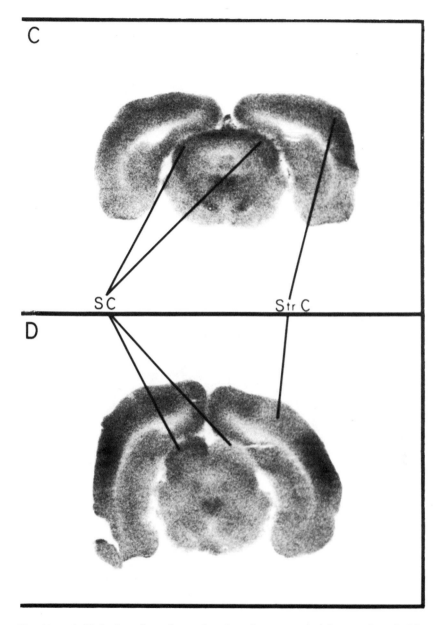

sides (A and C). In the unilaterally enucleated rat there are marked decreases in optical densities in the areas corresponding to these structures on the side contralateral to the enucleation (B and D). (From Kennedy *et al.*, 1975.)

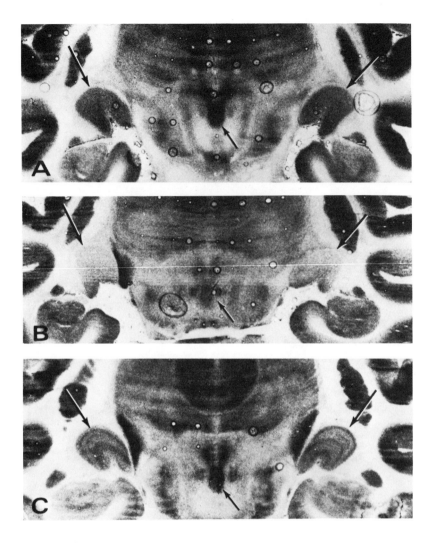

5.0mm

FIGURE 12. Autoradiography of coronal brain sections of monkey at the level of the lateral geniculate bodies. Large arrows point to the lateral geniculate bodies; small arrows point to oculomotor nuclear complex. (A) Animal with intact binocular vision. Note the bilateral symmetry and relative homogeneity of the lateral geniculate bodies and oculomotor nuclei. (B) Animal with bilateral visual occlusion. Note the reduced relative densities, the relative homogeneity, and the bilateral symmetry of the lateral geniculate bodies and oculomotor nuclei. (C) Animal with right eye occluded. The left side of the brain is on the left side of the photograph. Note the laminae and the inverse order of the dark and light bands in the two lateral geniculate bodies. Note also the lesser density of the oculomotor nuclear complex on the side contralateral to the occluded eye. (From Kennedy *et al.*, 1976.)

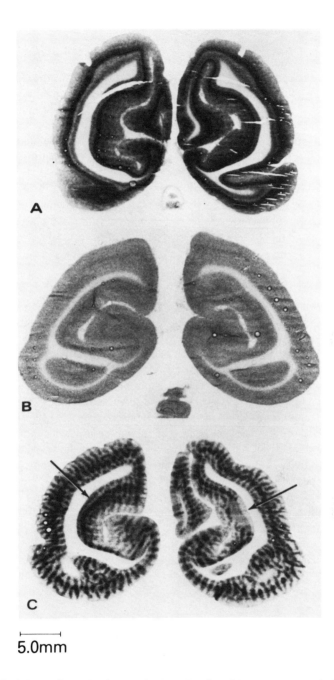

5.0mm

FIGURE 13. Autoradiographs of coronal brain sections from Rhesus monkeys at the level of the striate cortex. (A) Animal with normal binocular vision. Note the laminar distribution of the density; the dark band corresponds to Layer IV. (B) Animal with bilateral visual deprivation. Note the almost uniform and reduced relative density, especially the virtual disappearance of the

the nasal half of each retina cannot transmit to this region of the contralateral striate cortex, which therefore receives its sole input from an area in the temporal half of the ipsilateral retina. Occlusion of one eye deprives this region of the ipsilateral striate cortex of all input while the corresponding region of the contralateral striate cortex retains uninterrupted input from the intact eye. The metabolic reflection of this ipsilateral monocular input is seen in the autoradiograph in Figure 13C.

The results of these studies with the $[^{14}C]$-DG method in the binocular visual system of the monkey represent the most dramatic demonstration of the close relationship between physiological changes in functional activity and the rate of energy metabolism in specific components of the central nervous system.

8. MECHANISM OF COUPLING OF LOCAL FUNCTIONAL ACTIVITY AND ENERGY METABOLISM

In tissues, such as heart muscle, skeletal muscle, and kidney, which do recognizable physical work, there is a clear quantitative relationship between the work performed and the rate of energy metabolism. Presumably, at least part of the energy derived from metabolism is equivalent to the energy expenditure associated with the physical work and serves to resynthesize high energy phosphate bonds consumed in the process. It is less clear what type of physical work is performed by nervous tissue. The finding of a close coupling between local functional activity and glucose utilization suggests, however, that neural functional activity is associated with some energy-consuming physical and/or chemical processes.

Electrical activity appears to be the physical process most intimately involved with functional activity in nervous tissue. Action potentials are generated by the movement of ions, mainly Na^+ and K^+, across cell membranes down ionic gradients, and energy must be consumed to restore the ionic gradients to their resting levels. Increased electrical activity, i.e., increased fre-

---

(*Continued from p. 57*)

dark band corresponding to Layer IV. (C) Animal with right eye occluded. The half-brain on the left side of the photograph represents the left hemisphere contralateral to the occluded eye. Note the alternate dark and light striations, each approximately 0.3–0.4 mm in width that represent the ocular dominance columns. These columns are most apparent in the dark band corresponding to Layer IV but extend through the entire thickness of the cortex. The arrows point to regions of bilateral asymmetry where the ocular dominance columns are absent. These are presumably areas with normally only monocular input. The one on the left, contralateral to occluded eye, has a continuous dark lamina corresponding to Layer IV which is completely absent on the side ipsilateral to the occluded eye. These regions are believed to be the loci of the cortical representations of the blind spots. (From Kennedy *et al.*, 1976.)

quency of action potentials, might be expected to lead to greater ionic fluxes and therefore require more energy to restore the ionic gradients. Indeed, Yarowsky *et al.* (1979) have recently found in the superior cervical ganglion *in vivo* a direct linear relationship between the frequency of the electrical spike input and the rate of glucose utilization (see next paragraph). The energy required to transport the ions back across the cell membrane to restore the ionic gradients is presumably derived from the splitting of ATP by Na^+,K^+-ATPase (Albers, 1967; Caldwell, 1968). Once ATP is split, there are adequate biochemical mechanisms to explain the increased glucose utilization and energy metabolism. It has been estimated that more than 40% of the brain's energy consumption is used for the maintenance and restoration of ionic gradients and membrane potentials (Whittam, 1962).

This hypothesis implies that the Na^+,K^+-ATPase is a key link in the coupling of glucose utilization to functional activity. To test this hypothesis, Mata *et al.* (1980) have used the [^{14}C]-DG technique *in vitro* with electrically stimulated preparations of rat posterior pituitary. Electrical stimulation led to increased glucose utilization which was blocked by ouabain, an inhibitor of the Na^+,K^+-ATPase but not of the spike activity or the release of vasopressin by the gland. It is noteworthy that veratridine, an alkaloid that opens Na^+ channels, depolarizes the cell membranes and therefore activates Na^+,K^+-ATPase activity, also stimulated glucose utilization in the posterior pituitary. This effect was also blocked by ouabain or tetrodotoxin. These results strongly support the hypothesis that energy metabolism is coupled to functional activity through the activity of the Na^+,K^+-ATPase.

The posterior pituitary is highly enriched with axon terminals, which account for greater than 42% of the gland's total volume (Nordmann, 1977). The gland contains, therefore, an extraordinarily high content of elements with large areas of membrane surface relative to their volumes. Such structures are likely to suffer relatively large changes in ionic concentration gradients for a given amount of electrical spike activity. The increased glucose utilization observed by Mata *et al.* (1980) in the electrically stimulated posterior pituitary *in vitro* probably reflected mainly the metabolic activity of the axonal terminals. Schwartz *et al.* (1979) have studied the entire hypothalamo-hypophysial pathway *in vivo* by means of the [^{14}C]-DG method. Stimulation of this pathway physiologically by salt-loading also led to markedly increased glucose utilization in the posterior pituitary, but surprisingly, there were no detectable effects in the supraoptic and paraventricular nuclei (the loci of the cell bodies with projections to the posterior pituitary). Obviously the pathway had been activated by the osmotic stimulation. The discrepancy in the effects in the cell bodies and in the regions of termination of their projections may well reflect the greater sensitivity of axonal terminals and/or synaptic elements than that of perikarya to metabolic activation. Indeed, the results of the studies on the binocular system of the monkey described above also lend support to this possibility. In the animals with both eyes open, Layer IVB, the layer with predominantly neuropil and axodendritic connections, is clearly the most metabolically active portion of the striate cortex (Kennedy *et al.,* 1976) (Figure 13A). It is precisely this region which shows the greatest reduction in glucose utilization when both eyes are patched; the other layers also exhibit some reductions in metabolism but much less so and Layer IVB can hardly be distinguished from the other layers in the autoradiographs (Figure 13B). It seems likely then that the changes in local cerebral glucose utilization in response to altered functional activity revealed by the $[^{14}C]$-DG method represent mainly alterations in the metabolic activity of synaptic terminals triggered by changes in Na^+,K^+-ATPase activity.

9. APPLICATIONS OF THE DEOXYGLUCOSE METHOD

The results of studies like those described in Section 8 on the effects of experimentally induced focal alterations of functional activity on local glucose utilization have demonstrated a close coupling between local functional activity and energy metabolism in the central nervous system. The effects are often so pronounced that they can be visualized directly on the autoradiographs, which provide pictorial representations of the relative rates of glucose utilization throughout the brain. This technique of autoradiographic visualization of evoked metabolic response offers a powerful tool with which to map functional neural pathways simultaneously in all anatomical components of the central nervous system; extensive use has been made of it for this purpose (Plum *et al.,* 1976). The results have clearly demonstrated the effectiveness of metabolic responses, either positive or negative, in identifying regions of the central nervous system involved in specific functions.

The method has been used most extensively in qualitative studies in which regions of altered functional activity are identified by the change in their visual appearance relative to other regions in the autoradiographs. Such qualitative studies are effective only when the effects are lateralized to one side or when only a few discrete regions are affected; other regions serve as the controls. Quantitative comparisons cannot, however, be made for equivalent regions between two or more animals. To make quantitative comparisons between animals, the fully quantitative method must be used, which takes into account the various factors, particularly the plasma glucose level, that influence the magnitude of labeling of the tissues. The method must be used quantitatively when the experimental procedure produces systemic effects and alters metabolism in many regions of the brain.

A comprehensive review of the many qualitative and quantitative applications of the method is beyond the scope of this report. Only some of the many neurophysiological, neuroanatomical, pharmacological, and pathophysiological applications of the method will be briefly noted merely to illustrate the broad extent of its potential usefulness.

9.1. Neurophysiological and Neuroanatomical Applications

Many of the physiological applications of the $[^{14}C]$-DG method were in studies designed to test the method and to examine the relationship between local cerebral functional and metabolic activities. These applications have been described in Section 8. The most dramatic results have been obtained in the visual systems of the monkey and the rat. The method has, for example, been used to define the nature, conformation, and distribution of the ocular dominance columns in the striate cortex of the monkey (Figure 13C) (Kennedy *et al.*, 1976). It has been used by Hubel *et al.* (1978) to do the same for the orientation columns in the striate cortex of the monkey. A by-product of the studies of the ocular dominance columns was the identification of the loci of the visual cortical representation of the blind spots of the visual fields (Figure 13C) (Kennedy *et al.*, 1976). Studies are currently in progress to map the pathways of higher visual functions beyond the striate cortex; the results thus far demonstrate extensive areas of involvement of the inferior temporal cortex in visual processing (Jarvis *et al.*, 1978). Des Rosiers *et al.* (1978) have used the method to demonstrate functional plasticity in the striate cortex of the infant monkey. The ocular dominance columns are already present on the first day of life, but if one eye is kept patched for three months, the columns representing the open eye broaden and completely take over the adjacent regions of cortex containing the columns for the eye that had been patched. Inasmuch as there is no longer any cortical representation for the patched eye, the animal becomes functionally blind in one eye. This phenomenon is almost certainly the basis for the cortical blindness or amblyopia that often occurs in children with uncorrected strabismus.

There have also been extensive studies of the visual system of the rat. This species has little if any binocular vision and therefore lacks the ocular dominance columns. Batipps *et al.* (1981) have compared the rates of local cerebral glucose utilization in albino and Norway brown rats. The rates were essentially the same throughout the brain except in the components of the primary visual system. The metabolic rates in the superior colliculus, lateral geniculate, and visual cortex of the albino rat were significantly lower than those in the pigmented rat.

Miyaoka *et al.* (1979a) have studied the influence of the intensity of retinal stimulation with randomly spaced light flashes on the metabolic rates in the visual systems of the two strains. In dark-adapted animals there is relatively little difference between the two strains. With increasing intensity of light, the rates of glucose utilization first increase in the primary projection areas of the retina, e.g., superficial layer of the superior colliculus and lateral geniculate body, and the slopes of the increase are steeper in the albino rat. At 7 lux, however, the metabolic rates peak in the albino rat and then decrease with increasing light intensity. In contrast, the metabolic rates in the pigmented rat rise until they reach a plateau at about 700 lux, approximately the ambient light intensity in the laboratory. At this level the metabolic rates in the visual structures of the albino rat are considerably below those of the pigmented rat. These results are consistent with the greater intensity of light reaching the visual cells of the retina in the albino rats because of lack of pigment and the subsequent damage to the rods at higher light intensities. It is of considerable interest that the rates of glucose utilization in these visual structures obey the Weber–Fechner Law, i.e., the metabolic rate is directly proportional to the logarithm of the intensity of stimulation (Miyaoka *et al.*, 1979*a*). Inasmuch as this law was first developed from behavioral manifestations, these results imply that there is a quantitative relationship between behavioral and metabolic responses.

The method has also been applied, although less extensively, to other sensory systems. Studies of the olfactory system (Sharp *et al.*, 1975) have been discussed above. In addition to the experiments in the auditory system described in Section 7.2.1 (Figure 10), there have been studies of tonotopic representation in the auditory system. Webster *et al.* (1978) have obtained clear evidence of selective regions of metabolic activation in the cochlear nucleus, superior olivary complex, nuclei of the lateral lemnisci, and the inferior colliculus in cats in response to different frequencies of auditory stimulation. Similar results have been obtained by Silverman *et al.* (1977) in the rat and guinea pig. Studies of the sensory cortex have demonstrated metabolic activation of the "whisker barrels" by stimulation of the whiskers in the rat (Durham and Woolsey, 1977; Hand *et al.*, 1978). Each whisker is represented in a discrete region of the sensory cortex; their precise location and extent have been elegantly mapped by Hand *et al.* (1978) by means of the [^{14}C]-DG method.

Thus far, there has been relatively little application of the method to the physiology of motor functions. In their studies of higher visual functions in the monkey, however, Jarvis *et al.* (1978) studied monkeys that were conditioned to perform a task with one hand in response to visual cues; in the monkeys that were performing they observed metabolic activation in the appropriate areas of the motor as well as the sensory cortex.

An interesting physiological application of the [^{14}C]-DG method has been to the study of circadian rhythms in the central nervous system. Schwartz and his co-workers (1977, 1980) found that the suprachiasmatic nucleus in the rat exhibits circadian rhythmicity in metabolic activity, high during the day and low during the night. None of the other structures in the brain that they examined showed rhythmic activity. The normally low activity present in the nucleus in the dark could be markedly increased by light, but darkness did not reduce the glucose utilization during the day. The rhythm is entrained to light; reversal of the light–dark cycle leads to reversal of the rhythm not only in running activity but also in the cycle of metabolic activity in the suprachiasmatic nucleus. These studies lend support to a role of the suprachiasmatic nucleus in the organization of circadian rhythms in the central nervous system.

Much of our knowledge of neurophysiology has been derived from studies of the electrical activity of the nervous system. Indeed, from the heavy emphasis that has been placed on electrophysiology one might gather that the brain is really an electric organ rather than a chemical one that functions mainly by the release of chemical transmitters at synapses. Nevertheless, electrical activity is unquestionably fundamental to the process of conduction, and it is appropriate to inquire how the local metabolic activities revealed by the [^{14}C]-DG method are related to the electrical activity of the nervous system. This question is currently being examined by Yarowsky et al. (1979) in the superior cervical ganglion of the rat. The advantage of this structure is that its preganglionic input and postganglionic output can be isolated and electrically stimulated and/or monitored in vivo. The results thus far indicate a clear relationship between electrical input to the ganglion and its metabolic activity. In normal conscious rats its rate of glucose utilization equals approximately 35 μmol/100 g per min. This rate is markedly depressed by anesthesia or denervation and enhanced by electrical stimulation of the afferent nerves. The metabolic activation is frequency dependent in the range of 5–15 Hz, increasing linearly in magnitude with increasing frequency of the stimulation. Similar effects of electrical stimulation on the oxygen and glucose consumption of the excised ganglion studied in vitro have been observed (Larrabee, 1958; Horowitz and Larrabee, 1958; Friedli, 1977). Recent studies have also shown that antidromic stimulation of the postganglionic efferent pathways from the ganglion has similar effects; stimulation of the external carotid nerve antidromically activates glucose utilization in the region of distribution of the cell bodies of this efferent pathway, indicating that not only the preganglionic axonal terminals are metabolically activated, but also the postganglionic cell bodies as well (Yarowsky et al., 1980). As in the neurohypophysial pathway (Mata et al., 1980), the effects of electrical stimulation on energy metabolism in the superior cervical ganglion are probably due to the ionic currents associated with the spike activity and the consequent activation of the Na^+,K^+-ATPase activity to restore the ionic gradients. Electrical stimulation of the afferents to sympathetic ganglia has been shown to increase extracellular K^+ concentration (Friedli, 1977; Galvan et al., 1979). Each spike is normally associated with a sharp transient rise in extracellular K^+ concentration, which then rapidly falls and transiently undershoots before returning to the normal level (Galvan *et al.*, 1979); ouabain slows the decline in K^+ concentration after the spike and eliminates the undershoot. Continuous stimulation at a frequency of 6 Hz produces a sustained increase in cellular K^+ concentration (Galvan *et al.*, 1979). It is likely that the increased extracellular K^+ concentration and, almost certainly, increased intracellular Na^+ concentration activate the Na^+,K^+-ATPase, which in turn leads to the increased glucose utilization.

9.2. Pharmacological Applications

The ability of the $[^{14}C]$-DG method to map the entire brain for localized regions of altered functional activity on the basis of changes in energy metabolism offers a potent tool to identify the neural sites of action of agents with neuropharmacological and psychopharmacological actions. It does not, however, discriminate between the direct and indirect effects of the drug. An entire pathway may be activated even though the direct action of the drug may be exerted only at the origin of the pathway. This is of advantage in relating behavioral effects to central actions, but it is a disadvantage if the goal is to identify the primary site of action of the drug. To discriminate between direct and indirect actions of a drug the $[^{14}C]$-DG method must be combined with selectively placed lesions in the central nervous system that interrupt afferent pathways to the structure in question. If the metabolic effect of the drug then remains, it is due to direct action; if it is lost, the effect is likely to be indirect and mediated via the interrupted pathway. Nevertheless, the method has proved to be useful in a number of pharmacological studies.

9.2.1. Effects of Carbon Dioxide

The inhalation of 5–10% CO_2, which increases cerebral blood flow and produces desynchronization and a shift to higher frequency activity in the electroencephalogram, causes in the conscious rat moderate but diffuse reductions in local cerebral glucose utilization (Des Rosiers *et al.*, 1976).

9.2.2. Effects of γ-Butyrolactone

γ-Hydroxybutyrate and γ-butyrolactone (hydrolyzed to γ-hydroxybutyrate in plasma) produce trancelike behavioral states associated with marked suppresion of electroencephalographic activity (Roth and Giarman, 1966). These effects are reversible, and these drugs have been used clinically as anesthetic adjuvants. There is evidence that these agents lower neuronal activity in the nigrostriatal pathway and may act by inhibition of dopaminergic synapses (Roth, 1976). Studies in rats with the $[^{14}C]$-DG technique have demonstrated that γ-butyrolactone produces profound dose-dependent reductions of glucose utilization throughout the brain (Wolfson *et al.,* 1977). At the highest doses studied, 600 mg/kg of body weight, glucose utilization was reduced by approximately 75% in gray matter and 33% in white matter, but there was no obvious further specificity with respect to the local cerebral structures affected. The reversibility of the effects and the magnitude and diffuseness of the depression of cerebral metabolic rate suggests that this drug might be considered as a chemical substitute for hypothermia in conditions in which profound reversible reduction of cerebral metabolism is desired.

9.2.3. Effects of D-Lysergic Acid Diethylamide

The effects of the potent psychotomimetic agent, D-lysergic acid diethylamide, have been examined in the rat (Shinohara *et al.,* 1976). In doses of 12.5 to 125 μg/kg, it caused dose-dependent reductions in glucose utilization in a number of cerebral structures. With increasing dosage more structures were affected and to a greater degree. There was no pattern in the distribution of the effects—at least none discernible at the present level of resolution—that might contribute to the understanding of the drug's psychotomimetic actions.

9.2.4. Effects of Morphine Addiction and Withdrawal

Acute morphine administration depresses glucose utilization in many areas of the brain, but the specific effects of morphine could not be distinguished from those of the hypercapnia produced by the associated respiratory depression (Sakurada *et al.,* 1976). In contrast, morphine addiction, produced within 24 hr by a single subcutaneous injection of 150 mg/kg of morphine base in an oil emulsion, reduces glucose utilization in a large number of gray structures and in the absence of changes in arterial P_{CO_2}. White matter appears to be unaffected. Naloxone (1 mg/kg subcutaneously) reduces glucose utilization in a number of structures when administered to normal rats, but when given to the morphine-addicted animals produces an acute withdrawal syndrome and reverses the reductions of glucose utilization in several structures, most strikingly in the habenula (Sakurada *et al.,* 1976).

9.2.5. Pharmacological Studies of Dopaminergic Systems

The most extensive applications of the [^{14}C]-DG method to pharmacology have been in studies of dopaminergic systems. Ascending dopaminergic pathways appear to have a potent influence on glucose utilization in the forebrain of rats. Electrolytic lesions placed unilaterally in the lateral hypothalamus or pars compacta of the substantia nigra caused marked ipsilateral reductions of glucose metabolism in numerous forebrain structures rostral to the lesion, particularly the frontal cerebral cortex, caudate–putamen, and parts of the thalamus (Schwartz *et al.,* 1976; Schwartz, 1978). Similar lesions in the locus coeruleus had no such effects.

Enhancement of dopaminergic synaptic activity by administration of the agonist of dopamine, apomorphine (Brown and Wolfson, 1978), or of amphetamine (Wechsler *et al.,* 1979), which stimulates release of dopamine at the synapse, produces marked increases in glucose consumption in some of the components of the extrapyramidal system known or suspected to contain dopamine-receptive cells. With both drugs the greatest increases noted were in the zona reticulata of the substantia nigra and the subthalamic nucleus. Surprisingly, none of the components of the dopaminergic mesolimbic system appeared to be affected.

The studies with amphetamine (Wechsler *et al.,* 1979) were carried out with the fully quantitative $[^{14}C]$-DG method. The results in Table 5 illustrate the comprehensiveness with which this method surveys the entire brain for sites of altered activity resulting from actions of the drug. It also allows for quantitative comparison of the relative potencies of related drugs. For example, in Table 5, the comparative effects of *d*-amphetamine and the less potent dopaminergic agent, *l*-amphetamine, are compared; the quantitative results clearly reveal that the effects of *l*-amphetamine on local cerebral glucose utilization are more limited in distribution and of lesser magnitude than those of *d*-amphetamine. Indeed, in similar quantitative studies with apomorphine, McCulloch and co-workers (J. McCulloch, H. Savaki, A. Pert, W. Bunney, and L. Sokoloff, unpublished observations) have been able to generate the complete dose–response curves for the effects of the drug on the rates of glucose utilization in the various components of the dopaminergic systems. They have also demonstrated metabolically the development of supersensitivity to apomorphine in rats maintained chronically on the dopamine antagonist haloperidol.

9.2.6. Effects of α- and β-Adrenergic Blocking Agents

Savaki *et al.* (1978) have studied the effects of the α-adrenergic blocking agent, phentolamine, and the β-adrenergic blocking agent, propranolol. Both drugs produced widespread dose-dependent depressions of glucose utilization throughout the brain, but exhibit particularly striking and opposite effects in the complete auditory pathway from the cochlear nucleus to the auditory cortex. Propranolol markedly depressed and phentolamine markedly enhanced glucose utilization in this pathway. The functional significance of these effects is unknown but they seem to correlate with corresponding effects on the electrophysiological responsiveness of this sensory system. Propranolol depresses

TABLE 5. Effects of d-Amphetamine and l-Amphetamine on Local Cerebral Glucose Utilization in the Conscious Rat[a,b]

Structure	Control	d-Amphetamine	l-Amphetamine
Gray matter			
Visual cortex	102 ± 8	135 ± 11[c]	105 ± 8
Auditory cortex	160 ± 11	162 ± 6	141 ± 6
Parietal cortex	109 ± 9	125 ± 10	116 ± 4
Sensorimotor cortex	118 ± 8	139 ± 9	111 ± 4
Olfactory cortex	100 ± 6	93 ± 5	94 ± 3
Frontal cortex	109 ± 10	130 ± 8	105 ± 4
Prefrontal cortex	146 ± 10	166 ± 7	154 ± 4
Thalamus			
Lateral nucleus	97 ± 5	114 ± 8	117 ± 6
Ventral nucleus	85 ± 7	108 ± 6[c]	96 ± 4
Habenula	118 ± 10	71 ± 5[d]	82 ± 2[d]
Dorsomedial nucleus	92 ± 6	111 ± 8	106 ± 6
Medial geniculate	116 ± 5	119 ± 4	116 ± 4
Lateral geniculate	79 ± 5	88 ± 5	84 ± 4
Hypothalamus	54 ± 5	56 ± 3	52 ± 3
Suprachiasmatic nucleus	94 ± 4	75 ± 4[d]	67 ± 1[d]
Mamillary body	117 ± 8	134 ± 5	142 ± 5[c]
Lateral olfactory nucleus[e]	92 ± 6	95 ± 5	99 ± 6
A$_{13}$	71 ± 4	91 ± 4[d]	81 ± 4
Hippocampus			
Ammon's Horn	79 ± 5	73 ± 2	81 ± 6
Dentate gyrus	60 ± 4	55 ± 3	67 ± 7
Amygdala	46 ± 3	46 ± 3	44 ± 2
Septal nucleus	56 ± 3	55 ± 2	54 ± 3
Caudate nucleus	109 ± 5	132 ± 8[c]	127 ± 3[c]
Nucleus accumbens	76 ± 5	80 ± 3	78 ± 3
Globus pallidus	53 ± 3	64 ± 2[c]	65 ± 3[c]
Subthalamic nucleus	89 ± 6	149 ± 10[d]	107 ± 2
Substantia nigra			
Zona reticulata	58 ± 2	105 ± 4[d]	72 ± 4
Zona compacta	65 ± 4	88 ± 6[d]	72 ± 3
Red nucleus	76 ± 5	94 ± 5[c]	86 ± 2
Vestibular nucleus	121 ± 11	137 ± 5	130 ± 4
Cochlear nucleus	139 ± 6	126 ± 1	141 ± 5
Superior olivary nucleus	144 ± 4	143 ± 4	147 ± 6
Lateral lemniscus	107 ± 3	96 ± 5	98 ± 3
Inferior colliculus	193 ± 10	169 ± 5	150 ± 8[d]
Dorsal tegmental nucleus	109 ± 5	112 ± 7	122 ± 6
Superior colliculus	80 ± 5	89 ± 3	91 ± 3
Pontine gray	58 ± 4	65 ± 3	60 ± 1
Cerebellar flocculus	124 ± 10	146 ± 15	153 ± 10
Cerebellar hemispheres	55 ± 3	68 ± 6	64 ± 2
Cerebellar nuclei	102 ± 4	105 ± 8	110 ± 3

(Continued)

TABLE 5. (Continued)

Structure	Control	d-Amphetamine	l-Amphetamine
White matter			
Corpus callosum	23 ± 3	24 ± 2	23 ± 1
Genu of corpus callosum	29 ± 2	30 ± 2	26 ± 2
Internal capsule	21 ± 1	24 ± 2	19 ± 2
Cerebellar white	28 ± 1	31 ± 2	31 ± 2

[a] From Wechsler et al. (1979).
[b] All values are the means ± standard error of the mean for five animals.
[c] Significant difference from the control at the $p < 0.05$ level.
[d] Significant difference from the control at the $p < 0.01$ level.
[e] It was not possible to correlate precisely this area on autoradiographs with a specific structure in the rat brain. It is, however, most likely the lateral olfactory nucleus.

and phentolamine enhances the amplitude of all components of evoked auditory responses (T. Furlow and J. Hallenbeck, personal communication).

9.3. Pathophysiological Applications

The application of the [^{14}C]-DG method to the study of pathological states has been limited because of uncertainties about the values for the lumped and rate constants to be used. There are, however, pathophysiological states in which there is no structural damage to the tissue and the standard values of the constants can be used. Several of these conditions have been and are continuing to be studied by the [^{14}C]-DG technique, both qualitatively and quantitatively.

9.3.1. Convulsive States

The local injection of penicillin into the motor cortex produces focal seizures manifested in specific regions of the body contralaterally. The [^{14}C]-DG method has been used to map the spread of seizure activity within the brain and to identify the structures with altered functional activity during the seizure. The partial results of one such experiment in the monkey are illustrated in Figure 9. Discrete regions of markedly increased glucose utilization, sometimes as much as 200%, are observed ipsilaterally in the motor cortex, basal ganglia (particularly the globus pallidus), and thalamic nuclei, and contralaterally in the cerebellar cortex (Kennedy et al., 1975). Kato et al. (1980), Caveness et al. (1980), Hosokawa et al. (1980), and Caveness (1980) have carried out the most extensive studies of the propagation of the seizure activity in new-born and pubescent monkeys. The results indicate that the brain of the new-born monkey exhibits similar increases of glucose utilization in specific struc-tures, but the pattern of distribution of the effects is less well-defined than in the pubescent monkeys. Collins *et al.* (1976) have carried out similar studies in the rat with similar results but also obtained evidence on the basis of a local stimulation of glucose utilization of a "mirror focus" in the motor cortex con-tralateral to the side with the penicillin-induced epileptogenic focus.

Engel *et al.* (1978) have used the [^{14}C]-DG method to study seizures kin-dled in rats by daily electroconvulsive shocks. After a period of such treatment, the animals exhibit spontaneous seizures. Their results show marked increases in the limbic system, particularly the amygdala. The daily administration of the local anesthetic, lidocaine, effects similar seizures in rats. Post *et al.* (1979) have obtained similar results in such seizures with particularly pronounced increases in glucose utilization in the amygdala, hippocampus, and entero-rhinal cortex.

9.3.2. Spreading Cortical Depression

Shinohara *et al.* (1979) studied the effects of local applications of KCl on the dura overlying the parietal cortex of conscious rats or directly on the pial surface of the parietal cortex of anesthetized rats in order to determine if K$^+$ stimulates cerebral energy metabolism *in vivo* as it is well-known to do *in vitro*. The results demonstrate a marked increase in cerebral cortical glucose utili-zation in response to the application of KCl; NaCl has no such effect (Figure 14). Such application of KCl, however, also produces the phenomenon of spreading cortical depression. This condition is characterized by a spread of transient intense neuronal activity followed by membrane depolarization, elec-trical depression, and a negative shift in the cortical DC potential in all direc-tions from the site of initiation at a rate of 2–5 mm/min. The depressed cortex also exhibits a number of chemical changes, including an increase in extracel-lular K$^+$ presumably lost from the cells. At the same time as the increase in cortical glucose utilization, most subcortical structures that are functionally connected to the depressed cortex exhibit decreased rates of glucose utilization. During recovery from the spreading cortical depression, the glucose utilization in the cortex is still increased, but it is distributed in columns oriented perpen-dicularly through the cortex. This columnar arrangement may reflect the columnar functional and morphological arrangement of the cerebral cortex. It is likely that the increased glucose utilization in the cortex during spreading cortical depression is the consequence of the increased extracellular K$^+$ and activation of the Na$^+$,K$^+$-ATPase.

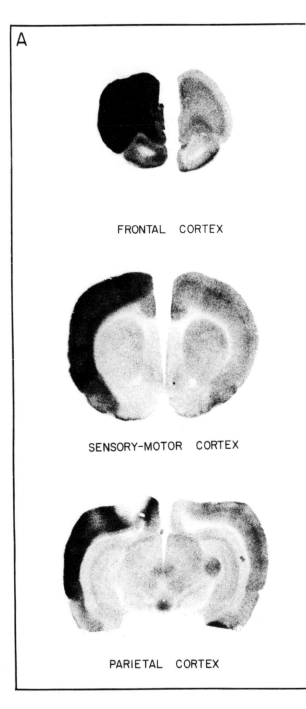

FRONTAL CORTEX

SENSORY-MOTOR CORTEX

PARIETAL CORTEX

FIGURE 14. Autoradiographs of sections of rat brains during spreading cortical depression and during recovery. The autoradiographs are pictorial representations of the relative rates of glucose

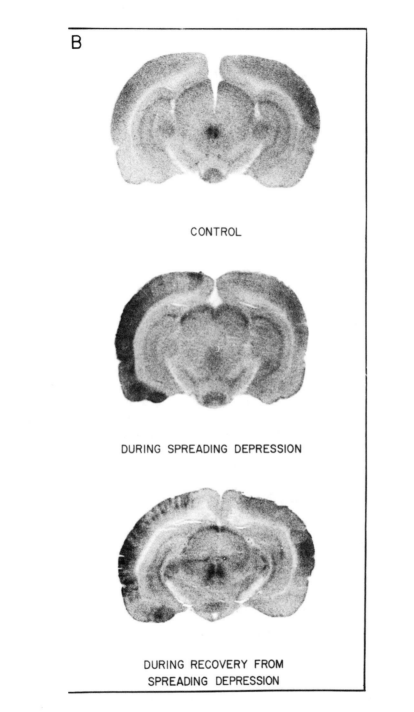

B

CONTROL

DURING SPREADING DEPRESSION

DURING RECOVERY FROM
SPREADING DEPRESSION

utilization in various parts of the brain; the greater the density, the greater the rate of glucose utilization. The left sides of the brain are represented by the left hemispheres in the autoradi-

9.3.3. Opening of Blood–Brain Barrier

Unilateral opening of the blood–brain barrier in rats by unilateral carotid injection with a hyperosmotic mannitol solution leads to widely distributed discrete regions of intensely increased glucose utilization in the ipsilateral hemisphere (Pappius *et al.,* 1979). These focal regions of hypermetabolism may reflect local regions of seizure activity. The prior administration of diazepam prevents in most cases the appearance of these areas of increased metabolism (Pappius *et al.,* 1979). Electroencephalographic recordings under similar experimental conditions reveal evidence of seizure activity (C. Fieschi, personal communication).

9.3.4. Hypoxemia

Pulsinelli and Duffy (1979) have studied the effects of controlled hypoxemia on local cerebral glucose utilization by means of the qualitative [^{14}C]-DG method. Hypoxemia was achieved by artificial ventilation of the animals with a mixture of N_2, N_2O, and O_2, adjusted to maintain the arterial P_{O_2} between 28 and 32 mm Hg. All the animals had had one common carotid artery ligated to limit the increase in cerebral blood flow and the amount of O_2 delivered to the brain. Their autoradiographs provide striking evidence of marked and disparate changes in glucose utilization in the various structural components of the brain. The hemisphere ipsilateral to the carotid ligation was not unexpectedly more severely affected. The most striking effects were markedly higher increases in glucose utilization in white matter than in gray matter, presumably because of the Pasteur effect, and the appearance of transverse cortical columns of high activity alternating with columns of low activity. By studies with black plastic microspheres, they were able to show that the cortical columns

---

(Continued from p. 71)

ographs. In all the experiments illustrated, the control hemisphere was treated the same as the experimental side except that equivalent concentrations of NaCl rather than KCl were used. The NaCl did not lead to any detectable differences from hemispheres over which the skull was left intact and no NaCl was applied. (A) Autoradiographs of sections of brain at different levels of cerebral cortex from a conscious rat during spreading cortical depression induced on the left side by application of 5 *M* KCl to the intact dura overlying the left parietal cortex. The spreading depression was sustained by repeated applications of the KCl at 15- to 20-min intervals throughout the experimental period. (B) Autoradiographs from sections of brain at the level of the parietal cortex from three animals under barbiturate anesthesia. The top section is from a normal anesthetized animal; the middle section is from an animal during unilateral spreading cortical depression induced and sustained by repeated applications of 80 m*M* KCl in artificial cerebrospinal fluid directly on the surface of the left parietooccipital cortex. At the bottom is a comparable section from an animal studied immediately after the return of cortical DC potential to normal after a single wave of spreading depression induced by a single application of 80 m*M* KCl to the parietooccipital cortex of the left side. (From Shinohara *et al.,* 1978.)

were anatomically related to penetrating cortical arteries with the columns of high metabolic activity lying between the arteries.

Miyaoka *et al.* (1979*b*) have also studied the effects of moderate hypoxemia in normal, spontaneously-breathing, conscious rats without carotid ligation. The hypoxemia was produced by lowering the O_2 in the inspired air to approximately 7%. Although this procedure reduced arterial P_{O_2} to approximately 30 mm Hg, the cerebral hypoxia was probably less than in the studies of Pulsinelli and Duffy (1979) because of the intact cerebral circulation. The animals remained fully conscious under these experimental conditions although they appeared subdued and less active. The quantitative [^{14}C]-DG method was employed and the rates of glucose utilization were determined. The results revealed many similarities to those of Pulsinelli and Duffy (1979). There was a complete redistribution of the local rates of glucose utilization from the normal pattern. Metabolism in white matter was markedly increased. Many areas showed decreased rates of metabolism. Columns were seen in the cerebral cortex, and the caudate nucleus exhibited a strange lacelike heterogeneity quite distinct from its normal homogeneity. Despite the widespread changes, however, overall average glucose utilization remained unchanged. These results are of relevance to the studies by Kety and Schmidt (1984*b*), who found in man that the breathing of 10% O_2 produced a wide variety of mental symptoms without altering the average O_2 consumption of the brain as a whole. The mental symptoms were probably the result of metabolic and functional changes in specific regions of the brain detectable only by methods like the [^{14}C]-DG method that measure metabolic rate in the structural components of the brain.

9.3.5. Normal Aging

Although, strictly speaking, aging is not a pathophysiological condition, many of its behavioral consequences are directly attributable to decrements in functions of the central nervous system (Birren *et al.*, 1963). Normal human aging has been found to be associated with a decrease in average glucose utilization of the brain as a whole (Sokoloff, 1966). Smith *et al.* (1980) have employed the quantitative [^{14}C]-DG method to study normal aging in Sprague-Dawley rats of between 5–6 and 36 months. Their results show widespread but not homogeneous reductions of local cerebral glucose utilization with age. The sensory systems, particularly auditory and visual, are particularly severely affected. The caudate nucleus is metabolically depressed; preliminary experiments indicate that it loses responsivity to dopamine agonists, such as apomorphine, with age. A striking effect was the loss of metabolically active neuropil in the cerebral cortex; Layer 4 is markedly decreased in metabolic activity and extent. Some of these changes may be related to specific functional disabilities that develop in old age.

10. RECENT TECHNOLOGICAL DEVELOPMENTS

Several recent technological developments, both completed and in progress, have simplified and increased the usefulness of the [^{14}C]-DG method, extended its level of resolution in animals, and adapted it for use in man.

10.1. Sequential Double-Label Modification

As originally designed, the [^{14}C]-DG method requires the killing of the animal at the end of the experimental period in order to measure the final concentrations of ^{14}C in the cerebral structures. This requirement leads to the limitation that only a single determination is possible in any one animal. There may be circumstances when it is advantageous to carry out two determinations, e.g., under control and experimental conditions, in the same animal. Altenau and Agranoff (1978) have designed an ingenious procedure which allows two sequential determinations of local cerebral glucose utilization. The procedure requires the use of both [^{14}C]-DG and [^{3}H]-DG. The [^{3}H]-DG is administered as a pulse at the beginning of a control period, and at a reasonable interval of time later, preferably 30–45 min, the [^{14}C]-DG is similarly administered at the beginning of the experimental period. The animal is killed 30–45 min later, the brain is autoradiographed for ^{14}C concentration, and selected brain samples are punched out and assayed for ^{3}H by liquid scintillation counting. The ^{3}H/^{14}C ratio provides an index of the relative rates of glucose utilization in the control and experimental period, provided systemic conditions, such as arterial plasma glucose concentrations and the time courses of the plasma clearance curve of DG, remain similar in the two periods. If the experiment can, however, be designed to provide asymmetrical changes on the two sides of the brain, then the control side serves to control for changes in this function and makes possible interpretation of changes in the opposite or experimental side.

10.2. Computerized Color-Coded Image Processing

The autoradiographs provide pictorial representations of only the relative and not the actual rates of glucose utilization in all the structures of the nervous system. Furthermore, the resolution of differences in relative rates is limited by the ability of the human eye to recognize differences in shades of gray. Manual densitometric analysis permits the computation of actual rates of glucose utilization with a fair degree of resolution. However, this generates enormous tables of data that fail to convey the tremendous heterogeneity of metabolic rates, even within anatomic structures, or the full information contained within the autoradiographs. Goochee *et al.* (1980) have developed a computerized image processing system to analyze and transform the autoradiographs into color-coded maps of the distribution of the actual rates of glucose utilization exactly where they are located throughout the central nervous system. The autoradiographs are scanned automatically by a computer-controlled scanning microdensitometer. The optical density of each spot in the autoradiograph, from 25 to 100 μm as selected, is stored in a computer, converted to ^{14}C concentration on the basis of the optical densities of the calibrated ^{14}C plastic standards, and then converted to local rates of glucose utilization by solution of the operational equation of the method. Colors are assigned to narrow ranges of the rates of glucose utilization, and the autoradiographs are then displayed on a color TV monitor along with a calibrated color scale for identifying the rate of glucose utilization in each spot of the autoradiograph from its color. Representative illustrations of such color maps are presented in Figure 15. These color maps add a third dimension, the rate of glucose utilization on a color scale, to the spatial dimensions already present on the autoradiographs.

10.3. Microscopic Resolution

The resolution of the present [^{14}C]-DG method is at best approximately 100 μm. The use of [^{3}H]-DG does not greatly improve the resolution when the standard autoradiographic procedure is used. The limiting factor is the diffusion and migration of the water-soluble labeled compound in the tissue during the freezing of the brain and the cutting of the brain sections. Des Rosiers and Descarries (1978) have been working to extend the resolution of the method to light and electron microscopic levels. They use [^{3}H]-DG and dipping emulsion techniques. They have reported that fixation, postfixation, dehydration, and embedding of the brain by perfusion *in situ* results in negligible loss or migration of the label in the tissue. They can localize grain counts over individual cells or portions of them. The method is at present only qualitative, but prospects to make it quantitative are promising.

10.4. The [^{18}F] Fluorodeoxyglucose Technique

Because the [^{14}C]-DG method requires the measurement of local concentrations of radioactivity in the individual components of the brain, it cannot be applied as originally designed to man. Recent developments in computerized emission tomography, however, have made it possible to measure local concentrations of labeled compounds *in vivo* in man. Emission tomography requires the use of γ radiation, preferably annihilation γ rays derived from positron emission. A positron-emitting derivative of DG, 2-[^{18}F]fluoro-2-deoxy-D-glucose, has been synthesized and found to retain the necessary biochemical properties of 2-DG (Reivich *et al.*, 1979). The method has therefore been adapted for use in man with [^{18}F]fluorodeoxyglucose and positron-emission tomography (Reivich *et al.*, 1979; Phelps *et al.*, 1979). The resolution of the method is still relatively limited (approximately 1 cm) but it is already proving to be useful in studies of clinical conditions, such as focal epilepsy (Kuhl *et al.*, 1979). This technique is of immense potential usefulness for studies of human local cerebral energy metabolism in normal states and in neurological and psychiatric disorders.

11. CONCLUDING REMARKS

The [^{14}C]-DG method provides the means to determine quantitatively the rates of glucose utilization simultaneously in all structural and functional components of the central nervous system and to display them pictorially superimposed on the anatomical structures in which they occur. Because of the close relationship between local functional activity and energy metabolism, the method makes it possible to identify all structures with increased or decreased functional activity in various physiological, pharmacological, and physiopathological states. The images provided by the method do resemble histological sections of nervous tissue, and therefore the method is sometimes misconstrued to be a neuroanatomical method and contrasted with physiological methods, such as electrophysiological recording. This classification obscures the most significant and unique feature of the method. The images are not of structure but of a dynamic biochemical process, i.e., glucose utilization, which is as physiological as electrical activity. In most situations changes in functional activity result in changes in energy metabolism, and the color-coded images can be used to visualize and identify the sites of altered activity. The images are, therefore, analogous to infrared maps; they record quantitatively the rates of a kinetic process and display them pictorially exactly where they exist. The fact that they depict the anatomical structures is fortuitous; it indicates that the rates of glucose utilization are distributed according to structure, and specific functions in the nervous system are associated with specific anatomical structures. The [^{14}C]-DG method therefore represents, in a real sense, a new type of encephalography, metabolic encephalography. At the very least, it should serve as a valuable supplement to more conventional types, such as electroencephalography. However, because it provides a new means to examine another aspect of function simultaneously in all parts of the brain, it is hoped that it and its derivative, the [^{18}F]fluorodeoxyglucose technique, will open new roads to the understanding of how the brain works in health and disease.

ACKNOWLEDGMENT

The author is indebted to Mrs. Ruth Bower for her outstanding editorial and bibliographic assistance in the preparation of this manuscript.

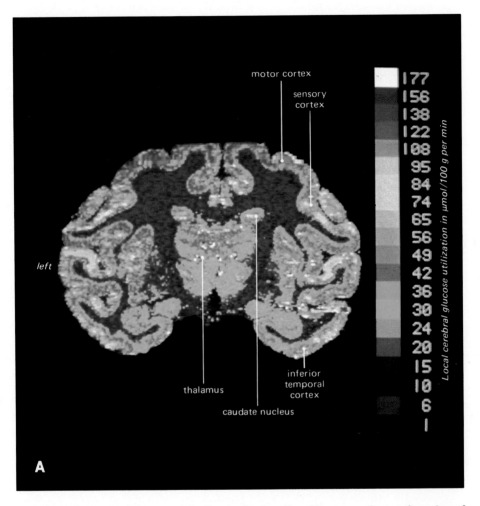

FIGURE 15. Brain metabolism in a visually stimulated monkey. Shown are color transformations of autoradiographs of coronal sections of monkey brain in which each color represents the rate of local cerebral glucose utilization in μmol/100 g per min according to the calibration scales on the right of the autoradiograph. Local cerebral glucose utilization was measured by the [14C]deoxyglucose method. Sections were taken at the same level, and include sensory and motor cortex, temporal cortex, thalamus, hypothalamus, and tails of caudate nuclei. The left side of the brain is on the left in the autoradiograph. (A) This section was obtained from a normal conscious monkey with an intact visual system that was stimulated by an illuminated moving black and white geometric pattern.

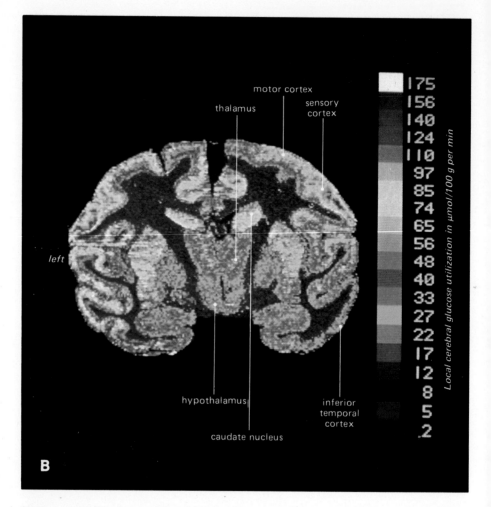

(B) Brain metabolism in a conditioned monkey being visually stimulated while using its left hand. The section is from a monkey with a transected right optic tract that was also stimulated visually while pulling a lever with its left hand. Note the decreased metabolic activity in the right inferior temporal cortex resulting from the optic tract section and the increased metabolic activity in the hand regions of the right sensory and motor cortex in correspondence with movements of the left hand. Unpublished experiments performed by C. Kennedy, M. Shinohara, M. Miyaoka, C. Jarvis, and M. Mishkin. Color transformations were carried out by the computerized technique of Goochee *et al.* (1980).

12. REFERENCES

Albers, R. W., 1967, Biochemical aspects of active transport, *Annu. Rev. Biochem.* **36**:727–756.

Altenau, L. L., and Agranoff, B. W., 1978, A sequential double-label 2-deoxyglucose method for measuring regional cerebral metabolism, *Brain Res.* **153**:375–381.

Bachelard, H. S., 1971, Specificity and kinetic properties of monosaccharide uptake into guinea pig cerebral cortex *in vitro, J. Neurochem.* **18**:213–222.

Bachelard, H. S., Clark, A. G., and Thompson, M. F., 1971, Cerebral-cortex hexokinases. Elucidation of reaction mechanisms by substrate and dead-end inhibitor kinetic analysis, *Biochem. J.* **123**:707–715.

Ballas, L. M., and Arion, W. J., 1977, Measurement of glucose 6-phosphate penetration into liver microsomes. Confirmation of substrate transport in the glucose-6-phosphatase system, *J. Biol. Chem.* **252**:8512–8518.

Batipps, M., Miyaoka, M., Shinohara, M., Sokoloff, L., and Kennedy, C., 1981, Comparative rates of local cerebral glucose utilization in the visual system of conscious albino and pigmented rats, *Neurology* **31**:58–62.

Bidder, T. G., 1968, Hexose translocation across the blood–brain interface: Configurational aspects, *J. Neurochem.* **15**:867–874.

Birren, J. E., Butler, R. N., Greenhouse, S. W., Sokoloff, L., and Yarrow, M. R. (eds.), 1963, *Human Aging: A Biological and Behavioral Study,* Public Health Service Publication No. 986, US Government Printing Office, Washington DC.

Brown, L., and Wolfson, L., 1978, Apomorphine increases glucose utilization in the substantia nigra, subthalamic nucleus, and corpus striatum of the rat, *Brain Res.* **148**:188–193.

Caldwell, P. C., 1968, Factors governing movement and distribution of inorganic ions in nerve and muscle, *Physiol. Rev.* **48**:1–64.

Caveness, W. F., 1969, Ontogeny of focal seizures, in: *Basic Mechanisms of the Epilepsies* (H. H. Jasper, A. A. Ward, and A. Pope, eds.), pp. 517–534, Little, Brown and Co., Boston.

Caveness, W. F., 1980, Appendix: Tables of local cerebral glucose utilization in various experimental preparations, *Ann. Neurol.* **7**:230–237.

Caveness, W. F., Kato, M., Malamut, B. L., Hosokawa, S., Wakisaka, S., and O'Neill, R. R., 1980, Propagation of focal motor seizures in the pubescent moneky, *Ann. Neurol.* **7**:213–221.

Collins, R. C., Kennedy, C., Sokoloff, L., and Plum, F., 1976, Metabolic anatomy of focal motor seizures, *Arch. Neurol. (Chicago)* **33**:536–542.

Des Rosiers, M. H., Kennedy, C., Shinohara, M., and Sokoloff, L., 1976, Effects of CO_2 on local cerebral glucose utilization in the conscious rat, *Neurology* **26**:346.

Des Rosiers, M. H., Sakurada, O., Jehle, J., Shinohara, M., Kennedy, C., and Sokoloff, L., 1978, Functional plasticity in the immature striate cortex of the monkey shown by the [^{14}C]deoxyglucose method, *Science* **200**:447–449.

Des Rosiers, M. H., and Descarries, L., 1978, Adaptation de la méthode au désoxyglucose à l'échelle cellulaire: préparation histologique du système nerveux central en vue de la radioautographie à haute résolution, *C. R. Acad. Sci. Ser. D* **287**:153–156.

Dixon, M., and Webb, E. C., 1964, *Enzymes,* 2nd ed., pp. 84–87, Academic Press, New York.

Duffy, T. E., Cavazzuti, M., Gregoire, N. M., Cruz, N. F., Kennedy, C., and Sokoloff, L., 1979, Regional cerebral glucose metabolism in newborn beagle dogs, *Trans. Am. Soc. Neurochem.* **10**:171.

Durham, D., and Woolsey, T. A., 1977, Barrels and columnar cortical organization: Evidence from 2-deoxyglucose (2-DG) experiments, *Brain Res.* **137**:169–174.

Eklöf, B., Lassen, N. A., Nilsson, L., Norberg, K., and Siesjö, B. K., 1973, Blood flow and metabolic rate for oxygen in the cerebral cortex of the rat, *Acta Physiol. Scand.* **88**:587–589.

Engel, J., Jr., Wolfson, L., and Brown, L., 1978, Anatomical correlates of electrical and behavioral events related to amygdaloid kindling, *Ann. Neurol.* 3:538–544.

Freygang, W. H., Jr., and Sokoloff, L., 1958, Quantitative measurement of regional circulation in the central nervous system by the use of radioactive inert gas, *Adv. Biol. Med. Phys.* 6:263–279.

Friedli, C., 1977, Kinetics of changes in pO_2 and extracellular potassium activity in stimulated rat sympathetic ganglia, in: *Advances in Experimental Medicine and Biology, Oxygen Transport to Tissue III* (I. A. Silver, M. Erecinska and H. I. Bicher, eds.), pp. 747–754, Plenum Press, New York.

Galvan, M., Ten Bruggencate, G., and Senekowitsch, R., 1979, The effects of neuronal stimulation and oubain upon extracellular K^+ and Ca^{2+} levels in rat isolated sympathetic ganglia, *Brain Res.* 160:544–548.

Gjedde, A., Caronna, J. J., Hindfelt, B., and Plum, F., 1975, Whole-brain blood flow and oxygen metabolism in the rat during nitrous oxide anesthesia, *Am. J. Physiol.* 229:113–118.

Goochee, C., Rasband, W., and Sokoloff, L., 1980, Computerized densitometry and color coding of [^{14}C]deoxyglucose autoradiographs, *Ann. Neurol.* 7:359–370.

Hand, P. J., Greenberg, J. H., Miselis, R. R., Weller, W. L., and Reivich, M., 1978, A normal and altered cortical column: a quantitative and qualitative (^{14}C)-2 deoxyglucose (2DG) mapping study, *Neurosci. Abstr.* 4:553.

Hawkins, R. A., and Miller, A. L., 1978, Loss of radioactive 2-deoxy-D-glucose-6-phosphate from brains of conscious rats: Implications for quantitative autoradiographic determination of regional glucose utilization, *Neuroscience* 3:251–258.

Hawkins, R. A., Miller, A. L., Cremer, J. E., and Veech, R. L., 1974, Measurement of the rate of glucose utilization by rat brain *in vivo*, *J. Neurochem.* 23:917–923.

Hers, H. G., 1957, *Le Métabolisme du Fructose*, p. 102, Arscia, Brussels.

Hers, H. G., and deDuve, C., 1950, Le système hexose-phosphatasique. II. Repartition de l'activite glucose-6-phosphatasique dans les tissus, *Bull. Soc. Chim. Biol.* 32:20–29.

Horowicz, P., and Larrabee, M. G., 1958, Glucose consumption and lactate production in a mammalian sympathetic ganglion at rest and in activity, *J. Neurochem.* 2:102–118.

Horton, R. W., Meldrum, B. S., and Bachelard, H. S., 1973, Enzymic and cerebral metabolic effects of 2-deoxy-D-glucose, *J. Neurochem.* 21:507–520.

Hosokawa, S., Iguchi, T., Caveness, W. F., Kato, M., O'Neill, R. R., Wakisaka, S., and Malamut, B. L., 1980, Effects of manipulation of the sensorimotor system on focal motor seizures in the monkey, *Ann. Neurol.* 7:222–229.

Hubel, D. H., and Wiesel, T. N., 1968, Receptive fields and functional architecture of monkey striate cortex, *J. Physiol.* 195:215–243.

Hubel, D. H., and Wiesel, T. N., 1972, Laminar and columnar distribution of geniculo-cortical fibers in the Macaque monkey, *J. Comp. Neurol.* 146:421–450.

Hubel, D. H., Wiesel, T. N., and Stryker, M. P., 1978, Anatomical demonstration of orientation columns in macaque monkey, *J. Comp. Neurol.* 177:361–380.

Jarvis, C. D., Mishkin, M., Shinohara, M., Sakurada, O., Miyaoka, M., and Kennedy, C., 1978, Mapping the primate visual system with the [^{14}C]2-deoxyglucose technique, *Neurosci. Abstr.* 4:632.

Kato, M., Malamut, B. L., Caveness, W. F., Hosokawa, S., Wakisaka, S., and O'Neill, R. R., 1980, Local cerebral glucose utilization in newborn and pubescent monkeys during focal motor seizures, *Ann. Neurol.* 7:204–212.

Kennedy, C., Des Rosiers, M., Jehle, J. W., Reivich, M., Sharp, F., and Sokoloff, L., 1975, Mapping of functional neural pathways by autoradiographic survey of local metabolic rate with [^{14}C]deoxyglucose, *Science* 187:850–853.

Kennedy, C., Des Rosiers, M. H., Sakurada, O., Shinohara, M., Reivich, M., Jehle, J. W., and Sokoloff, L., 1976, Metabolic mapping of the primary visual system of the monkey by means of the autoradiographic [¹⁴C]deoxyglucose technique, *Proc. Natl. Acad. Sci. USA* **73**:4230–4234.

Kennedy, C., Sakurada, O., Shinohara, M., Jehle, J., and Sokoloff, L., 1978, Local cerebral glucose utilization in the normal conscious Macaque monkey, *Ann. Neurol.* **4**:293–301.

Kety, S. S., 1950, Circulation and metabolism of the human brain in health and disease, *Am. J. Med.* **8**:205–217.

Kety, S. S., 1957, The general metabolism of the brain *in vivo*, in: *Metabolism of the Nervous System* (D. Richter, ed.), pp. 221–237, Pergamon Press, London.

Kety, S. S., 1960, Measurement of local blood flow by the exchange of an inert, diffusible substance, *Methods Med. Res.* **8**:228–236.

Kety, S. S., and Schmidt, C. F., 1948a, The nitrous oxide method for the quantitative determination of cerebral blood flow in man: theory, procedure, and normal values, *J. Clin. Invest.* **27**:476–483.

Kety, S. S., and Schmidt, C. F., 1948b, Effects of altered arterial tensions of carbon dioxide and oxygen on cerebral blood flow and cerebral oxygen consumption of normal young men, *J. Clin. Invest.* **27**:484–492.

Knott, G. D., and Reece, D. K., 1972, MLAB: A civilized curve-fitting system, in: *Proceedings of the* ONLINE *'72 International Conference,* Vol. 1, pp. 497–526, Brunel University, England.

Knott, G. D., and Shrager, R. I., 1972, On-line modeling by curve-fitting, in: *Computer Graphics: Proceedings of the* SIGGRAPH *Computers in Medicine Symposium,* Vol. 6, No. 4, pp. 138–151, Association for Computing Machinery, SIGGRAPH Notices.

Kuhl, D., Engel, J., Phelps, M., and Selin, C., 1979, Patterns of local cerebral metabolism and perfusion in partial epilepsy by emission computed tomography of ¹⁸F-flurodeoxyglucose and ¹³N-ammonia, *Acta Neurol. Scand. Suppl.* **60**:538–539.

Landau, B. R., and Lubs, H. A., 1958, Animal response to 2-deoxy-D-glucose administration, *Proc. Soc. Exp. Biol.* **99**:124–127.

Landau, W. M., Freygang, W. H., Jr., Rowland, L. P., Sokoloff, L., and Kety, S. S., 1955, The local circulation of the living brain; Values in the unanesthetized and anesthetized cat, *Trans. Am. Neurol. Assoc.* **80**:125–129.

Larrabee, M. G., 1958, Oxygen consumption of excised sympathetic ganglia at rest and in activity, *J. Neurochem.* **2**:81–101.

Lashley, K. S., 1934, The mechanism of vision. VII. The projection of the retina upon the primary optic centers of the rat, *J. Comp. Neurol.* **59**:341–373.

Lassen, N. A., 1959, Cerebral blood flow and oxygen consumption in man, *Physiol. Rev.* **39**:183–238.

Lassen, N. A., and Munck, O., 1955, The cerebral blood flow in man determined by the use of radioactive krypton, *Acta Physiol. Scand.* **33**:30–49.

Mata, M., Fink, D. J., Gainer, H., Smith, C. B., Davidsen, L., Savaki, H., Schwartz, W. J., and Sokoloff, L., 1980, Activity-dependent energy metabolism in rat posterior pituitary reflects sodium pump activity, *J. Neurochem.* **34**:213–215.

Meldrum, B. S., and Horton, R. W., 1973, Cerebral functional effects of 2-deoxy-D-glucose and 3-O-methylglucose in Rhesus monkeys, *Electroencephalogr. Clin. Neurophysiol.* **35**:59–66.

Miyaoka, M., Shinohara, M., Batipps, M., Pettigrew, K. D., Kennedy, C., and Sokoloff, L., *1979a,* The relationship between the intensity of the stimulus and the metabolic response in the visual system of the rat, *Acta Neurol. Scand. Suppl.* **60**:16–17.

Miyaoka, M., Shinohara, M., Kennedy, C., and Sokoloff, L., *1979b,* Alterations in local cerebral glucose utilization (LCGU) in rat brain during hypoxemia, *Trans. Am. Neurol. Assoc.* **104**:151–154.

Montero, V. M., and Guillery, R. W., 1968, Degeneration in the dorsal lateral geniculate nucleus of the rat following interruption of the retinal or cortical connections, *J. Comp. Neurol.* **134**:211–242.

Nordlie, R. C., 1971, Glucose-6-phosphatase, hydrolytic and synthetic activities, in: *The Enzymes* 3rd ed., Vol. IV (P. D. Boyer, ed.), pp. 543–610, Academic Press, New York.

Nordlie, R. C., 1974, Metabolic regulation by multifunctional glucose-6-phosphatase, *Curr. Top. Cell Regul.* **8**:33–117.

Nordmann, J. J., 1977, Ultrastructural morphometry of the rat neurohypophysis, *J. Anat.* **123**:213–218.

Oldendorf, W. H., 1971, Brain uptake of radiolabeled amino acids, amines, and hexoses after arterial injection, *Am. J. Physiol.* **221**:1629–1638.

Pappius, H. M., Savaki, H. E., Fieschi, C., Rapoport, S. I., and Sokoloff, L., 1979, Osmotic opening of the blood-brain barrier and local cerebral glucose utilization, *Ann. Neurol.* **5**:211–219.

Patlak, C. S., and Pettigrew, K. D., 1976, A method to obtain infusion schedules for prescribed blood concentration time courses, *J. Appl. Physiol.* **40**:458–463.

Phelps, M. E., Huang, S. C., Hoffman, E. J., Selin, C., Sokoloff, L., and Kuhl, D. E., 1979, Tomographic measurement of local cerebral glucose metabolic rate in humans with (F-18)2-fluoro-2-deoxy-d-glucose: Validation of method, *Ann. Neurol.* **6**:371–388.

Plum, F., Gjedde, A., and Samson, F. E., 1976, Neuroanatomical mapping by the radioactive 2-deoxy-D-glucose method, *Neurosci. Res. Program Bull.* **14**:457–518.

Post, R. M., Kennedy, C., Shinohara, M., Squillace, K., Miyaoka, M., Suda, S., Ingvar, D. H., and Sokoloff, L., 1979, Local cerebral glucose utilization in lidocaine-kindled seizures, *Neurosci. Abstr.* **5**:196.

Prasannan, K. G., and Subrahmanyam, K., 1968, Effect of insulin on the synthesis of glucogen in cerebral cortical slices of alloxan diabetic rats, *Endocrinology* **82**:1–6.

Pulsinelli, W. A., and Duffy, T. E., 1979, Local cerebral glucose metabolism during controlled hypoxemia in rats, *Science* **204**:626–629.

Raggi, F., Kronfeld, D. S., and Kleiber, M., 1960, Glucose-6-phosphatase activity in various sheep tissues, *Proc. Soc. Exp. Biol. Med.* **105**:485–486.

Rakic, P.,1976, Prenatal genesis of connections subserving ocular dominance in the rhesus monkey, *Nature* **261**:467–471.

Reivich, M., Jehle, J., Sokoloff, L., and Kety, S. S., 1969, Measurement of regional cerebral blood flow with antipyrine-[¹⁴C] in awake cats, *J. Appl. Physiol.* **27**:296–300.

Reivich, M., Kuhl, D., Wolf, A., Greenberg, J., Phelps, M., Ido, T., Cassella, V., Fowler, J., Hoffman, E., Alavi, A., Som, P., and Sokoloff, L., 1979, The [¹⁸F]fluoro-deoxyglucose method for the measurement of local cerebral glucose utilization in man, *Circ. Res.* **44**:127–137.

Roth, R. H., 1976, Striatal dopamine and gamma-hydroxybutyrate, *Pharmacol. Ther.* **2**:71–88.

Roth, R. H., and Giarman, N. J., 1966, γ-Butyrolactone and γ-hydroxybutyric acid—I. Distribution and metabolism, *Biochem. Pharmacol.* **15**:1333–1348.

Sacks, W., 1957, Cerebral metabolism of isotopic glucose in normal human subjects, *J. Appl. Physiol.* **10**:37–44.

Sakurada, O., Shinohara, M., Klee, W. A., Kennedy, C., and Sokoloff, L., 1976, Local cerebral glucose utilization following acute chronic morphine administration and withdrawal, *Neurosci. Abstr.* **2**:613.

Savaki, H. E., Kadekaro, M., Jehle, J., and Sokoloff, L., 1978, α- and β-adrenoreceptor blockers have opposite effects on energy metabolism of the central auditory system, *Nature* **276**:521–523.

Savaki, H. E., Davidsen, L., Smith, C., and Sokoloff, L., 1980, Measurement of free glucose turnover in brain, *J. Neurochem.* **35**:495–502.

Scheinberg, P., and Stead, E. A., Jr., 1949, The cerebral blood flow in male subjects as measured by the nitrous oxide technique. Normal values for blood flow, oxygen utilization, and peripheral resistance, with observations on the effect of tilting and anxiety, *J. Clin. Invest.* **28**:1163–1171.

Schwartz, W. J., 1978, A role for the dopaminergic nigrostriatal bundle in the pathogenesis of altered brain glucose consumption after lateral hypothalamic lesions. Evidence using the ¹⁴C-labeled deoxyglucose technique, *Brain Res.* **158**:129–147.

Schwartz, W. J., and Gainer, H., 1977, Suprachiasmatic nucleus: use of ¹⁴C-labeled deoxyglucose uptake as a functional marker, *Science* **197**:1089–1091.

Schwartz, W. J., Sharp, F. R., Gunn, R. H., and Evarts, E. V., 1976, Lesions of ascending dopaminergic pathways decrease forebrain glucose uptake, *Nature (London)* **261**:155–157.

Schwartz, W. J., Smith, C. B., Davidsen, L., Savaki, H., Sokoloff, L., Mata, M., Fink, D. J., and Gainer, H., 1979, Metabolic mapping of functional activity in the hypothalamoneurohypophysial system of the rat, *Science* **205**:723–725.

Schwartz, W. J., Davidsen, L. C., and Smith, C. B., 1980, *In vivo* metabolic activity of a putative circadian oscillator, the rat suprachiasmatic nucleus, *J. Comp. Neurol.* **189**:157–167.

Shapiro, H. M., Greenberg, J. H., Reivich, M., Shipko, E., Van Horn, K., and Sokoloff, L., 1975, Local cerebral glucose utilization during anesthesia, in: *Blood Flow and Metabolism in the Brain* (A. M. Harper, W. B. Jennett, J. D. Miller and J. O. Rowan, eds.), pp. 9.42–9.43, Churchill Livingstone, Edinburgh.

Sharp, F. R., Kauer, J. S., and Shepherd, G. M., 1975, Local sites of activity-related glucose metabolism in rat olfactory bulb during olfactory stimulation, *Brain Res.* **98**:596–600.

Shinohara, M., Sakurada, O., Jehle, J., and Sokoloff, L., 1976, Effects of D-lysergic acid diethylamide on local cerebral glucose utilization in the rat, *Neurosci. Abstr.* **2**:615.

Shinohara, M., Dollinger, B., Brown, G., Rapoport, S., and Sokoloff, L., 1979, Cerebral glucose utlization: Local changes during and after recovery from spreading cortical depression, *Science* **203**:188–190.

Silverman, M. S., Hendrickson, A. E., and Clopton, B. M., 1977, Mapping of the tonotopic organization of the auditory system by uptake of radioactive metabolities, *Neurosci. Abstr.* **3**:11.

Smith, C. B., Goochee, C., Rapoport, S. I., and Sokoloff, L., 1980, Effects of ageing on local rates of cerebral glucose utilization in the rat, *Brain* **103**:351–365.

Sokoloff, L., 1960, Metabolism of the central nervous system *in vivo,* in: *Handbook of Physiology-Neurophysiology,* Vol. III (J. Field, H. W. Magoun and V. E. Hall, eds.) pp. 1843–1864, American Physiological Society, Washington, D.C.

Sokoloff, L., 1966, Cerebral circulatory and metabolic changes associated with aging, *Res. Publ. Res. Assoc. Nerv. Ment. Dis.* **41**:237–254.

Sokoloff, L., 1969, Cerebral circulation and behavior in man: strategy and findings, in: *Psychochemical Research in Man* (A. J. Mandell and M. P. Mandell, eds.), pp. 237–252, Academic Press, New York.

Sokoloff, L., 1976, Circulation and energy metabolism of the brain, in: *Basic Neurochemistry* 2nd ed. (G. J. Siegel, R. W. Albers, R. Katzman, and B. W. Agranoff, eds.), pp. 388–413, Little, Brown and Company, Boston.

Sokoloff, L., 1977, Relation between physiological function and energy metabolism in the central nervous system, *J. Neurochem.* **29**:13–26.

Sokoloff, L., 1978, Mapping cerebral functional activity with radioactive deoxyglucose, *Trends Neurosci.* **1**(3):75–79.

Sokoloff, L., 1979, The [¹⁴C]deoxyglucose method: four years later, *Acta Neurol. Scand. Suppl.* **60**:640–649.

Sokoloff, L., Reivich, M., Kennedy, C., Des Rosiers, M. H., Patlak, C. S., Pettigrew, K. D., Sakurada, O., and Shinohara, M., 1977, The [¹⁴C]deoxyglucose method for the measurement of local cerebral glucose utilization: theory, procedure, and normal values in the conscious and anesthetized albino rat, *J. Neurochem.* **28**:897–916.

Sols, A., and Crane, R. K., 1954, Substrate specificity of brain hexokinase, *J. Biol. Chem.* **210**:581–595.

Tower, D. B., 1958, The effects of 2-deoxy-D-glucose on metabolism of slices of cerebral cortex incubated *in vitro, J. Neurochem.* **3**:185–205.

Webster, W. R., Serviere, J., Batini, C., and LaPlante, S., 1978, Autoradiographic demonstration with 2-[^{14}C]deoxyglucose of frequency selectivity in the auditory system of cats under conditions of functional activity, *Neurosci. Lett.* **10**:43–48.

Wechsler, L. R., Savaki, H. E., and Sokoloff, L., 1979, Effects of *d-* and *l-*amphetamine on local cerebral glucose utilization in the conscious rat, *J. Neurochem.* **32**:15–22.

Whittam, R., 1962, The dependence of the respiration of brain cortex on active cation transport, *Biochem. J.* **82**:205–212.

Wick, A. N., Drury, D. R., Nakada, H. I., and Wolfe, J. B., 1957, Localization of the primary metabolic block produced by 2-deoxyglucose, *J. Biol. Chem.* **224**:963–969.

Wiesel, T. N., Hubel, D. H., and Lam, D. M. K., 1974, Autoradiographic demonstration of ocular dominance columns in the monkey striate cortex by means of transneuronal transport, *Brain Res.* **79**:273–279.

Wolfson, L. I., Sakurada, O., and Sokoloff, L., 1977, Effects of γ-butyrolactone on local cerebral glucose utilization in the rat, *J. Neurochem.* **29**:777–783.

Yarowsky, P. J., Jehle, J., Ingvar, D. H., and Sokoloff, L., 1979, Relationship between functional activity and glucose utilization in the rat superior cervical ganglion *in vivo, Neurosci. Abstr.* **5**:421.

Yarowsky, P. J., Crane, A. M., and Sokoloff, L., 1980, Stimulation of neuronal glucose utilization by antidromic electrical stimulation in the superior cervical ganglion of the rat, *Neurosci. Abstr.* **6**:340.

BIOSYNTHESIS AND FUNCTION OF UNCONJUGATED PTERINS IN MAMMALIAN TISSUES

E. MARTIN GÁL

Neurochemical Research Laboratories
Department of Psychiatry
University of Iowa
Iowa City, Iowa

Chance favors the prepared mind
LOUIS PASTEUR (1822–1895)

1. INTRODUCTION

Sometime, somewhere in the very distant biological past, possibly at the time of the primordial "ooze" with the arrival of purine nucleotides, other condensed pyrimidine rings might have also appeared. Of the condensed pyrimidines, the bicyclic nitrogen-containing ring termed pyrimido-(4,5-b)-pyrazine is the central cast of our story. This story is as old as modern science itself.

It was the restless and creative curiosity of Sir Frederick G. Hopkins (1889) which led him to study the nature of the pigments of butterfly wings.

He made scientists aware of the presence of the pyrimidopyrazine ring in living organisms. Between 1889 and 1895 Hopkins, in four distinct reports, opened the way to the understanding of the compounds which are in part responsible for the splendid colors (e.g., red, yellow, and brown) of butterfly wings. Wieland and Schöpf (1925) who isolated these pigments named them pterins after the Greek word *pteros,* meaning wing. The pigments revealed the same fundamental ring structure, thus the form "pteridine" was introduced to denote the pyrimido-(4,5-b)-pyrazines. Pfleiderer (1964) suggested that the term "pterin" should be reserved for derivatives of 2-amino-4-hydroxypterines only. Accordingly, "pteridine" and "pterin" will be used in this chapter with this distinction in mind.

Nature never surrenders her secrets lightly, thus the research on the elucidation of the identity of butterfly pigments by Purrmann (1940) became one of arduous task and withal a milestone in organic chemistry. Of course, butterfly wings are by no means the exclusive source of pteridines. Analysis of bacteria, molds, plants, protozoa, and metazoa all revealed their presence. Pterins occur unconjugated or conjugated like folic acid. In this chapter, no attempt will be made to review the available data on folic acid and its derivatives as ample literature exists, represented by scholarly surveys of the chemistry and biology of folates (Stokstad and Koch, 1967; Blakley, 1969; Iwai *et al.,* 1970; Shiota, 1971; Brown, 1971; Pfleiderer, 1975).

As intimated in the preceding paragraph, a great deal of information exists concerning the chemistry and occurrence of pterins particularly as they relate to species other than mammals. As recently as 1969 Blakley, in his book *The Biochemistry of Folic Acid and Related Pteridines,* noted that "little is known of the occurrence of pterins in mammalian species."

This chapter will attempt to fill this gap in our information. The accomplishments of the last twenty years of research on the function and biosynthesis of pterins in mammals will be reviewed and assessed. Interest in pteridines is something more than contemplation of the eye-pleasing, esthetic effects of colors. It is rather a profound preoccupation to comprehend their role in the mechanism of cell life.

2. CHEMISTRY AND ISOLATION

2.1. Chemistry

The basic structure of the pteridine ring, pyrimido-[4,5-b]-pyrazine, is given with the generally accepted numbering (1). The structures of naturally occurring pteridines with 2-amino-4-hydroxy groups, as mentioned in Section 1, are referred to as pterins (2). Examination of the tautomer forms 2 and 3

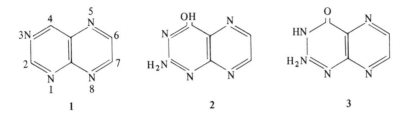

indicated that structure **3**, the oxoform, is the prevalent tautomer (Pfleiderer *et al.,* 1960; Brown and Jacobsen, 1961). The hydrogenated derivatives such as dihydro and tetrahydro forms are of importance as naturally occurring compounds which participate in biocatalytic reactions. The reduction of the pteridines in biological systems accords well with the nature of the two diazines of which the pyrazine ring is reduced with ease while the pyrimidine ring is rather resistant to hydrogenation, particularly at pH 7.0 and above. Interestingly, electron donor substituents such as NH_2 and OH (those in pterins) increase the stability of the parent compounds but decrease it in the reduced derivatives. For example, pteridine is quite unstable but its 5,6,7,8-tetrahydro derivative is stable to 1 *N* HCl, to 1 *N* NaOH, to light, and to most oxidizing agents. Tetrahydropterin (**4**) is rapidly oxidized (it is light sensitive) to the 7,8-dihydropterin, (**5**) which is further oxidized to the parent pterin (**3**) in acid or alkaline solution. The biochemical importance of the biological oxidation of reduced pterins will be treated more extensively in Sections 4 and 7.

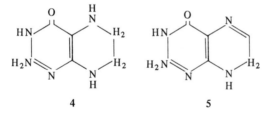

Electrophilic substitution at C atoms of pteridines, except for chlorine, is not known for these compounds. The chlorine atom, however, becomes very reactive, being next to nitrogen, and thus it is prone to nucleophilic displacement by NH_2, SH, or OH groups. Alkylation of the ring was extensively reported. The nature and the site of alkylation will depend on the substitutions and side chains of the pteridine ring. Structurally, the pteridine ring, as shown by X-ray studies (Hamor and Robertson, 1956), possesses planar arrangement of its atoms. Bond angle and bond distance measurements revealed no central symmetry of structure.

Knowledge of the ionization constants of pteridines (Table 1) is one of the best ways of determining the major tautomer form at equilibrium. The unsub-

TABLE 1.   Ionization of Some Pterins in Water

Compound	pK_a Basic	pK_a Acidic
6,7-Dimethylpterin	2.6	8.9
7,8-Dihydro-6,7-dimethylpterin	4.2	11.1
5,6,7,8-Tetrahydro-6,7-dimethylpterin	5.6	10.4
6-Methylpterin	2.8	8.3
7,8-Dihydro-6-methylpterin	4.2	10.9
5,6,7,8-Tetrahydro-6-methylpterin	5.4	10.5
Biopterin	2.4	7.7
Dihydrobiopterin	4.1	10.2
5,6,7,8-Tetrahydrobiopterin	5.3	10.4
Sepiapterin	2.4	7.7

stituted pteridine is a weak base (pK_a 4.1) without acidic properties. Introduction of an OH group at the 2,4, or 7 carbon positions brings about a decrease in basic strength. The acidic pK_a of pterins is therefore due to the 4-OH or 3-NH group. Hydrogenation of the pyrazine ring leads to an increase in basic strength due to decreased aromatization. Protonation at N-5 was shown to cause the basic pK_a of tetrahydropterins (Whiteley and Huennekens, 1967).

Polarography is another approach to gain important insights into the structure of pteridines (Rembold, 1964; Lund, 1975). Their half-wave potential is useful in deducing certain configurational characteristics. Proton resonance spectroscopy is another technique for resolving structures (Philipsborn et al., 1964). The proton resonance spectra are informative, especially when the compounds are deuterated. Nuclear magnetic resonance studies of some biologically active 7,8-dihydropterins have been reported (Fukushima and Akino, 1968).

Valuable information can also be obtained from the ultraviolet spectra of pteridines although the ultraviolet spectrum alone is insufficient for identification. It is apparent from the ultraviolet spectra (Table 2) that there are several maxima, frequently greater than 300 nm. These are distinguishing parameters of the pterins when compared to pyrimidines and pyrazines. Some pterins, such as sepiapterin and erythropterin, have maxima above 400 nm. Hydrogenation of pterins shifts their spectra to shorter ultraviolet wave lengths with the exception of the reduced forms of pterin-6-carboxylic acid which has a maximum at 380 nm.

Another area in analytical techniques is the measurement of the fluorescence properties of pteridines, which aids in their characterization and detection from biological sources. A fairly comprehensive study (Uyeda and Rabi-

TABLE 2. Ultraviolet Spectra of Some Pterins

Compound	Maxima (nm)	E_{max} (mol) × 10^{-3}	pH
6-Methylpterin	248, 324	10.3, 8.2	1
7,8,-Dihydro-6-methylpterin	253, 365	22.8, 7.5	13
7,8-Dihydro-6-methylpterin (6-MPH$_2$)	252, 361	18.6, 5.1	1
5,6,7,8-Tetrahydro-6-methylpterin (6-MPH$_4$)	229, 279, 324	25.7, 10.5, 5.6	7
	261, 303	16.0	1
6,7-Dimethylpterin	250, 355	21.9, 9.5	7
7,8-Dihydro-6,7-dimethylpterin (DMPH$_2$)	252, 280, 350	17.4, 11.2, 7.5	13
5,6,7,8-Tetrahydro-6,7-dimethylpterin (DMPH$_4$)	227, 266, 318	25.1, 8.3, 8.7	1
	231, 281, 318	14.5, 17.8, 6.2	7
6-(L-Erythro-1',2'-dihydroxypropryl)pterin-biopterin (mol. wt. 237)	220, 297, 290	17.0, 10.0, 6.2	12
	247, 322	15.6, 7.4	1
7,8-Dihydrobiopterin (BH$_2$)	254, 363	21.1, 6.6	13
	255, 354	13.6, 6.3	7.6
5,6,7,8-Tetrahydrobiopterin (BH$_4$)	256, 275, 314	12.9, 7.5, 5.6	1
	284, 330	9.5, 7.3	13
6-(D-Erythro-1',2',3'-trihydroxypropyl)pterin-neopterin	247, 321	14.1, 4.6	1
Sepiapterin	281, 410	10.4, 8.0	1
	267, 423	16.1, 10.3	5
	268, 440	15.8, 12.1	11

nowitz, 1963) described maximal excitation between 350 and 380 nm and emission about 450 nm for pterins. This fluorescence is markedly pH dependent. The fluorescence intensity of the parent compound gradually decreases upon di- or tetrahydrogenation of the pyrazine ring (Table 3).

Of course, the study of the naturally occurring pteridines was greatly enhanced by the rapid development of their synthesis. Of significance was the recognition (Purrmann, 1941) that condensation of 4,5-diaminopyrimidines with α-keto acids was pH dependent. The NH_2 groups on carbon atoms 4 and 5 of the pyrimidine nucleus possess different nucleophilic potentials (Pfleiderer, 1957), thus as condensation products, 7-substituted pteridines arise in neutral, weakly acidic, or organic solvents. Protonation of the more basic NH_2 groups at C-5 yields 6-substituted pteridines at strongly acidic pH. In general, the condensation product represents a mixture of the 6 and 7 substituted forms which can be separated by chromatography. Procedures of asymmetric syntheses have been reported for biopterins (Andrews *et al.*, 1969; Taylor and Jacobi, 1974, 1977) that lead unambiguously to 6-substituted products. For details of the chemistry of pteridines the reader is referred to reviews (Pfleiderer and Taylor, 1964; Elderfield and Mehta, 1967).

A few words need to be said about the reduction of pteridines to their dihydro or tetrahydro forms. Some of the 7,8-dihydropteridines can be directly synthesized by condensation of 4-chloro-5-nitropyrimidines with α-amino-diazo ketones or aldehydes (Boon and Jones, 1951). The prevalent practice, however, is the reduction of the various pteridines by zinc dust in alkali or in acid, by $NaBH_4$ or by dithionate. Catalytic hydrogenation with platinum, palladium, or Raney-nickel is another technique of reduction. There is some variation in the efficiency of these reducing agents depending on pH, temperature, and ring substitutions. As alluded to before, most reductions take place in the

TABLE 3. Fluorescence Properties of Some Pterins

| Compound | Fluorescence (nm) | | |
	Activation max	Emission max	Relative T(%)
Biopterin	350	435	40.6
7,8-BH_2	275	570	7.2
q-BH_2	270	430	6.4
5,6,7,8-BH_4	350	420	0.02
6-Methylpterin	355	450	37.9
6-MPH_2	290	550	6.0
q-6-MPH_2	270	435	6.2
6-MPH_4	350	420	0.09

pyrazine ring. Pyrimidines are resistant to reduction particularly in alkaline medium. Catalytic hydrogenation, for the most part, yields 5,6,7,8-tetrahydro forms, while zinc gives 7,8-dihydro derivatives. Reduction with sodium borohydride often results in a mixture of the dihydro and tetrahydro forms. Sodium or potassium amalgam is at times capable of removing side chains from C-6 position (Nawa *et al.*, 1953). Oxidation of some dihydropterins in trifluoroacetic acid by H_2O_2 has given rise to free radicals (Ehrenberg *et al.*, 1967). In solution, at low temperatures, pteridines can form charge-transfer complexes with indole derivatives, for instance with tryptophan and 5-hydroxytryptamine. These complexes which are free radicals (Fujimori, 1959) only take place with the parent compound but not with the reduced pteridines. Free radicals are assumed to be intermediates formed during oxidation of reduced pterins by O_2, H_2O, or Fe^{3+} as 5,6,7,8-tetrahydropterin (4) is oxidized to quinonoid dihydropterin (6). (See Section 5.) The quinonoid slowly tautomerizes to 7,8-dihydropterin, 5 (Vonderschmitt and Scrimgeour, 1967). It was suggested that reaction between the quinonoid dihydropterin (6) and 7,8-dihydropterin (5) results in the formation of pterin and 5,6,7,8-tetrahydropterin.

In general, 7,8-dihydropterin forms adducts with ammonia, bisulphite, cyanide, thiols, and carbanions with active hydrogen. However, nucleophilic addition to 6-alkyl-7,8-dihydropterins are only known for bisulphite (Vonderschmitt *et al.*, 1967). The reduced forms of C-6-substituted pterins become even more photolabile and oxidizable than those without C-6 or C-7 substitution. Reduced biopterin or neopterin, for instance, were observed to lose the di- or trihydroxypropyl side chain at C-6 in boiling water (Rembold *et al.*, 1969).

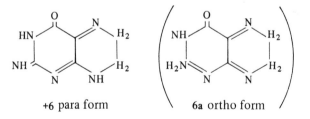

+6 para form   6a ortho form

2.2. Isolation

The micro amounts of pterins in biological material reflect the quasi vitaminlike or cofactorial role they play in cell life. There are several procedures for the isolation of pteridines from microbial, plant, or animal tissues. The method of choice will be contingent on the nature of the pteridine, particularly on its stability and solubility. In general, it is recommended that all manipulation involving pteridines should be conducted under dim light or preferably in darkness. Removal of protein or peptides by trichloroacetic acid (Rembold and Buschmann, 1962) or $Al_2(SO_4)_3/Ba(OH)_2$ has been extensively used.

Sephadex-G-25 was also employed to recover protein free fractions containing folic acid and biopterin (Dewey and Kidder, 1967). Recently a mixture of proteolytic enzymes (pronase and papain) were used to predigest the animal tissues (Gál et al., 1976) followed by addition of 0.3 N Ba(OH)$_2$ containing 1% mercaptoethanol and ethanol. Proteolysis permitted release of any protein-bound pteridine thus obviating extraction by alkaline reagents which are often destructive to reduced pteridines. The protein free extracts serve for separation, recovery, and purification of pteridines by column chromatography using DOWEX-1 and -50 (Rembold and Buschmann, 1962). Phosphocellulose or Ecteola cellulose was also put to good use to effect separation (Rembold and Buschmann, 1962). Paper chromatography was one of the earliest techniques of separation (Hadorn and Mitchell, 1951) and it is still a good one for identification of pteridines. Separation of pterins has been achieved by thin layer chromatography (Nicolaus, 1960; Bertino et al., 1965; Descimon and Barial, 1973). Electrophoresis on cellulose acetate (Gerhart and MacIntyre, 1970; Loo and Adamson, 1965; Hillcoat and Blakley, 1964) as well as isoelectrofocusing (Eugster et al., 1970) are other techniques which were employed for separation of pteridines. Recently high pressure liquid chromatography (HPLC) using SCX column was successfully applied to separation of pteridines (Bailey and Ayling, 1975). The isolation of as small an amount as 25 pg of biopterin and neopterin by HPLC was reported (Gál and Sherman, 1977a).

Several methods exist for identification of the isolated pteridines. Some of these methods like chromatography provide us with characteristic R_fs while ultraviolet or fluorescence analyses provide us with characteristic absorption or emission spectra. There are color tests (McNutt, 1964) and a specific pterin-dependent enzyme test (Guroff et al., 1967). However, the most sensitive method of identification is gas chromatography (Haug, 1970; Lloyd et al., 1971; Gál and Sherman, 1977a). Generally, heptafluorobutyric anhydride (HFB) or bistrimethylsilyltrifluoroacetamide (TMS) are used to derivatize pteridines for gas chromatography. The choice of one or the other reagent or their combination will, of course, depend on the nature of reactive substitutions of the parent ring. As little as 0.1 pmol of derivatized pterins could be detected (Gál and Sherman, 1977a). These derivatives of pteridines because of their greatly increased volatility enabled their mass spectroscopic identification (Haug, 1970; Lloyd et al., 1971). The above-mentioned techniques not only aid in identification but, when properly executed, also serve for quantitation of pteridines.

One would be remiss not to mention the *Crithidia fasciculata* or *Tetrahymena pyriformis* growth tests (Dewey and Kidder, 1971). These biological tests employ the calibrated growth response of these protozoa to pterins. However, the biological assay alone is insufficient proof for the identity of a particular pterin, since 2,4,5-triamino-6-hydroxypyrimidine will substitute for pterins for the growth of *Crithidia* (Dewey *et al.*, 1959). A biosynthetic product like biopterin from D-erythrodihydroneopterin triphosphate was shown to be positive by *Crithidia* assay but different in its chromatographic properties (Eto *et al.*, 1976). The assignment of absolute structure and identification requires a combination of the techniques described in this section. The selection of various techniques will have to depend on the scale of isolation whether for preparative or for analytical purposes.

3. OCCURRENCE OF PTERINS

Although several reviews are available on pteridines found in microbes (Forrest and van Baalen, 1970), insects (Ziegler and Harmsen, 1969), and lower vertebrates (Hama, 1953; Ortiz *et al.*, 1962), a brief survey might nevertheless serve as a useful corollary.

The pterins from butterfly wing, white leucopterin (**7**), yellow xanthopterin (**8**), and orange red erythropterin (**9**), yielded our earliest knowledge of pterins.

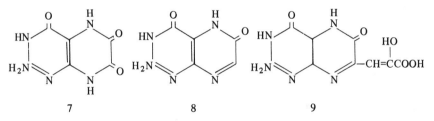

In the eyes of fruit flies (Drosophilae) and of honey bees, other pterins such as biopterin (**10**), sepiapterin (**11**), and neopterin (**12**) have also been detected. These pterins have been proved to be of biochemical importance for some enzyme catalyzed reactions (Shiota, 1971). All three pterins have C-6 alkyl chain in common. It should be noted that the structures of biopterin and neopterin (Rembold and Buschmann, 1963) are given here without reference to their proper configuration. Biopterin was first isolated and shown to be growth promoting in *Crithidia fasciculata* (Patterson *et al.*, 1955). In addition

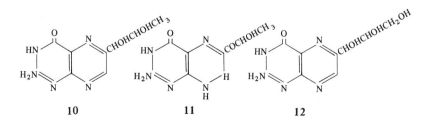

to the above structures several others, such as chrysopterin, ekapterin, and lepidopterin, have been isolated. The function of pterins in insects is unclear. Presumably they participate as light filters (Viscontini and Schmidt, 1965) and in sex recognition by insects, e.g., bees and ants.

Biopterin and sepiapterin occur in the skin of red carp, of goldfish, and of many other fishes along with the violet-fluorescing isoxanthopterin-6-carboxylic acid (13) and ichtiopterin (14) which are both absent from insects, amphibia, or reptiles. Unconjugated pterins have also been isolated from the skin and eyes of amphibia. They appear to be linked with specific chromatophores like xanthophores which are rich in pterins, and melanophores which

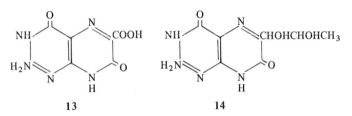

13   14

possess only traces of pterins (Bagnara, 1961; Bagnara and Obika, 1965). Pterin content of amphibia undergoes marked changes during metamorphosis (Hama, 1963) both in content and structural differentiation. During development biopterin and isoxanthopterin appear first with the melanophores, while later only sepiapterin and isosepiapterin are present in the xanthophores. Ranachrome 3 (probably 6-hydroxylmethylpterin) puts in appearance still later in the erythrophores.

The skin of reptiles and turtles also contains various pterins, particularly biopterin and pterin-6-carboxylic acid (a possible metabolite of biopterin or neopterin). It is thought that the pterins are of importance in the synthesis of melanin in fish, amphibia, and reptiles (Ziegler, 1964) since during the course of melanin formation pterins exist in their reduced form to act as cofactors in the synthesis of tyrosine. This amino acid represents the initial substance needed for melanin synthesis. In adult animals, with cessation of melanin formation, pterins are present in their metabolically inert form.

Pterins were found in chicken liver (Fukushima *et al.*, 1977) showing that they also occur in other avian organs. The pterin content of chicken blood and serum corresponds to 76 ng/ml and 300 ng/ml, respectively, by *Crithidia* assay (Frank *et al.*, 1963).

During the last 40 yr the presence of pterins in the mammalian organs has been finally established. The information on distribution, and chemical profile of pterins from mammalian sources is still not extensive but enough to gain a picture of their ubiquity. The first attempt to identify a sulfur-containing pigment, urothione (**15**), as a pterin in human urine was unsuccessful (Koschara, 1936). The structure of this compound is now presumed to be

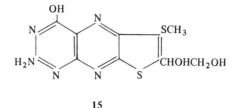

15

Most of the reported quantitation of pterins in the serum, blood, or tissues of mammals (Frank *et al.,* 1963) relied on the *Crithidia* assay (Rembold and Metzger, 1967*a*; Baker *et al.,* 1974; Leeming *et al.,* 1976*a,b*). *Pseudomonas* phenylalanine hydroxylase assay (Guroff *et al.,* 1967) permitted quantitation of tetrahydrobiopterin (BH$_4$). Recent advances in methodology based on HPLC and GC now allow the simultaneous assessment of picomole amounts of biopterin, neopterin, and their reduced forms in mammalian organs (Gál and Sherman, 1977*a*). A listing, albeit not too extensive, illustrates the occurrence and level of pterins in the organs and blood of various mammals (Table 4). Determination of the pterin content in mammalian tissue by the *Crithidia* test resulted in a scatter of values. The biopterin level of human blood was reported to be 48 ng/ml by one group of investigators and 4 ng/ml by another; a similar spread occurred in the values for human sera. The values are apparently functional to the expertise of the investigators. There is much better concordance between the values obtained by *Pseudomonas* assay and HPLC–GC.

The levels of biopterins in various areas of human brain from two fresh autopsy materials are presented in Table 5 to demonstrate the major existing pools. The pons and the colliculi revealed an elevated level of reduced biopterins (unpublished observations). The pattern of distribution of biopterins in human brain and in rat brain was not critically divergent. Again, the largest pool of BH$_2$ and BH$_4$ was recoverable from the pontine region (Table 6A), while in the cerebellum biopterin was the predominant form. The ratio of the sum of BH$_2$ and BH$_4$ to B ranged from 20:1 in the pons to 1:1 in the small brain.

Measurement of the pool sizes in the subcellular fractions of the brain (Table 6B) revealed that most of the biopterins concentrated in the postmitochondrial fractions. Sucrose density gradient separation of the crude mitochondria yielded 66% of its pterins in the synaptosomes and 34% in the mitochondrial pellet. None was recovered from the myelin or the sucrose layers. Biopterins in the synaptosomes constituted 6% of the cerebral pool.

A study of the pool sizes and turnover rates following intraperitoneal

TABLE 4. Distribution of Pterins in the Organs of Mammals

Species	Organ or fluid	Pterin[b]	(μg/g) or (ml)	Assay[a]	Reference
Cattle	Blood		0.51		Frank et al. (1963)
	Serum		0.12		Frank et al. (1963)
Horse	Blood		0.80		Frank et al. (1963)
	Serum		0.12		Frank et al. (1963)
Human	Blood		0.048		Frank et al. (1963)
	Blood		0.002		Baker et al. (1974)
	Blood		0.004		Leeming et al. (1976a)
Children	Blood		0.002		Leeming et al. (1976)
	Serum		0.027		Frank et al. (1963)
Females	Serum		0.003		Fleming and Broquist (1967)
	Serum		0.002		Leeming et al. (1976a)
	Erythrocytes		0.0078		Leeming et al. (1976a)
	Plasma		0.0009		Baker et al. (1974)
Children with PKU	Plasma		0.0018		Leeming et al. (1976b)
	Plasma		0.0049		Leeming et al. (1976b)
Adult	Brain:				
	White matter		0.046		Leeming et al. (1976b)
	Gray matter		0.025		Leeming et al. (1976b)
	Substantia nigra		0.23		Leeming et al. (1976b)
	CSF		0.0019		Leeming et al. (1976b)
	CSF		0.0004		Leeming et al. (1976b)
	Urine		0.75		Fukushima et al. (1978)
	Brain	BH_2	0.11	HPLC-GC	Gál and Sherman (unpublished)
	Brain	BH_4	0.24	HPLC-GC	Gál and Sherman (unpublished)
	Brain		0.21	HPLC-GC	Gál and Sherman (unpublished)
	Liver		0.52		Baker et al. (1974)
Mouse	Blood		0.20		Fukushima et al. (1978)

	Tissue	Form	Value	Method	Reference
Rat	Serum		0.45		Frank et al. (1974)
	Blood		0.046		Baker et al. (1974)
	Serum		0.2		Rembold and Metzger (1967 a,b)
	Plasma	BH_2	0.08	HPLC-GC	Gál et al. (1966)
	Plasma	BH_4	0.11	HPLC-GC	Gál et al. (1966)
	Plasma		0.34	HPLC-GC	Gál et al. (1966)
	Brain		0.20		Rembold and Metzger (1967a,b)
	Brain		0.08		Baker et al. (1974)
	Brain	BH_2 and BH_4	0.75	Pseudomonas	Guroff et al. (1967)
	Brain	BH_2	0.12	HPLC-GC	Gál et al. (1977)
	Brain		0.20	HPLC-GC	Gál et al. (1977)
	Brain	BH_4	0.33	HPLC-GC	Gál et al. (1977)
	Liver		2.3		Baker et al. (1974)
	Liver		0.39	HPLC-GC	Gál and Sherman (1977)
	Liver	BH_2	11.7	HPLC-GC	Gál and Sherman (1977)
	Liver	BH_4	0.38	HPLC-GC	Gál and Sherman (1977)
	Liver	BH_2 and BH_4	13.0	Pseudomonas	Guroff et al. (1967)
	Liver		6.0		Rembold and Metzger (1967a,b)
	Adrenals		4.8		Rembold and Metzger (1967a,b)
	Bone marrow		0.60		Rembold and Metzger (1967 a,b)
	Eyes		0.02		Rembold and Metzger (1967a,b)
	Heart		0.20		Rembold and Metzger (1967a,b)
	Kidneys		1.20		Rembold and Metzger (1967a,b)
	Lungs		0.90		Rembold and Metzger (1967a,b)
	Spleen		3.00		Rembold and Metzger (1967a,b)
	Adrenals		0.95	HPLC	Fukishima and Nixon (1980)
	Brain		0.09	HPLC-GC	Fukishima and Nixon (1980)
	Kidney		0.16	HPLC-GC	Fukishima and Nixon (1980)
	Liver		1.6	HPLC-GC	Fukishima and Nixon (1980)
	Pineal gland		12.5	HPLC-GC	Fukishima and Nixon (1980)

a Done by Crithidia assay unless otherwise stated.
b Pterin denotes biopterin (B) unless otherwise indicated.

TABLE 5. Levels of Biopterins in Various Areas of Human Brain ($\mu g/g$)

Areas	B	BH$_2$	BH$_4$
Neocortex			
Frontal	0.10	0.20	0.17
Parietal	0.09	0.13	0.18
Occipital	0.15	0.16	0.15
Pons	0.07	0.60	0.24
Medulla	0.13	0.18	0.21
Cerebellum	0.07	0.17	0.11
Colliculi	0.25	0.65	0.62
Thalamus	0.08	0.19	0.16
Hypothalamus	0.05	0.14	0.25
Striatum	0.24	0.17	0.17
Septum	0.20	0.12	0.24
Caudate	0.07	0.12	0.09

TABLE 6. Regional Levels and Subcellular Distribution of Biopterins in Rat Brain

	B	BH$_2$	BH$_4$
A. Area[a]			
Neocortex	0.09	0.12	0.18
Subcortex	0.05	0.13	0.44
Cerebellum	0.29	0.08	0.26
Colliculi	0.15	0.19	0.25
Pons	0.09	0.79	1.03
B. Fraction[b]			
Nuclear	0.10	0.19	0.30
Microsomal	0.31	0.36	0.50
Supernatant	0.47	0.94	1.44
Myelin[c]	—	—	—
Synaptosomal	0.04	0.13	0.16
Mitochondrial	0.03	0.09	0.15

[a] Units in $\mu g/g$ wet weight
[b] Units in nmol/fraction. A nanomole of biopterin is 0.237 μg.
[c] Crude mitochondrial pellets were used in toto for gradient separation; hence values were not available.

injection of [^{14}C]biopterin and reduced biopterins showed that in the liver BH$_2$ was the major form of biopterin whereas in the plasma and brain it was BH$_4$ (Gál et al., 1976). In the brain, biopterins have rapid turnover rates. The total pool of BH$_2$ plus BH$_4$ was 0.62 $\mu g/g$ and 0.56 nmol/g per hr turnover rate (Table 7). This turnover rate implied replacement of the cerebral pool in 0.5 hr, an indication of very active cerebral synthesis of BH$_2$. This was eventually born out by experimental evidence (Gál and Sherman, 1976; Kidder et al., 1964).

It was mentioned earlier that the flagellate Crithidia fasciculata required biopterin for growth. However, the growth requirement could be equally met by high concentration of folic acid (Broquist and Albrecht, 1955; Patterson et al., 1955). On feeding [^{14}C]folic acid to Crithidia cultures [^{14}C]biopterin was recovered (Kidder et al., 1964). This was adduced as evidence that biopterin in mammals may have derived from folic acid. However, clinical observations (Fleming and Broquist, 1967) and experiments consistently failed to confirm biopterin as the catabolic product of folic acid in mammalian tissues (Pabst and Rembold, 1966; Gál and Sherman, 1976).

TABLE 7. Summary of Data on Efflux Rates and Turnover
by Isotope Dilution

Parameter	BH_2	B	BH_4
		Brain	
$T_{1/2}$ (hr)	1.29	1.26	1.73
K	0.54	0.55	0.40
Pool ($\mu g/g$)	0.19	0.11	0.32
Turnover (nmol/g per hr)	0.43	0.25	0.53
		Liver	
$T_{1/2}$ (hr)	4.44	2.64	4.30
K	0.16	0.26	0.16
Pool ($\mu g/g$)	11.58	0.41	0.40
Turnover (nmol/g per hr)	7.84	0.47	0.28
		Plasma	
$T_{1/2}$ (hr)	0.93	0.92	1.59
K	0.75	0.75	0.44
Pool ($\mu g/ml$)	0.12	0.08	0.37
Turnover (nmol/ml per hr)	0.36	0.25	0.66

4. METABOLISM

4.1. Biosynthesis of Pterins in Vivo

Until recently, the biogenesis of biopterin in mammals was not well understood. There were some indirect observations which implied the existence of a
biosynthetic mechanism for biopterins. Among the most salient facts which
attested to such a mechanism were the following: (1) biopterin appeared as a
normal urinary constituent (Patterson et al., 1955; Fukushima and Shiota,
1972; Röthler and Karobath, 1976); (2) biopterin-free diet had no growth-
retarding effect in young rats (Kraut et al., 1963) and its excretion continued
even in sulfonamide-treated animals at doses of this drug which arrested the
growth of intestinal flora; (3) dietary folate or riboflavin was also excluded as
the source of biopterin since rats and chicks deficient in these vitamins continued to excrete biopterin in normal amounts (Pabst and Rembold, 1966; Fleming and Broquist, 1967). Feeding biopterin-deficient diet containing 2,4-dia-
mino-6-hydroxypyrimidine (1% by dry weight of diet) through nine weeks

lowered urinary output of biopterin by 80% without influencing the growth of the rats (Pabst and Rembold, 1966). These authors rightly concluded that the biopterin needed for growth and maintenance was lower than indicated by its urinary levels (about 30 μg daily excretion). Consequently, they suggested that the results of their experiments indicated a "*de novo* synthesis of biopterin" in rats. Much the same conclusion was drawn from measurements of serum biopterin and folic acid levels in 85 patients with or without pregnancy anemia. In 31 patients with megaloblastic anemia due to folic acid deficiency, the serum levels of biopterin were from normal to very high:1.2–31.8 ng/ml (1.2–5.5 ng/ml in nonanemic women) (Fleming and Broquist, 1967). In brief, there was no correlation between levels of folic acid and biopterin, consequently disproving a precursor–product relationship. In all, mammals cannot synthesize folic acid. Folic acid levels of blood and tissues were significantly lower than the levels of biopterin (Frank *et al.,* 1963).

Whence, then, does biopterin originate in the mammalian body? It was noted that preparations of guanosine contained a contaminant which by analysis appeared to be biopterin (Nathan and Cowperthwaite, 1955). The structural similarity between this purine and the pterins made it attractive to speculate on the existence of a biochemical conversion. Indeed, the feasibility of transformation of purines into pterins involving the loss of C-8 as formic acid was soon demonstrated (Albert, 1957). Several studies with microbes, insects, and lower vertebrates confirmed the conversion of purines into pterins. These studies were reviewed (Shiota, 1971). Tissue slices of tadpole skins, when incubated in a media containing [2,4-^{14}C] guanine, synthesized labeled biopterin (about 35.5 μg/mg of skin) and pterin-6-carboxylic acid (Levy, 1964; Sugiura and Goto, 1968). Experiments with guanosine monophosphate (GMP) and guanosine triphosphate (GTP) have borne out the participation of the ribose moiety of these nucleotides in providing carbons C-6 and C-7 of the pyrazine ring (Krumdieck *et al.,* 1966). These observations served as foundation of a tentative biosynthetic pathway of the GTP conversion to 6-hydroxymethyldihydropterin via dihydroneopterin triphosphate (Weygand *et al.,* 1961; Krumdieck *et al.,* 1966). Nevertheless, the origin of the 6-alkyl side chain remained for sometime a matter of contention. Isosepiapterin synthesized from reduced pterin and 2-ketobutyric acid led to the assumption that reduced pterin was the common intermediate for 6-substituted naturally occurring pterins (Forrest and Nawa, 1964). Experimental confirmation of this proposal was apparently supplied by the incorporation of [^{14}C] reduced pterin into sepiapterin and biopterin from *Drosophila melanogaster* and from skin of bullfrog tadpoles (Okada and Goto, 1965; Sugiura and Goto, 1967). Research on the biosynthesis of pterins received great impetus by the proof that neopterin was produced from GTP (Guroff and Strenkoski, 1966) and by the isolation of an enzyme from *E. coli* which converts GTP to dihydroneopterin triphosphate and formic acid (Burg and Brown, 1968). These results encouraged the reexamination of the problem concerning the origin of the C-6-alkyl side chain of some pterins. Bullfrogs were injected with $[U-C^{14}]$-GTP (10μCi) and carboxy-labeled 6-pterincarboxylic acid (30 μCi). A negligible amount of label was recoverable in biopterin (14 cpm/μmol). Most of the label was found in isoxanthopterin (96.00 cpm/μmol) derived from pterin-6-carboxylic acid, while from labeled GTP significant incorporation took place in biopterin and in sepiapterin (Fukushima, 1970).

Even though the stage was now set, there were no reports as yet on the biosynthesis of pterins in mammals. At long last in 1973 the first communication appeared in which the data revealed the appearance of ^{14}C in urinary biopterin from $[U-^{14}C]$-GTP-injected male rats and mice (Sugiura and Goto, 1973). In these experiments the animals received intravenous (i.v.) injection of 2 μCi of GTP at a time. The urine samples were collected for 7 days, pooled, and were given 4 μmol of nonradioactive biopterin. Biopterin was isolated and purified on a DEAE-Sephadex column, followed by two dimensional paper chromatography and charcoal treatment. An aliquot of biopterin, thus recovered, was oxidized by alkali permanganate to 6-carboxypterin. The specific activities of the recovered $[^{14}C]$biopterin and 6-carboxypterin were low, yet sufficient to show that the label in the pterin ring and in the side chain derived directly from GTP. Data reported by others (Buff and Dairman, 1975*a,b*) confirmed the urinary excretion of $[^{14}C]$biopterin from $[2-$$^{14}C]$guanine and the lack of it from $[8-^{14}C]$guanine in germfree animals. These authors, however, could not demonstrate synthesis of biopterin as such in any of the tissues examined. The difficulty rested mainly with the emphasis on the isolation of biopterin (B) rather than the isolation of dihydrobiopterin (BH$_2$). Compounding this difficulty was the dilution of the labeled pterin by carrier biopterin or by the existing large pools of GTP and biopterins in the tissues. For the most part, however, this difficulty could be traced to the limitations of the experimental procedure imposing inherently low recoveries of pterins.

However, these researchers were more successful in demonstrating biosynthesis of pterins in mammalian cell cultures. Mouse neuroblastoma clones (N-18 and N-1E) grown for 1–2 days in medium containing 40 μCi of either $[2-^{14}C]$- or $[8-^{14}C]$guanosine were capable of synthesizing C-6-substituted pterins. Biopterin and 6-carboxypterin were recovered by paper chromatography. In spite of the low recoveries of label, the presence of ^{14}C in the pterins from $[2-^{14}C]$guanosine was unequivocal. Again there was no radioactivity incorporated from $[8-^{14}C]$guanosine (Buff and Dairman, 1975*a*). The biosynthesis of biopterin was demonstrated in Chinese hamster ovary (CHO KI) cell cultures (Fukushima and Shiota, 1974). Addition of $[2-^{14}C]$folic acid to these cultures resulted in the appearance of 6-hydroxymethylpterin and 6-carboxypterin but not of biopterin. When the cells were grown in presence of $[2-$

[14]C]guanine, labeled biopterin along with other pterins could be recovered. In cells grown on biopterin-free medium with [2-^{14}C]guanine, the specific radioactivities of the biopterin formed and the GMP derived from RNA were in good accord. Experiments with [U-^{14}C]guanosine revealed that only 10% of the radioactivity found in GMP appeared in its ribose. This experiment failed to yield unequivocal answers as to the role of the ribosyl moiety of GMP in biopterin synthesis, particularly since the label appeared in the ribose of nucleotides other than GMP. When [6-^{14}C]glucose was added to the cell cultures most of the label in biopterin appeared in the side chain and in C-5 of the ribose of GMP derived from RNA. These results implied that one of the phosphorylated derivatives of guanosine might be a precursor for biopterin synthesis. Addition of sepiapterin along with [2-^{14}C]guanine to the cultures reduced the label content of biopterin but increased its absolute amount. The investigators (Fukushima and Shiota, 1974) adduced this as evidence for sepiapterin as a possible intermediate in the pathway of biopterin synthesis. These data, on the basis of the observations by others (Weygand *et al.*, 1961), accorded well with the proposal that guanine nucleotides may serve as precursors for biopterin synthesis (Kaufman, 1967*b*). However, there existed arguments counter to this hypothesis (Rembold and Gyure, 1972) because of the negligible incorporations of purines and their derivatives into biopterin. These authors failed to take into account the dilutive effect of the nucleotide pool and the low yield of biopterin from GTP. Another point of objection arose from the observation that injection of labeled neopterin or labeled tetrahydroneopterin failed to yield labeled biopterin (Rembold *et al.*, 1971*b*). Yet injections of actinomycin D, which leads to increased levels of cellular nucleotides, brought about increased levels of biopterin (Rembold and Gyure, 1972).

Be that as it may, labeled BH_2 has been retrieved after intracerebral injection of labeled 7,8-D-erythrodihydroneopterin triphosphate (unpublished observation). It is to be noted, however, that this BH_2 did not originate from the biologically dominant quinonoid D-erythrodihydroneopterin triphosphate. Therefore, the synthetic product of this experiment was L-erythro-7,8-dihydrobiopterin with a mixture of q-BH_2 derived from the oxidation of the BH_4 pool.

Up to this point, none of the studies cited have unequivocally resolved the derivation of the 6-alkyl side chain of biopterin. How is one to account for the L-erythro configuration of the 1',2'-hydroxypropyl side chain in biopterin by starting with D-ribose through D-erythroneopterin? This and other problems like the nature of the intermediates were left unresolved by the experiments with cell cultures. However, followup experiments employing homogenates of different organs from Syrian golden hamsters successfully demonstrated the synthesis of D-erythrodihydroneopterin triphosphate ($NPTH_2$-P_3) and the appearance of a "*Crithidia*-active" substance from GTP and GDP (Fukushima *et al.*, 1975*a,b*).

This was the extent of our knowledge in 1975 when it was established that the amounts of biopterin or its reduced forms, which penetrated the brain from the periphery, could not account for the size or turnover of the cerebral pool (Gál et al., 1976). The data suggested independent cerebral synthesis of dihydrobiopterin. Intraventricular injection of [U-14C]-GTP and [8-14C]-GTP has, indeed, brought to light the existence of active cerebral synthesis of BH_2. These experiments, because of the significant methodological improvements (Gál and Sherman, 1976, 1977a), also permitted isolation of many of the intermediates in the pathway from [U-14C]-GTP to [14C]-BH_2. Among these intermediates 2-amino-4-hydroxy-5(or 6)-formamido-6-ribosylaminopyrimidine triphosphate and dihydroneopterin triphosphate need be mentioned. This was the first unequivocal proof of the enzymatic synthesis of BH_2 and some of the intermediates from GTP in any mammalian tissue *in vivo* (Gál and Sherman, 1976). As measured by the added labeled BH_2 more than 80% of pterins were recovered from the tissues. Intraventricular injection of 300-ng quantities of GTP (containing 4×10^5 dpm of [U-14C]-GTP) led to the recovery of about 1.2 ng labeled BH_2. No label was detectable in any of the pterins from injected quantities of [8-14C]-GTP or [U-14C] deoxyguanosine triphosphate (dGTP). The identity of [14C]-BH_2 from the brain was also confirmed by mass fragmentography (Gál and Sherman, 1976). GTP appeared to serve as a better precursor than GDP for biopterin synthesis (Table 8). Dihydrobiopterin, isolated from the liver of rats and injected intraventricularly with labeled [U-

TABLE 8. Cerebral Synthesis
of [14C]-L-BH_1 from Various
[U-14C] Guanine Nucleotides *in Vivo*[a]

	Recovered as [14C]-BH_2	
Nucleotide[b,d]	Total (dpm)	Label (%)
GMP (2)	171	0.01
GDP (2)	764	0.19
GTP (6)	3156[c]	0.26
8-GTP (2)	0	0.00
dGTP (2)	0	0.00

[a] Nucleotides (0.54 μg or 1.2×10^6 dpm) were intraventricularly injected.
[b] Rats given GDP were killed in 90 min, all others 2 hr later.
[c] The specific activity of the recovered [14C]-BH_2 was calculated as 91% of the injected [U-14C]-GTP.
[d] Number of animals are in parentheses.

^{14}C]-GTP (1.2 $\times$ 10^6 dpm), contained no radioactivity. The absence of label was due to large hepatic pools and turnover rates of GTP and BH$_2$ (11.6 μg/ g) and to the slow rate of labeled GTP reaching the liver from the brain. However, intraperitoneally administered [U-^{14}C]-GTP (2.2 $\times$ 10^7 dpm) to 200-g rats resulted in the appearance of label in BH$_2$ from the liver. In 30 min the label of BH$_2$ corresponded to 0.025% of the [U-^{14}C]-GTP (unpublished observation).

The rate of synthesis of labeled BH$_2$ from [U-^{14}C]-GTP *in vivo* corresponded to a linear curve within 2 hr, thereafter the rate declined rapidly owing to the decrease of [^{14}C]-GTP pool (Figure 1). The rate of BH$_2$ synthesis was calculated to be 0.53 nmol/g wet brain per hr. This rate of synthesis was found not to be altered in the brains of animals kept on folate-deficient diet for 16 days. The rate of cerebral synthesis of BH$_2$ was consistent with its estimated turnover rate and pool size (Table 7).

These experiments *in vivo* also revealed the presence of two hitherto undetected metabolites of GTP in mammalian tissues, i.e., D-erythroneopterin (6 ng/g), isolated as neopterin, and 2-amino-6-(5'-triphosphoribosyl)-amino-5(or 6)-formamido-6-hydroxypyrimidine triphosphate (FPyd-P$_3$) (1–2 ng/g). Both compounds were verified by gas chromatography. They are isographic with the synthetic samples.

At this point a brief overview of the story of FPyd-P$_3$ would be in order. However, it will be recounted in Section 4.2.

A study of selective inhibition has proved to be a remarkably successful tool in studying the sequential nature of metabolic pathways. Of the potential inhibitors 2,4-diamino-6-hydroxypyrimidine (DAOPyr), when administered intraventricularly, caused about 83% inhibition in the conversion of intraventricularly injected [U-^{14}C]-GTP into [^{14}C]-BH$_2$ (Table 9) with a concomitant accumulation of cerebral FPyd-P$_3$ (Gál and Sherman, 1976). A diet of 1% DAOPyr fed to rats for 2 weeks produced only limited inhibition of cerebral BH$_2$ synthesis. Another inhibitor studied was dGTP. The effect of dGTP was as a result of its enzymatic conversion to dFPyd-P$_3$. The deoxy analog of FPyd-P$_3$ cannot undergo cyclization to dihydroneopterin triphosphate. Following intraventricular administration of the deoxy derivative, competitive inhibition of BH$_2$ synthesis occurred in rats. Intraventricularly injected [^{14}C]-dFPyd-P$_3$ had a half-life of about 14 min in the brain. Therefore, to achieve a concentration of its K_I (5 $\times$ 10^{-7} M) at 90 min, which was the time maximal synthesis of [^{14}C]-BH$_2$ from [U-^{14}C]-GTP took place, 70 μg of dFPyd-P$_3$ was intraventricularly injected in a solution containing labeled GTP (1 $\times$ 10^6 dpm). After 90 min there was 78% inhibition of BH$_2$ synthesis. Repeated doses of dFPyd-P$_3$ (70 μg) caused 99.5% inhibition of cerebral BH$_2$ synthesis at 180 min with a simultaneous tenfold increase in FPyd-P$_3$ (Sherman and Gál, 1979). Based upon these findings, there is scarcely any doubt that the synthesis of BH$_2$ from

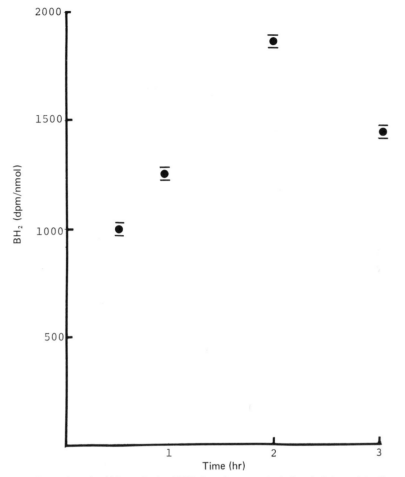

FIGURE 1. Rate of cerebral biosynthesis of BH$_2$ from intraventricularly administered [U-^{14}C]-GTP. Each point represents the mean ($\pm$ S.E.M.) for 4 animals.

GTP in mammalian tissues *in vivo* proceeds from GTP via FPyd-P$_3$ and NPTH$_2$-P$_3$ to BH$_2$ (Figure 2). Presence of sepiapterin was not observed. These enzyme-catalyzed steps were found to be irreversible. Starting from [U-^{14}C]-GTP, the specific radioactivities of FPyd-P$_3$, NPTH$_2$-P$_3$, and BH$_2$ revealed that the carbon skeleton of the purine base (except for C-8) and that of the ribose of GTP were carried through unchanged along the biosynthetic pathway to BH$_2$.

TABLE 9. Inhibition of Cerebral Synthesis of BH_2 *in Vivo*

Inhibitor[c]	Total (dpm)	Label (%)	dpm/nmol	Inhibition (%)
Control[a] (3)	3405	0.28	2481	0
dFPyd-P_3 (4)	75	0.008	335	86
2,4-Diamino-6-hydroxypyrimidine (2)	561	0.05	421	83
2,4-Diamino-6-hydroxypyrimidine[b](3)	1486	0.12	1666	33
2,4,6-Triaminopyrimidine (3)	1809	0.15	1887	24
8-Mercaptoguanosine (2)	3030	0.25	2273	8
6-Mercaptoguanosine (3)	1884	0.16	1413	43

[a] Injected intraventricularly with [U-^{14}C]-GTP (0.54 μg or 1.2 × 10^6 dpm). Inhibitors (300 μg) except dFPyd-P_3 (200 μg) were administered by the same route in the solution containing [U-^{14}C]-GTP.
[b] Inhibitor was given with the folate-deficient diet.
[c] Number of animals are in parentheses.

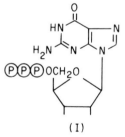
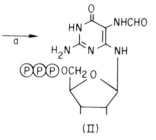

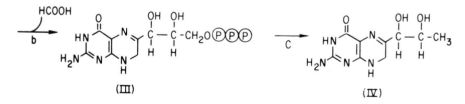

FIGURE 2. Simplified pathway of the metabolic conversion of GTP to 7,8-BH_2 in mammalian brain. (I) Guanosine triphosphate; (II) formamidopyrimidine ribotide (FPyd-P_3); (III) D-erythro-7,8-NPTH$_2$-P_3; (IV) 7,8-BH_2. Enzymes involved are: a—GTP cyclohydrolase A-I or A-II; b—D-erythro-7,8-dihydroneopterin triphosphate synthetase; c—isomerase and dephosphorylase.

The syntheses of BH_2 and, therefore, those of B and of BH_4 were regulated by the concentration of GTP (0.66 μmol/g wet brain) channeled into the synthesis of FPyd-P_3. The rate of this reaction was 0.5 $\pm$ 0.05 nmol/g per hr *in vivo* and is the rate limiting step of the biosynthetic pathway to BH_2. This reaction rate will also depend on competitive concentrations of adenine nucleotides and deoxyribonucleotides, and especially on the availability of dATP and dGTP to the cell (Gál and Sherman, 1977*b*). The conversion of FPyd-P_3 via $NPTH_2$-P_3 to BH_2 had an estimated rate of 1.17 $\pm$ 0.03 nmol/g per hr *in vivo*. The rate of conversion of the active form FPyd-P_3 to $NPTH_2$-P_3 will be greatly influenced by the degree of phosphorylation of this enzyme (D-erythro-q-BH_2-P_3 synthetase) (Gál and Sherman, 1978*a,b*) and by the presence of dGTP or dFPyd-P_3. The rate of conversion of intraventricularly injected [U-^{14}C]-D-erythro-7,8-dihydroneopterin triphosphate (7,8-$NPTH_2$-P_3) to [^{14}C]-BH_2 was calculated to be 1.4 nmol/g per hr. This fast rate of conversion explains the low cerebral pool concentration of $NPTH_2$-P_3 found *in vivo*. However, one should bear in mind that it is the quinonoid NPTH-P_3 which is the natural intermediate (Gál *et al.*, 1978*a*, 1979*a*) and not 7,8-$NPTH_2$-P_3, consequently this rate is an approximation.

The nature of the four enzymes involved in the synthesis of BH_2 from GTP, GTP-cyclohydrolase A-I and A-II, D-erythrodihydroneopterin synthetase and L-erythrodihydrobiopterin synthetase, will be dealt with under the metabolic aspects of BH_2 synthesis *in vitro*. These enzymes from mammalian tissues, though they catalyze some of the reactions observed with the microbial enzymes, are divergent in many of their physicochemical and molecular parameters.

4.2. Biosynthesis of Pterins *in Vitro*

As experiments *in vivo* are important in their ultimate relevance, the complexity of simultaneous and multiple reactions preclude understanding of an individual reaction in a chain of biological events. The biochemical mosaic of cell life is best comprehended through the synthesis of the results of studies *in vitro* which unfold the molecular kinetic and quantal nature of reactions and the relationships among them. An amalgam of these results with those observations *in vivo* will thus lead to a balanced view of natural phenomena.

As already mentioned in Section 4.1, crude homogenates of Syrian golden hamster organs revealed synthesis of biopterin *in vitro* (Eto *et al.*, 1976) when [U-^{14}C]-D-$NPTH_2$-P_3 was used as precursor. Homogenates of brain, kidney, lung, and liver of hamsters synthesized 0.14–0.54 nmol/mg protein of biopterin using dialyzed extracts of these organs. In these experiments the extracts of kidney were the most active while in the earlier experiments when organ extracts were incubated with GTP the liver preparations yielded the highest equivalents of "*Crithidia*-active" substances (Fukushima *et al.*, 1975*a*). This activity of the organ extracts was markedly stimulated by the addition of a mixture of pyridine nucleotides (NADPH$_2$ and NADP). These data also confirmed those obtained from experiments *in vivo* and confirmed that the alkyl side chain of L-erythrodihydrobiopterin in fact derived from the original alkyl side chain of D-erythro-NPTH$_2$-P$_3$. The lack of conversion of nonphosphorylated dihydroneopterin to biopterin implied that phosphates required in the primary step of conversion to BH$_2$ and the involvement of nonspecific phosphatases might be discounted. Of particular interest was the dependence of this reaction on pyridine nucleotides with an enzyme from hamster kidneys (Eto *et al.*, 1976) and with a soluble rat brain fraction (Lee *et al.*, 1979). This dependence was not observed with 96% pure (by terminal amino acid analysis) enzyme preparations from rat and guinea pig brain and livers (Gál *et al.*, 1978*a*), nor was the presence of sepiapterin ever detected in any of our experiments *in vivo* or *in vitro*. However, the Ultrogel AcA-34 enzyme from golden hamster kidneys and the rat brain fraction (Lee *et al.*, 1979) were crude preparations. Thus the participation of pyridine nucleotides in the conversion of NPTH$_2$-P$_3$ to BH$_2$ was not proven unequivocally (Eto *et al.*, 1976). The hypothetical scheme offered by these authors for the enzymatic synthesis of biopterin from GTP consequently remains tenuous.

Unquestionably the synthesis of BH$_2$ from GTP now represents a well-documented biochemical event in the mammalian tissue. Contrary to a recent statement (Lee *et al.*, 1979), incubation of postmitochondrial fractions of cerebral tissue from several species with GTP resulted in the synthesis of BH$_2$ *in vitro;* it was markedly elevated in pig and ox brain (Gál *et al.*, 1978*a*). This synthetic capacity displayed marked regional variation (Table 10). Subcellular fractionation of tissues solubilized the synthetic enzymes of the GTP to BH$_2$ pathway with only 10–15% remaining in the crude mitochondrial pellet. The presence of these enzymes was also demonstrated in the synaptosomes (Gál and Sherman, 1976). The method of preparation of the synaptosomes had decided bearing on their synthetic activity (Gál *et al.*, 1978*b*). The sucrose gradient, in contrast to the Ficoll gradient, yielded synaptosomes highly contaminated by mitochondria of pericaryal origin which synthesized 12 pmol/mg per hr BH$_2$. The synaptosomes isolated by Ficoll density gradient revealed very low synthesis of BH$_2$ (0.8 pmol/mg per hr). This significant drop in synthetic activity was not owing to synaptosomal disintegration since the synaptosomes prepared by the Ficoll method showed an active uptake of [^{14}C]biopterin with respect to time. This and the retention of endogenous BH$_2$ were indications of the functional integrity of the Ficoll preparations.

Perhaps in no other organ are the cell types as functionally differentiated as are the glia and neurons in the brain. It appeared plausible, therefore, that cerebral synthesis of BH$_2$ might have localized in one or both of these cell

TABLE 10.   Regional Biosynthetic
Capacity in Rat Brain[a]

Area[b]	BH$_2$ (dpm/g per hr)
Cerebellum	12,110 ± 2440
Pons	5,760 ± 1480
Colliculi	1,550 ± 525
Thalamus	952 ± 76
Globus pallidus	851 ± 266
Hypothalamus	483 ± 33
Neocortex	194 ± 21

[a] Values are mean ± S.D. from 3 rats.
[b] Areas incubated with 110,000 dpm (49 ng) [^{14}C]-GTP for 1 hr in supernatant obtained after homogenization of the area in 2 volumes of 0.05 M Tris-Ac, pH 8.0, and centrifugation at 16,000 g.

types. Both glial and neuronal fractions from neocortices of 8-month-old rabbits were capable of BH$_2$ synthesis from GTP (Gál *et al.*, 1978*b*) although the glia seemed to be about four times as active as the neurons. Incidentally, the cortical and medullary layers of adrenals were also capable of BH$_2$ synthesis (unpublished observations).

5.   ENZYMOLOGY OF BIOPTERIN BIOSYNTHESIS

In the above sections evidence was brought forth which supported the biosynthesis of BH$_2$ from GTP *in vivo* and *in vitro* in mammalian tissues. Reference was made to an enzyme from kidneys of Syrian golden hamsters which converted D-erythrodihydroneopterin triphosphate to L-erythrodihydrobiopterin as identified by *Crithidia* test and thin layer chromatography.

Until the present little was known about the number and the nature of the enzymes which participate in the reactions subsequent to the ring opening of GTP, and the enzymes which lead to ring closure of a pyrimidine to a pterine and formic acid. Recently these enzymes have been purified from mammalian tissues and some of their properties have been investigated (Gál *et al.*, 1978*a*; Gál and Sherman, 1978*a,b*). In this section, a somewhat detailed presentation will be attempted of the synthesis of each intermediate as well as the nature and properties, as presently known, of each participating enzyme.

5.1. Reaction of GTP to FPyd-P$_3$

It is apparent that enzymatic cleavage of the imidazole carbon (C-8) of GTP was needed to produce a formamidated pyrimidine which ultimately hydrolyzed to HCOOH and Pyd-P$_3$. The same reaction occurred with dGTP as substrate. This reaction is catalyzed in the mammalian tissue by GTP-cyclohydrolase (A-I and A-II). In many respects these enzymes are not similar to the GTP-cyclohydrolases isolated from *E. coli* and *Lactobacillus plantarum* (Burg and Brown, 1968; Yim and Brown, 1976;Jackson and Shiota, 1971) and to the Mg^{2+}-dependent enzyme (Brown *et al.,* 1975, Cone and Guroff, 1971). There appears to be little doubt as to the mechanism of the first reaction. However, the mammalian GTP-cyclohydrolases, A-I and A-II, unlike the enzymes from microbial or plant origin, selectively catalyze the first reaction only and are unable to convert FPyd-P$_3$ to NPTH$_2$-P$_3$. This step of ring closure is catalyzed by another enzyme in the mammalian tissues.

Stoichiometric cleavage of GTP to 2,5-diamino-6-(5-triphosphoriboryl)amino-4-hydroxypyrimidine and formic acid by microbial enzymes has been described. This pyrimidine was identified by its condensation with glyoxal to pteridine (Shiota *et al.,* 1969). It was observed by Shiota *et al.* (1967) that when GTP was incubated for 1 hr at 37°C, in presence of 0.7 *M* mercaptoethanol and 0.01 *M* FeSO$_4$ in 0.3 *M* Tris buffer at pH 8.0, a nonenzymatic cleavage of GTP at C-8 took place. The yield of the chemically prepared FPyd-P$_3$ and FPyd was about 15%. FPyd-P$_3$ was purified from a dark purple brown mixture by DuPont 841 HPLC first on a SAX (anion-exchange column) and second, for further separation from FPyd, on a silica column (Gál *et al.,* 1978*a*). Separation of dFPyd-P$_3$ from dGTP was effected by the same process. There is little doubt to the identity of FPyd-P$_3$ obtained either by mammalian GTP-cyclohydrolases or by chemical hydrolysis. The chemically or enzymatically prepared FPyd-P$_3$ displayed isochromatography of their heptafluorobutyryl derivatives by TLC or gas chromatography (Gál *et al.,* 1978*a*). Above all, the imidazole cleavage of [U-^{14}C]-GTP resulted in the transfer of all labeled carbon into FPyd-P$_3$. Significantly, [U-^{14}C]-FPyd-P$_3$ did not undergo ring closure in various buffers at pH 7.6–8.0 or in presence of GTP-cyclohydrolases A-I or A-II from mammalian brain or liver (Gál *et al.,* 1978*a*; Gál and Sherman, 1978*b*). Phosphate (α, β, or γ) reappeared in FPyd-P$_3$ when it was prepared from ^{32}P-(α, β, or γ)-GTP.

Direct evidence of the expulsion of C-8 from [8-^{14}C]-GTP by mammalian tissue was also obtained from experiments *in vivo* (Gál and Sherman, 1976) and *in vitro* (Fukushima *et al.,* 1975*a,b*; Gál and Sherman, 1976 Gál *et al.,* 1978*a*). The formyl group did not cleave off FPyd-P$_3$ or FPyd during the enzymatic attack on GTP by GTP-cyclohydrolase (mammalian sources). Controlled degradation procedure permitted the assignment of the formyl substituent of the scissioned GTP to position N-5 thus yielding a structure of 2-amino-5-formamido-6(5'-triphosphoribosyl)-amino-4-hydroxypyrimidine (FPyd-P_3) or the (5-triphosphodeoxyribosyl) analog from dGTP as dFPyd-P_3. The ultraviolet spectra of the samples of FPyd obtained by chemical and enzymatic synthesis were identical with the absorption spectra reported by others (Shiota *et al.*, 1967; Shiota *et al.*, 1969). Absorption maxima are at 272 nm in 0.1 *M* phosphate buffer (pH 7.0) and at 265 nm in 0.1 *N* HCl. The ultraviolet spectra of the chemically prepared formamidopyrimidine from GTP agreed well with the spectra of a fission product of guanilic acid obtained after exposure to high-energy electrons (4×10^6 *r*) and purified by paper chromatography (Hems, 1958).

It is almost certain that both enzymatic and chemical breakdown of GTP to the formamidopyrimidine required the presence of phosphate groups. The appearance of FPyd could have been due to partial hydrolysis by phosphatase impurities in the GTP-cyclohydrolase preparations from mammalian tissues, since this enzyme, unlike the GTP-cyclohydrolase from *E. coli* (Brown *et al.*, 1975), never gave a single homogeneous electrophoretic band. Shiota (1971) considered direct detection of these formamidopyrimidines "to be difficult since these intermediates may be enzyme bound or are extremely unstable."

Yet FPyd-P_3 and dFPyd-P_3 were easily isolated and remained stable at low-temperature storage for over a long period (Gál *et al.*, 1978a). The presence of FPyd-P_3 or rather FPyd, as mentioned earlier, could also be detected from samples of brain tissue. Its concentration increased *in vivo* in presence of inhibitors which prevented its enzymatic cyclization to D-erythrodihydroneopterin triphosphate.

GTP-cyclohydrolase (A-I) from mammalian tissues was purified 2000-fold. This enzyme, unlike GTP-cyclohydrolases reported by others (Brown *et al.*, 1975), was inhibited by its substrate at a concentration of about 5×10^{-6} *M* and was also competitively inhibited by dGTP, ATP, and dATP. It is heat stable with a $T_{1/2}$ of 11 min inactivation rate at 80°C. This enzyme was not activated by Mg^{2+}. GTP-cyclohydrolase A-I has an estimated molecular weight of 135,000 daltons by Sephadex-G-200 gel filtration. Its electrophoretic pattern on polyacrylamide gel displayed a strong (R_m 0.7) and a weak band. Only the major band possessed enzyme activity. The enzyme protein has a p*I* of 4.95. Kinetic studies revealed a V_{max} of 7.1 nmol/mg per hr and a K_m of 1.2 $\times 10^{-6}$ M for GTP. The cyclohydrolysis of GTP to FPyd-P_3 was linear to 90 min, showing a stoichiometric ratio of 1.0, i.e., the hydrolysis of 1 mol of GTP to 1 mol of FPyd-P_3. GTP-cyclohydrolase (A-I), like the enzyme from *E. coli* (Brown *et al.*, 1975), disaggregated into four subunits on a Sephadex column prepared with 0.3 *M* KCl as developing buffer. The four subunits of the enzyme lost their thermostability but hydrolyzed 10^{-6}–10^{-7} *M* solution of GTP prior to heat treatment. The subunits, which are thermolabile, did not require Mg^{2+} for the cyclohydrolysis. GTP-cyclohydrolase (A-I) did not catalyze the reversible reaction of FPyd-P$_3$ to GTP. As mentioned earlier, the transfer of labeled carbons and phosphates of GTP remained unbroken in FPyd-P$_3$. The large-scale preparation of FPyd-P$_3$ is best achieved with pure GTP-cyclohydrolase of *E. coli* (700 units/mg) (Brown *et al.,* 1975) and purified by the recommended HPLC procedure (Gál *et al.,* 1978*a*).

The Mg^{2+}-dependent GTP-cyclohydrolase (A-II) resembles the Mg^{2+}-dependent enzyme isolated from *E. coli* (Brown *et al.,* 1975). The mammalian GTP-cyclohydrolase (A-II) is thermolabile, has a molecular weight of 34,000 daltons, and has a pI of 6.65. On polyacrylamide gels the purified enzyme showed two bands of R_m 0.15 and R_m 0.18, both enzymatically active, and one weak inactive band of impurity at R_m 0.27. The K_m of GTP-cyclohydrolase (A-II) was 5.8×10^{-5} M and the V_{max} 12.2 nmol/mg per hr in the presence of 6.7×10^{-4} atom-equivalent of Mg^{2+}. GTP-cyclohydrolase (A-II), like (A-I), catalyzed in linear fashion the synthesis of FPyd-P$_3$; however, its stoichiometric ratio was 1 mol GTP to 0.0035 mol of product, apparently owing to the release of magnesium pyrophosphate, an inhibitor of (A-II). The optimal function of this enzyme was around pH 7.4.

If one lists the effectiveness of these enzymes according to their stoichiometric parameters consistent with the pool sizes of the reactants, GTP-cyclohydrolase (A-I) appears as the preferred catalyst of mammalian tissue in the synthesis of FPyd-P$_3$. This would indicate that for instance 6.6×10^{-6} M GTP of its 6.6×10^{-4} M cerebral pool concentration would be required for a 0.53 nmol/g per hr cerebral BH$_2$ synthesis. In contrast, GTP-cyclohydrolase (A-II) would necessitate the conversion of 1.3×10^{-3} M GTP to satisfy the same rate of BH$_2$ synthesis. The overall stoichiometry revealed by experimental data *in vivo* and *in vitro* were mutually supportive (Gál and Sherman, 1977*b*).

5.2. D-Erythro-q-Dihydroneopterin Triphosphate Synthetase*

It was suggested that the ring closure from FPyd-P$_3$ may be nonenzymatic (Shiota, 1971). Possibly a very slow nonenzymatic Amadori rearrangement could occur, although we have never observed it in the absence of the enzyme, D-erythro-q-dihydroneopterin triphosphate synthetase.

The first experimental proof for synthesis of neopterin from GTP by an extract of *Pseudomonas* was reported in 1966 (Guroff and Strenkoski, 1966) and with an extract of *E. coli* (Jones and Brown, 1967). These authors obtained formate and neopterin from [U-^{14}C]-GTP with GTP-cyclohydrolase. Purified extracts from *Lactobacillus plantarum* also converted [U-^{14}C]-GTP stoichiometrically to H^{14}COOH and labeled dihydroneopterin triphosphate. It was

---

*Where q is the abbreviated form of quinonoid.

recommended that this enzyme complex transforming GTP to dihydroneopterin-P_3 should be designated as dihydroneopterin triphosphate synthetase (Shiota *et al.*, 1970). It was recently reported (Gál and Sherman, 1977*b*; Gál *et al.*, 1978*a*; Gál and Sherman, 1978*b*) that there is a well-defined basic protein of small molecular weight in the mammalian tissue. This protein, D-erythro-q-dihydroneopterin triphosphate synthetase, performs the sole and crucial function of converting FPyd-P_3 into D-q-NPTH$_2$-P_3 and could not utilize GTP as substrate for the synthesis of dihydroneopterin-P_3. The isolation of this hitherto undescribed enzyme was successfully achieved from all mammalian tissues so far examined. This enzyme thus became an unquestionable link in the pathway of GTP to BH$_2$. The configuration of the product was confirmed as D-erythroneopterin since the following hydrolytic removal of phosphate labeled neopterin was isochromatographic with an authentic sample of D-erythroneopterin.

Preparations of D-erythrodihydroneopterin triphosphate from GTP or from FPyd-P_3 in reasonable yields were achieved with enzymes from mammalian tissues (Gál *et al.*, 1978*a*) or with partially purified preparation of *Lactobacillus plantarum* (Eto *et al.*, 1976). (It is to be stated that all procedures were performed in dimmed light to minimize photoinstability of the product.) The size of the enzyme catalyzing this reaction is 9177 daltons. This molecular weight makes D-erythro-q-dihydroneopterin triphosphate synthetase the smallest enzyme protein molecule known to date. The enzyme is a single filament and consists of 68 amino acid residues. An exception is the enzyme isolated from rat brain which has an extra aspartic acid (residue 7), which appears to impart additional catalytic properties (see Section 5). The enzyme possesses three active SH-groups at residues 19, 40, and 52. The enzyme in its most active form is phosphorylated at serine 66 or serine 67 in the rat brain enzyme. Phosphorylated and dephosphorylated forms of the enzyme from rat brain had the same R_m (0.47) by polyacrylamide gel electrophoresis. The dephosphorylation was particularly rapid in brain homogenates. The catalytic rate of the phosphorylated enzyme is close to the 0.1 μmol/mg per hr (*in vivo* rate) and appropriately fits the biological conditions in which the enzyme has to operate *in vivo* (Gál and Sherman, 1977*b*).

The phosphorylated enzyme has a V_{max} of 94 nmol/mg per hr and a K_m of 8.9×10^{-6} *M* for FPyd-P_3 (Gál and Sherman, 1978*b*). The enzyme from tissues other than rat brain showed an electrophoretic mobility of R_m 0.58 at pH 4.5. FPyd-P_3 is the specific substrate of this enzyme, not FPyd. The enzyme was inhibited by GTP or dGTP, or most effectively by dFPyd-P_3 (K_I 4.7×10^{-7} *M*) and 2,4-diamino-6-hydroxypyrimidine (K_I 1.1×10^{-5} *M*). The enzyme is heat labile and in the presence of 10^{-5} *M* DDT its $T_{1/2}$ of inactivation was 8 days at $-80°$C.

The structure of this enzyme was determined by sequencing the peptides isolated from mild acid, trypsin, and chymotrypsin digests by two dimensional TLC (Gál *et al.,* 1979*b*). Manual Edman degradation analysis has yielded the exact overlap of the peptides of known sequence into the complete sequence of D-erythro-q-dihydroneopterin triphosphate synthetase. Its structure (Gál *et al.,* 1979*b*) is as follows:

```
                   5                    10                   15
Ile-Ser-His-Gly-Phe-Arg-Tyr-Asp-Ala-Ile-Ala-Lys-Leu-Phe-Arg-
                  20                    25                   30
Pro-Phe-Phe-Cys-Gly-Asp-Gly-Tyr-Gly-His-Arg-Ile-Gly-Glu-Thr-
                  35                    40                   45
Val-Tyr-Tyr-Ala-Gly-Ser-Leu-Lys-Tyr-Cys-Ala-Arg-Ser-Phe-Asp-
                  50                    55                   60
Val-Gly-Ala-Glu-Ile-Ile-Cys-Lys-Gly-Phe-Tyr-Tyr-Phe-Gly-Ile-
                  65
Tyr-Lys-Arg-Arg-Val-Ser-Glu-Val
```

In immunological tests, this enzyme (antigen) revealed no precipitin lines against rabbit preimmunization serum, but a strong single band against the immune sera, and a single arc by immunoelectrophoresis. The antiserum against the enzyme from beef brain crossreacted with the enzyme samples prepared from brain and livers of other species.

Mammalian D-erythro-q-dihydroneopterin triphosphate synthetase is quite different, in all respects, from the enzyme recently isolated from avian liver (Fukushima *et al.,* 1977) which utilizes GTP as substrate. Traces of the FPyd-P_3-specific enzyme in chicken liver were found, but significant amounts of it only occur in the mammalian tissues. This could be an interesting philogenetic development of the FPyd-P_3-specific enzyme. An important characteristic of the mammalian D-erythro-q-dihydroneopterin triphosphate synthetase appeared to be the release of its product as the quinonoid tautomer of dihydroneopterin-P_3 which is ultimately converted into the quinonoid L-erythrodihydrobiopterin by the L-erythrodihydrobiopterin synthetase. The quinonoid dihydroneopterin and quinonoid BH_2 were identified and quantified by their ultraviolet spectra and fluorescence emission spectra through their time- and pH-dependent rearrangement to their 7,8-dihydro tautomers, also by gas chromatography of their rapidly synthesized trimethylsilyl derivatives (Gál *et al.,* 1979*a*). Direct proof for their enzymatic synthesis from FPyd-P_3 was obtained by isolation of the compound which was identical in all respects to q-BH_2 obtained by mild oxidation of BH_4 (Kaufman, 1961). Experiments *in vivo* also established that dihydrofolate reductase (DHFR) did not participate in the reduction of q-BH_2 to BH_4 when the former was synthesized *de novo* from [U-^{14}C]-GTP (Gál and Sherman, 1978*a*, 1979*a*). Incubation of [^{14}C]-FPyd-P_3 with the D-erythrodihydroneopterin triphosphate and L-erythrodihydrobiop-

TABLE 11. *De Novo* Synthesis of [^{14}C]-BH$_4$ from [^{14}C]-FPyd-P$_3$ in Presence of DHPR or DHFR[a]

	[^{14}C]-BH$_4$ (nmol) formed in incubation time		Calculated amount of q-BH$_2$[b] (nmol/hr)
	3 min	15 min	
Complete system + DHPR	0.026	0.13	0.52
Complete system + DHPR + MTX	0.025	0.12	
Complete system + DHFR	0	0.073	0.29[c]
Complete system + DHFR + MTX	0	0	

[a] The complete system contained in 0.6 ml of 0.05 M Tris-acetate buffer pH 7.6, are excess of 10 nmol FPyd-P$_3$ with 2×10^6 dpm of [^{14}C]-FPyd-P$_3$, 1.05 units (11.5 μg) of phosphorylated enzyme B, 1.21 units (80 μg) enzyme C, and NADH$_2$ 10^{-5} M. Additions: 15 μg DHPR or 15 μg DHFR; the methotrexate (MTX) concentration was 5×10^{-6} M. Incubation at 38°C in the dark. The reaction FPyd-P$_3$ to BH$_2$ is linear to 90 min (Gál *et al.*, 1978).
[b] One unit of enzyme B and C will synthesize 1 nmol of BH$_2$/hr.
[c] At this rate the total was 0.81 nmol including 0.29 nmol originally in the form of q-BH$_2$ tautomerized to 7,8-BH$_2$ during 15 min.

terin synthetases (Table 11) led to a product, q-BH$_2$, which was reducible to BH$_4$ by dihydropteridine reductase (DHPR) but not by DHFR. The reduction was not inhibited by addition of methotrexate, a powerful inhibitor of DHFR. The data confirmed that q-BH$_2$ is the product synthesized from GTP and regained as q-BH$_2$ after oxidation of BH$_4$ during cofactorial participation of BH$_4$ in the synthesis of, e.g., tyrosine, L-3,4-dihydroxyphenylalanine, or L-5-hydroxytryptophan.

q-BH$_2$ was converted readily to 7,8-BH$_2$ particularly in presence of phosphate ions (Kaufman, 1961; Archer *et al.*, 1972). Experimental evidence ruled out the 5,8- and the 5,6-dihydro structures (Kaufman, 1964). The structure of the paraquinonoid tautomer depicted earlier is now accepted as proposed by others (Kaufman, 1961; Viscontini and Bobst, 1965).

5.3. L-Erythrodihydrobiopterin Synthetase

During the studies of the biosynthetic pathway of q-BH$_2$ from GTP in the mammalian cell, the existence of an enzyme was noted which catalyzed the conversion of D-erythro-q-dihydroneopterin triphosphate to L-erythro-q-dihydrobiopterin. This enzyme was isolated from brain and liver of various species and purified to electrophoretic homogeneity (Gál *et al.*, 1978a). The enzyme is an acidic heat-labile protein of about 124,000 daltons with a pI of 4.9. It catalyzes the irreversible conversion of its specific substrates q-NPTH$_2$-P$_3$ or

7,8-NPTH$_2$-P$_3$ to q-BH$_2$ or 7,8-BH$_2$. It has an apparent K_m of 1.7×10^{-7} M and a V_{max} of 20 nmol/mg per hr. The stoichiometric ratio of BH$_2$ to NPTH$_2$-P$_3$ was 0.98. The nonphosphorylated dihydroneopterin was not converted to BH$_2$ but into a compound unisographic with BH$_2$ by GC, thus confirming similar findings (Eto et $al.$, 1976). The enzyme remained stable at $-80°$C for over two weeks in 10^{-3} M DTT. Essentially this enzyme catalyzes a fairly complicated mechanism of epimerization and dephosphorylation by an apparent hydrolytic reaction.

As mentioned earlier, three hypotheses were offered for the origin of the dihydroxypropyl side chain of biopterin from neopterin. One suggestion proposed that the side chain of dihydroneopterin was retained and merely underwent steric changes; our data with uniformly labeled NPTH$_2$-P$_3$ would support this suggestion. Other ideas postulated the removal of carbon atoms C-2′ and C-3′, followed by replacement by another two-carbon unit, or removal of the entire alkyl chain and its replacement by a new carbon chain.

Some reports cited previously support the contention for the transfer of intact ^{14}C-labeled alkyl side chain. These reports were based on experiments with nonmammalian systems.

To explain the change of the alkyl side chain of 6-substituted pterin, hitherto all the schemes proposed involved the participation of sepiapterin (or 6-lactyl-7,8-dihydropterin) as an intermediate to L-erythrodihydrobiopterin (Eto et $al.$, 1976). It was noted (Taira, 1961) that sepiapterin from $Drosophila$ was reduced to BH$_2$ by NADPH-dependent DHFR from chicken liver. It was ultimately observed (Matsubara and Akino, 1964; Matsubara et $al.$, 1966) that there were two distinct steps from sepiapterin to BH$_2$. One step involved the reduction of sepiapterin by DHFR to tetrahydrosepiapterin at pH 4.3 (Katoh et $al.$, 1970), the other in the reduction of sepiapterin to BH$_2$ by sepiapterin reductase and NADPH, measured by the concomitant decrease of the optical density at 420 nm, and by the isolation of 7,8-BH$_2$ (Nagai, 1968).

Sepiapterin, a structural isomer of biopterin, also possesses L-configuration (Iwanami and Akino, 1975). Sepiapterin reductase catalyzes the oxidation of BH$_2$ to sepiapterin, in presence of NADPH, but not that of D-erythrodihydroneopterin (Katoh et $al.$, 1970). Apart from sepiapterin, only isosepiapterin (6-propionyl pterin) was reduced by this enzyme at an appreciable rate. Sepiapterin reductase was purified from rat liver (Matsubara et $al.$, 1966; Nagai, 1968) and about 5000-fold from horse liver (Katoh, 1971). Its molecular weight is about 47,000 daltons. The enzyme was detectable in most tissues except the stomach, small intestine, and muscles. Several of the pterins inhibited it (Katoh, 1971). The equilibrium constant of the reversible reaction and the standard free-energy change were about 1×10^9 and -12 kcal/mol at $28°$C respectively. The equilibrium thus lies in favor of BH$_2$ synthesis. The significance of the role of sepiapterin reductase in brain awaits further examination since the presence of sepiapterin in the brain either *in vivo* or *in vitro* was not demonstrable. Most importantly, highly purified enzyme L-erythro-dihydrobiopterin synthetase did not require the addition of pyridine nucleotides during the synthesis of L-erythro-q-BH_2 or 7,8-BH_2 from q-$NPTH_2$-P_3 or 7,8-$NPTH_2$-P_3 (Gál *et al.*, 1978*a*).

Fifteen years ago the presence of 7,8-BH_2, a naturally occurring cofactor of phenylalanine hydroxylation in the rat liver, was demonstrated (Kaufman, 1963). Later the mechanism of conversion of 7,8-BH_2 to 5,6,7,8-BH_4, the ultimate cofactor of most hydroxylases, was revealed (Kaufman, 1964). In a coupled oxidative reaction BH_4 was oxidized to q-BH_2. The enzyme, quinonoid dihydropterin reductase (DHPR) (EC 1.6.99.7), which was first isolated from sheep liver (Kaufman, 1956; Craine *et al.*, 1972), catalyzes the reduction of q-BH_2 back to BH_4 in presence of $NADH_2$ or $NADPH_2$, thus enabling a continuous shuttle of a pair of hydrogens to the enzymic sites where the products are formed. DHPR is widely distributed in mammalian organs including the brain (Craine *et al.*, 1972; Musacchio *et al.*, 1972; Cheema *et al.*, 1973; Turner *et al.*, 1974; Snady and Musacchio, 1978*b*). The molecular weight of bovine cerebral DHPR was found to be 47,000 and 22,400 daltons respectively which implies that native DHPR is a dimer of two monomers of 22,400 daltons each (Cheema *et al.*, 1973; Snady and Musacchio, 1978*a*). The K_m for DHPR with $NADH_2$ was 5.5×10^{-5} M, and 4×10^{-4} M with $NADPH_2$ (Scrimgeour and Cheema, 1971). Rat and human liver DHPR with BH_4 had an apparent K_m 1.1×10^{-6} M and a V_{max} of 2.0–1.8 μmol/mg of enzyme per min respectively (Craine *et al.*, 1972). In all instances 2,4-diamino pteridines inhibited DHPR (Lind, 1972). Amethopterin (4-amino-10-methyl-4-deoxyfolic acid, methotrexate) a powerful noncompetitive inhibitor of dihydrofolate reductase, competitively inhibited DHPR with a K_I of 4×10^{-5} M (Craine *et al.*, 1972). Similarly aminopterin (4-amino-4-deoxyfolic acid) had a K_I of 2.4×10^{-4} M (Scrimgeour and Cheema, 1971). The regional and subcellular distribution of DHPR was also measured in the rat brain along with its subcellular distribution in the liver (Snady and Musacchio, 1978*a,b*). The activity of cerebral DHPR was lowest in the cerebral cortex and highest in the posterior colliculi. The enzyme displayed the greatest specific activity in the soluble fraction of the tissues. Regrettably, the reported data (Table 12) for DHPR activity (Turner *et al.*, 1974; Snady and Musacchio, 1978*b*; Bullard *et al.*, 1978) were obtained with 6,7-dimethyl-5,6,7,8-tetrahydropterin ($DMPH_4$) or 6-methyl-5,6,7,8-tetrahydropterin (6-MPH_4) instead of BH_4 and, therefore, they may not necessarily reflect the true biological values. Furthermore, the values representing regional DHPR activity in rat brain were significantly higher in one of the studies (Snady and Musacchio, 1978*b*).

Results of subcellular distribution of DHPR in rat brain indicated that its cellular profile was very similar to that of lactic dehydrogenase. Ranked in

TABLE 12. q-Dihydropterin Reductase Activity in Various Regions of Adult Rat Brain[a]

Region	Number of samples	Enzyme activity (μmol NADH oxidized/mg wet weight per min) ($\pm$ S.E.)
Cerebral cortex	8	0.14 $\pm$ 0.01
Hippocampus	7	0.33 $\pm$ 0.06
Caudate nucleus	8	0.62 $\pm$ 0.11
Thalamus	7	0.93 $\pm$ 0.07
Cerebellum	7	1.04 $\pm$ 0.12
Substantia nigra	6	1.16 $\pm$ 0.06
Hypothalamus	9	1.25 $\pm$ 0.12
Olfactory bulb	5	1.30 $\pm$ 0.46
Anterior colliculus	8	1.34 $\pm$ 0.12
Raphe nuclei	7	1.73 $\pm$ 0.22
Spinal cord	5	1.78 $\pm$ 0.29
Medulla–midbrain[a]	7	2.05 $\pm$ 0.21
Locus coeruleus	8	2.21 $\pm$ 0.42
Posterior colliculus	8	2.35 $\pm$ 0.37

[a] Reproduced with permission from Musacchio et al. (1972).
[b] This area is composed of all parts of the brain (excluding the locus coeruleus, substantia nigra, colliculi, and raphe nuclei) that come from a block of tissue between (1) the coronal plane, which cuts through the caudal edge of the mammilary bodies and the rostral edge of the anterior colliculus, and (2) the coronal plane, which cuts through the rostral edge of the spinal cord.

order of activities (μmol/mg protein per min) or in relative specific activities (RSA, defined as the ratio of the percentage of DHPR of the fraction, to the percentage of recovered protein in that fraction), DHPR was diluted in all fractions relative to the homogenate (0.13 SA and 1.00 RSA) except in the synaptosomes (0.38 SA and 3.04 RSA) and in the soluble fraction (0.29 SA and 2.31 RSA) (Snady and Musacchio, 1978b). Even the membrane synaptic vesicles had DHPR of 0.06 SA and 0.57 RSA. These data and others (Bullard et al., 1978) are not supportive of the assumption that the majority of DHPR activity is "extraneuronal and may serve in, as yet, unidentified hydroxylation reactions" (Turner, 1977). This was suggested to explain the lack of effect of 6-hydroxydopamine on rat cerebral DHPR (Turner et al., 1974).

In terms of the pool sizes of reduced biopterins of the various tissues, the estimated activities of DHPR are far in excess of the need to maintain a steady reduction of q-BH_2 to BH_4. Theoretically, the reduction of 10 nmol of BH_2 would take about 250 μs in the brain. This raises the question as to the nature of the biochemical factors that regulate the rate of reduction of q-BH_2 to BH_4 in vivo.

In discussing the various reductases one certainly should not gloss over DHFR. The scope of this review obviously precludes a detailed presentation of the nature and role of DHFR (EC 1.6.1.3) in the mammalian tissues. Nevertheless, it will be discussed briefly as this enzyme was surmised to participate in the reduction of 7,8-BH$_2$ *in vivo* (Stone, 1976; Spector *et al.*, 1977; Lynn *et al.*, 1977; Abelson *et al.*, 1978). This was a logical assumption which was reinforced first by the demonstration that DHFR specifically reduced 7,8-BH$_2$ to BH$_4$ *in vitro* (Kaufman, 1967a) and second by the isolation and identification of DHFR from brain (Spector *et al.*, 1977). It was suggested that the spontaneous rearrangement of q-BH$_2$ may occur *in vivo* leading to a "sink" for BH$_4$ and thus becoming an important step in the *de novo* synthesis of BH$_4$ enabling it to recycle to q-BH$_2$ (Stone, 1976). Recently it was demonstrated that DHFR did not participate in the reduction of BH$_2$ to BH$_4$ when the former was synthesized from GTP *de novo* (Gál *et al.*, 1979a).

Intraventricularly injected FPyd-P$_3$ was enzymatically converted to the quinonoid-D-erythro-dihydroneopterin triphosphate whence q-BH$_2$ was formed. Also, intraventricularly injected methotrexate at 5×10^{-6} *M* exerted no inhibition on the reduction of the biosynthetic q-BH$_2$ to BH$_4$ *in vivo*, yet completely inhibited the reduction of intraventricularly injected tritiated dihydrofolate to tetrahydrofolate (Table 13).

TABLE 13. Effect of Methotrexate on Cerebral Synthesis of Reduced Biopterins from [U-^{14}C]-GTP and Inhibition of Cerebral Dihydrofolate Reductase *in vivo*

A[a]	Total recovered (dpm ± S.D.)	
	[^{14}C]-BH$_2$	[^{14}C]-BH$_4$
Control (4)	1615 ± 71	456 ± 42
Methotrexate (4)	1570 ± 69	464 ± 58

B[b]	Recovered [^{3}H]-FH$_4$ (dpm ± S.D.)	Inhibition (%)
Control (4)	3,177,000 ± 193,000	—
Methotrexate (4)	37,000 ± 16,000	98.8

[a] Animals received 0.54μg (1.2 × 10^6 dpm) of [^{14}C]-GTP intraventricularly 1½ hr before sacrifice. Methotrexate (67 μg) was given simultaneously to the experimental group. Number of animals in brackets.

[b] Eight rats were injected with 10 μCi of [^{3}H]-dihydrofolic acid in 20 μl H$_2$O. Four of these animals also received 67 μg of methotrexate intraventricularly dissolved in the solution containing the dihydrofolic acid. Animals were killed 1½ hr later and the levels of FH$_4$ were measured by scintillation counting. Number of animals in brackets.

The studies *in vivo* are complicated since q-BH_2 can arise from BH_4 as the latter is oxidized during enzymatic hydroxylations. Admittedly, the nature of the product formed *de novo* in brain or in other tissues could only be determined after a single molecule of q-BH_2 was synthesized and consequently reduced to BH_4. At present, logistic obstacles prevent execution of such an experiment, therefore the evidence from experiments *in vivo* should be considered indirect. Yet it is difficult to explain how a pure enzyme will form one product *in vitro* and another one from the same substrate *in vivo*. The participation of DHFR in the metabolism of unconjugated pteridines *in vivo* perhaps is limited to reduction of a small amount of the biopterin pool to 7,8-BH_2 (Kaufman, 1967a). Corollary evidence for the absence of synthesis of BH_4 through DHFR came from the experiments *in vivo* with trimethoprin [2,4-diamino-5-(3′,4′,5′-trimethoxybenzyl)pyrimidine], a strong competitive inhibitor of DHFR (Burchall and Hitchings, 1965). Injection of 185–18.5 mg/kg rat with this inhibitor had no effect on the mean hepatic concentrations of BH_4 in the rat. It was concluded that this lack of effect was owing either to unavailability of the drug to the site of DHFR or to the fact that the reduction of 7,8-BH_2 to BH_4 did not contribute to the maintenance of BH_4 concentration (Stone, 1976). This author thus concluded that "this would indicate that there is no significant isomerization of quinonoid dihydrobiopterin to 7,8-dihydrobiopterin *in vivo* and that the biosynthesis of tetrahydrobiopterin in the rat is unlikely to involve reduction of 7,8-dihydrobiopterin." The data in Table 13 are completely consistent with this statement and indicate the position taken earlier by Gál and Sherman (1978a).

In a critical review (Cotton, 1977) this problem was further examined in its clinical framework. It was proposed that complete deficiency of DHFR would be lethal (Kaufman *et al.*, 1975). However, the reviewer (Cotton, 1977) refers to two clinical cases of DHFR deficiency with 0% and 25% residual activity showing normal Guthrie tests and HVE analysis of the urine (Tauro *et al.*, 1976). This problem will be discussed further in Section 7 of this review.

6. CATABOLISM OF PTERINS IN MAMMALIAN TISSUES

Understanding of the catabolism of pterins is largely as a result of the efforts of Rembold and his colleagues at the Max-Planck Institute, Munich, who in a series of reports on the "Catabolism of pteridine cofactors" recorded their findings. In general, catabolism is the biochemical pathway to elimination, exclusion, or excretion. Very often the nature or rate of catabolism of a compound will depend on whether it is of exogenous or endogenous origin. Pterins are no exceptions to this, as exogenous biopterin injected, let us say, intraperitoneally was excreted in a short time mostly unchanged. Injection of

[2-¹⁴C] biopterin into rats was recoverable after days from their urine as 20% biopterin, 45% pterin-6-carboxylic acid, 16% pterin, and 0.4% isoxanthopterin, to name but a few (Rembold, 1964). After intraperitoneal injection of 3.6 μCi (or 64 μg) [¹⁴C] biopterin or isobiopterin (7-dihydroxypropylpterin) into rats, 80–85% of these compounds were eliminated in the urine within 6 hr (Gál *et al.*, 1976). Elimination of exogenous reduced biopterins was much slower. The main catabolic product of neopterin and BH_4 metabolism *in vivo* and *in vitro* was 6-hydroxylumazine (**16**) (lumazine serves as sole source for the riboflavin synthesis in microorganisms), lumazine, and 7,8-dihydroxanthopterin.

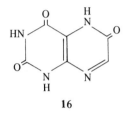

16

According to Rembold (1970) there are at least three major reactions in degradation of bio- and neopterin, namely (1) cleavage of the side chain, (2) deamination of the pterin ring, and (3) appearance of oxygen at position C-6. In general, the catabolic studies would indicate that terminal metabolites at reduced level of oxygen were xanthopterin and 6-hydroxylumazine, whereas at high tension of oxygen isoxanthopterin and 7-hydroxylumazine were predominating, which may be further oxidized enzymatically to leucopterin and 6,7-dihydroxylumazine. Reduced 6-polyhydroxyalkylpterin, like BH_4, in presence of iodine at acid pHs was recoverable as 33% biopterin while in presence of air without iodine only 4% was present as biopterin but 36% as dihydroxanthopterin and 36% pterin, respectively.

This section will be restricted to the enzymatically catalyzed degradation of pterins. For studies on chemical oxidation and degradation, the readers are referred to a specialized review (Rembold, 1970).

When BH_4 was incubated in a veronal–acetate buffer (pH 7.5) at 37°C under aerobic condition for 30 min with rat liver homogenates, the resulting mixture of compounds consisted mainly of xanthopterin, dihydroxanthopterin, pterin, biopterin, lumazine, and 6- and 7-hydroxylumazines. Lumazines which were formed by enzyme catalysis could be isolated in high yields (Rembold *et al.*, 1969). During longer incubation times, like 50 or 90 min, 6-hydroxylumazine increased at the expense of lumazine. These reactions were greatly dependent on oxygen concentration rather than that of the homogenate. Reincubation of 6-hydroxylumazine with fresh liver homogenate yielded 6,7-dihydroxylumazine which did not occur among the compounds of the primary incubation. Similarly reincubation of lumazine has led to the apperance of 7-

hydroxylumazine. Xanthine oxidase (EC 1.2.3.2) was suggested as the responsible enzyme for this second oxidation since 6-hydroxylumazine was one of its substrates (Bergmann and Kwietny, 1959). These authors showed that amino and hydroxypteridines were oxidized at carbon atoms 2, 4, and 7 of the pteridine ring. Reduced pteridines, however, like BH_4 or 5,6,7,8-tetrahydrolumazine were also oxidized at C-6, involving a covalently hydrated derivative of 7,8-dihydropteridine as an intermediate (Rembold and Gutensohn, 1968). Milk xanthine oxidase, incidentally, was found to oxidize 2-aminopteridines much more rapidly than 4-aminopteridines (Valerino and McCormack, 1969), whereas 4-hydroxypteridines were oxidized at a faster rate than the 2-hydroxypteridines. The kinetics of BH_4 degradation also apply to tetrahydroneopterin ($NPTH_4$).

Deamination of the pterin ring is also an enzyme catalyzed reaction. Pteridine deaminating enzymes have been detected in microbes, silkworm, and honeybee, also a specific pterin aminohydrolase in rat liver (Rembold and Simmersbach, 1969). In preparing this enzyme the experimental difficulty of its separation from guanine deaminase had to be overcome. The characteristics of pterin deaminase were the loss of activity in 2 wk, its inhibition by KCN and azaguanine, and some activation (35%) by p-chloromercuribenzoate. Its pH maximum was found to be 6.5, while that of the guanine deaminase is pH 9.2. The highest pterin deaminase activity was cytoplasmic. The deamination of tetrahydro- and dihydropterins actually occurred at a higher rate than that of pterin, which would place BH_2 and BH_4, through their degradation, among the prime substrates for pterin deaminase in vivo. Some pterins, such as xanthopterin, biopterin, neopterin, 6-hydroxymethylpterin, and pterin-6-carboxylic acid, were not deaminated by this enzyme (Rembold and Simmersbach, 1969). Overall, these data indicate that the catabolic reaction sequence, from BH_4 or $NPTH_4$ to 6-hydroxylumazine, must involve a deaminase and xanthine oxidase in vivo. Even under anaerobic conditions 60% of the 6-hydroxylumazine was synthesized from $NPTH_4$ within 30 min, in presence of a mixture of deaminase and xanthine oxidase. Incubation of $NPTH_4$ with xanthine oxidase alone resulted in a mixture of xanthopterin and 7,8-dihydroxanthopterin. Incidentally, xanthine oxidase degraded folic acid in a similar fashion. Tetrahydrofolic acid was oxidized by air to 17% xanthopterin (Blakley, 1957). It was suggested (Viscontini and Bobst, 1965) that air oxidation of tetrahydropteridines begins with a one-electron loss at N-5 followed by another electron and two protons to yield paraquinonoid dihydropteridines (II, VIc, and IXc), then followed by their rearrangement to 7,8-dihydropteridines. Paraquinonoid dihydroneopterin, for instance, with migration of the proton from C-6 yields $7,8\text{-}NPTH_2$ (III) which, after oxidation, becomes neopterin (IV). Similarly this is the pathway to pterin (VII) from tetrahydropterin (V) and of tetrahydrolumazine (X) to lumazine.

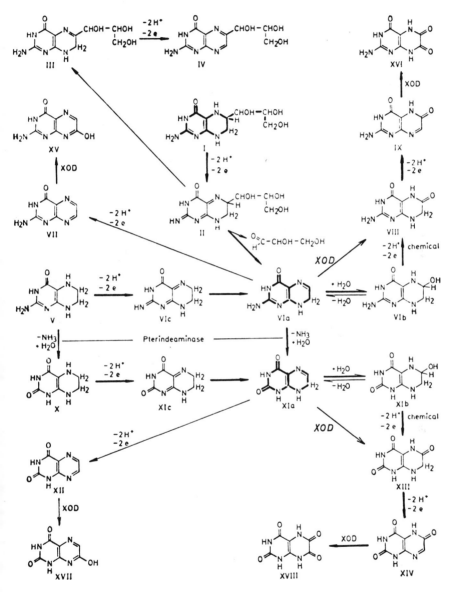

FIGURE 3. Scheme of pteridine catabolism, XOD = xanthine oxidase. (Rembold *et al.*, 1971*a*.)

Another pathway for the tautomerization of paraquinonoid dihydropteridine (II) was suggested by Rembold (1970) as being through the cleavage of the polyhydroxyalkyl chain as a positively charged residue, which would rapidly stabilize as glyceraldehyde and 7,8-dihydropterin (VIa) in equilibrium with its hydrated form VIb; oxidation would produce dihydroxanthopterin (VIII) and xanthopterin (IX). In contrast to this biochemical pathway, the 7,8-dihydroxanthopterin, produced by xanthine oxidase, did not require the dihydropterin hydrate (VIb). Xanthine oxidase is most likely to attack the unhydrated double bond of 7,8-dihydropterin (VIa).

In presence of deaminase the reactions proceeded from the pterin to lumazines. Here similar steps were observed. The oxidation of 7,8-dihydro-6-hydroxylumazine (XIII) to 6-hydroxylumazine (XIV) was extremely rapid and quantitative. Xanthine oxidase also produced metabolites from pteridines which were not in reduced state. Consequently pterin (V), xanthopterin (IX), lumazine (XII), and 6-hydroxylumazine (XIV) were converted to isoxanthopterin (XV), leucopterin (XVI), 7-hydroxylumazine (XVII), and 6,7-dihydroxylumazine (XVIII). All the above reactions are presented in the flowsheet "Scheme of Pterin Catabolism" (Rembold *et al.*, 1971*a*) and are reproduced through the permission of Professor H. Rembold (Figure 3). This scheme clearly assigns the importance of the two enzymes pterin deaminase and xanthine oxidase in the catabolism of pteridines. The significance of oxygen supply is particularly apparent for the nonenzymatic production of biopterin, neopterin, pterin, dihydroxanthopterin, and xanthopterin. The autooxidative conversions of tetrahydropteridines were recently discussed (Mager, 1975; Pearson and Blair, 1975).

7. COFACTORIAL FUNCTIONS

To do justice to the previous sections one is compelled to ask what are the functions of pteridines in the biochemical matrix of mammalian cell life. Questions of this nature are the consequence of scientific pragmatism! The reader's indulgence is asked, should he come across a somewhat repetitious narrative of a particular aspect already reviewed by others (Kaufman and Fisher, 1974). Preference will be given to the pertinent illustration of cofactorial functions in this limited framework.

Enzymatic reactions involving folic acid and its derivatives are numerous. In contrast the participation of unconjugated pteridines is well established for only L-erythro-5,6,7,8-BH$_4$, which serves as a natural cofactor in the enzymatic hydroxylation of phenylalanine, tyrosine, tryptophan, and some of their analogs.

7.1. Hydroxylases

About 20 years ago it was recognized that the enzymatic conversion of L-phenylalanine to L-tyrosine by rat liver phenylalanine hydroxylase (EC 1.14.3.1) required the presence of a new cofactor (Kaufman, 1958) in addition to $NADPH_2$. This investigator found that the new cofactor was extractable from rat liver but not from other tissues. It could be replaced by tetrahydrofolic acid in stimulating the hydroxylation of L-phenylalanine but some unconjugated pteridines appeared to be more active (Kaufman, 1959). 6,7-Dimethyl-5,6,7,8-tetrahydropterin ($DMPH_4$) or 6-methyl-5,6,7,8-tetrahydropterin (6-MPH_4) was prepared and used in these early studies. These revealed that $DMPH_4$ and phenylalanine hydroxylase were directly tied to synthesis of L-tyrosine while the pyridine nucleotides and sheep liver enzyme (later found to be q-dihydropterin reductase) assured continuous tetrahydrogenation of the pterin. These model compounds proved to be useful tools in elucidation of the basic nature of the reactions involved in the enzymatic hydroxylation of L-phenylalanine. Kinetic studies (Kaufman, 1961) with these compounds led to the recognition of the formation of a quinonoid intermediate. This intermediate was also prepared by oxidation of tetrahydropteridines with 2,6-dichlorophenolindophenol, peroxide, and Fe^{2+}.

In catalyzing phenylalanine hydroxylase, none of the model compounds was as active as the cofactor from rat liver extract except a reduced sample of synthetic biopterin (Kaufman, 1962). As mentioned earlier, the cofactor isolated from rat liver was identified as BH_2 (Kaufman, 1963); thus the results obtained with the synthetic reduced biopterin were fully confirmed. The mechanism of the BH_4-dependent phenylalanine hydroxylation was then proposed (Kaufman, 1964). Present knowledge of the synthesis of q-BH_2 from GTP *in vivo* permits the following modification of the hydroxylating process as it occurs. The two schemes can be linked as illustrated in Figure 4.

The interaction between BH_4 and the hydroxylase monooxygenase is possibly more complex, at least *in vitro*. A protein (PHS) was detected in rat liver that stimulated phenylalanine hydroxylase at high concentration of the enzyme, exclusively in presence of BH_4 (Kaufman, 1970). PHS increased the apparent affinity of the enzyme for BH_4 (K_m 2.5 $\times$ 10^{-6} *M*) without affecting the velocity of the reaction (Huang and Kaufman, 1973). In absence of PHS and L-phenylalanine, an assay mixture of low BH_4 concentration, phenylalanine hydroxylase, DHPR, and $NADH_2$ at pH 8.2 provided spectrophotometric evidence for the appearance of an intermediate of reduced biopterin. There was a characteristic marked increase in optical density between 240 and 260 nm upon addition of L-phenylalanine with concomitant increases at 270–275 nm corresponding to synthesis of L-tyrosine. Addition of PHS to the above assay mixture resulted in a rapid disappearance of the 245 nm peak inferring that the intermediate was a substrate of PHS (Kaufman, 1975). This mechanism assigned a hydroperoxide of BH_4 as the active agent of hydroxylation. There is some chemical proof for the appearance of hydroperoxides during nonenzymatic oxidation of tetrahydropteridines (Mager and Berends, 1965). At this stage, various schemes were proposed to explain this process. One of the hypotheses invoked the hydroperoxide of BH_4 (**17**) and an intermediate, a hydrated percursor of the q-BH_2. "This reaction would be non-rate limiting at pH 7.0 and rate limiting at pH 8.0 in the absence of PHS, hence the role of PHS in the hydroxylation reaction would be the catalysis of reaction . . . " of the hydrated form of q-BH_2 going to the dehydrated q-BH_2 (Kaufman, 1975). The other hypothesis advocated that the hydroperoxide of BH_4 itself, and not the hydroxylating agent, is the compound which undergoes a ring opening between N-5 and C-4a with the formation of an ozone. One molecule of this ozone would hydroxylate the substrate to product, while a cleaved pterin ring would represent a 2-amino-4,5-dioxopyrimidine. This compound would then, through ring closure, become the paraquinonoid dihydrobiopterin (Hamilton, 1974). At present, the validity of these schemes to the biochemistry of q-BH_2 $\rightleftharpoons BH_4$ *in vivo* remains questionable.

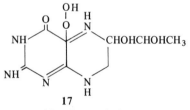

17

The nature of the enzyme kinetics and the response of the hydroxylases will greatly depend on whether the natural cofactor BH_4 or model (pseudo) cofactors are employed in the experiments. The use of the model cofactors has been of great benefit in the earlier exploratory studies that established the role pterins play in the biochemistry of hydroxylases. However, with the discovery of BH_4 as the natural cofactor, the use of model cofactors and their attendant disadvantages in the study of the properties of BH_4-dependent enzymes should have become rather obvious. In spite of critical reviews of this problem (Gál, 1974*b*), there are still too many researchers who use model cofactors and attempt to arrive at data which they interpret as relevant to the biochemical events *in vivo* and *in vitro*. Therefore, let us once more look at some properties of the hydroxylating enzymes which will appear in presence of BH_4 but not in presence of the model cofactors (such as 6-MPH_4 and 6,7-$DMPH_4$). Apart from the above-mentioned BH_4-dependent PHS for phenylalanine hydroxylase, one could single out the phosphorylated phenylalanine hydroxylase which is stimulated in presence of BH_4 (Abita *et al.*, 1976). Dephosphorylation of the enzyme leads to loss of activity in the presence of BH_4 but not with a model cofactor (Jedlicki *et al.*, 1977; Donlon and Kaufman, 1977). Yield of product, the specific activity of the enzyme, could be ten, twenty, or more times greater with BH_4 than with its analogs. Significant differences in the Michaelis–Menten curves for hydroxylation of phenylalanine existed whether one added BH_4 or $DMPH_4$ to the reaction mixture (Ayling and Helfand, 1975). Substrate and oxygen inhibition of the phenylalanine hydroxylase (25% inhibition at 21% oxygen) was observed in the presence of BH_4 *in vitro* (Fisher and Kaufman, 1972). *p*-Chlorophenylalanine became fifty times more inhibiting to phenylalanine hydroxylase *in vitro* with BH_4 as cofactor than 6,7-$DMPH_4$ (model cofactor) (Ayling and Helfand, 1975). Marked stimulation of rat liver phenylalanine hydroxylase (in presence of BH_4) by phospholipids such as lysolecithin and lysophosphatidylserine was noted by Fisher and Kaufman (1973 *b*).

Significant differences in the kinetics of hydroxylases were found recently even with the different diastereoisomers of BH_4 (Bailey and Ayling, 1978). Upon chemical reduction of BH_4 asymmetry at C-6 is created, namely *d,l*-L-erythro-5,6,7,8-BH_4. The enzymatically reduced 7,8-BH_2 by DHFR resulted in the *l*-L-erythro-BH_4 stereoisomer. This was verified by ORD (optical rotatory dispersion) and CD (circular dichroism) spectrography (Hasegawa *et al.*, 1978).

In experiments on nonenzymatic oxidation of BH_4, additions of catalase slowed down the rate of oxidation. This indicated that hydrogen peroxide (H_2O_2) was an aerobic oxidation product of tetrahydropterin and consequently q-dihydropterin formation was stimulated (Kaufman, 1961; Storm and Kaufman, 1968). Interestingly, catalase did not impede the rate of aerobic oxidation of tetrahydropteridin (Nielsen, 1969). Catalase could replace the glucose dehydrogenase only in presence of model cofactors but not on addition of BH_4. The dehydrogenase therefore contained a second factor only stimulatory to the oxidation of BH_4. This factor was called PHS from rat liver (Kaufman, 1970).

The role and function of BH_4 with phenylalanine hydroxylase has been discussed in more detail since phenylalanine hydroxylase, albeit absent from brain tissue, represents a hydroxylase which is well defined in most of its properties and extensively studied in its kinetic and regulatory relation to BH_4 (Kaufman, 1971). Phenylalanine hydroxylase was consequently chosen as the prototype for the discussions relative to the other two pterin-dependent monooxygenases, L-tyrosine hydroxylase and L-tryptophan hydroxylase.

Even though the role of cofactors in the function of tyrosine hydroxylase (EC 1.14.16.2) from the adrenal medulla was reviewed previously by Kaufman (1973), recent data on cerebral biopterin levels and distribution and functional roles for cerebral hydroxylases (Gál and Sherman, 1977*b*) may now dispel any "uncertainty about whether biopterin is cofactor for tyrosine hydroxylase in this tissue" (Kaufman, 1973). Tyrosine hydroxylase catalyzes mainly the conversion of L-tyrosine to L-3,4,-dihydroxyphenylalanine (L-DOPA) and under certain experimental conditions synthesizes L-tyrosine from L-phenylalanine (Ikeda *et al.*, 1965), and L-5-hydroxytryptophan from L-tryptophan (Gál, 1975). The dependence of this enzyme on $DMPH_4$ was known for sometime (Nagatsu *et al.*, 1964; Brenneman and Kaufman, 1964). Addition of reduced biopterin, instead of $6-MPH_4$, led to six-fold increase of DOPA synthesis. L-$NPTH_4$ (10^{-3} M) was less effective than $6-MPH_4$ in catalyzing conversion of L-tyrosine to L-DOPA; L-$NPTH_4$ produced 24 nmol L-DOPA while $6-MPH_4$ produced 72 nmol (Ellenbogen *et al.*, 1965). (It is likely that the D-$NPTH_4$ or its triphosphate would have been more active.) These studies also indicated that the reduced cofactors at 10^{-2} M or 2×10^{-2} M were strongly inhibitory. This inhibition, however, could be overcome in presence of 10^{-3} M Fe^{2+}. In fact the ion, Fe^{2+}, markedly stimulated tyrosine hydroxylase activity. Incidentally, the stimulation of phenylalanine and tryptophan hydroxylase by Fe^{2+} was also demonstrated; however, addition of catalase abolished this stimulation (Fisher *et al.*, 1972). The response of tyrosine hydroxylase, i.e., the stoichiometry of the reaction to various reduced pterins along with the substrate specificity dependent on the choice of the stereochemical structure of BH_4 (Numata *et al.*, 1977), accords well with that of phenylalanine hydroxylase. Again, tyrosine hydroxylase was inhibited by its substrate in the presence of BH_4 and, when phosphorylated, it responded to $6-MPH_4$ with a change in its affinity for this cofactor (Lovenberg *et al.*, 1975). Phosphatidylserine also stimulated tyrosine hydroxylase (Lloyd and Kaufman, 1974). The inhibition of tyrosine hydroxylase by DOPA (the reaction product) became much more pronounced in the presence of BH_4 than with $DMPH_4$. Evidently addition of BH_4 to the enzyme imparted important regulatory properties. It is to be noted that this selective relation of the enzyme to BH_4 applied to its soluble as well as to its "particulate" form.

Studies with tyrosine hydroxylase in rat brain homogenates suggested that, unlike in the adrenal tissue, the cerebral enzyme was particulate-bound and was insensitive to $30-1 \times 10^{-4}$ M $DMPH_4$ in the presence of $6 \times 10^{-2} M$ mercaptoethanol (McGeer *et al.*, 1967). This observation was consistent with the report that $DMPH_4$ and $NADPH_2$ had no effect on the particulate-bound tryptophan hydroxylase of rat brain (Gál *et al.*, 1966). Recently, solubilized tyrosine hydroxylase from brain tissue (Kuczenski and Mandell, 1972) had the same affinity as the particulate for $DMPH_4$ (K_m 1.5×10^{-5} M). In contrast to the solubilized enzyme the untreated soluble enzyme had a K_m of 7.4×10^{-4} M. The apparent K_m (1×10^{-4} M) of BH_4 for the enzyme from the adrenal medulla is the same as the K_m observed for $DMPH_4$ with the particulate tyrosine hydroxylase from human adrenals, or with the particulate enzyme of pheochromocytoma (Nagatsu *et al.*, 1972*b*). The apparent K_ms of the soluble enzyme were lower, 4.1×10^{-5} M for the adrenal and 6.5×10^{-5} M for the tumor. Partially purified tyrosine hydroxylase from bovine adrenal medulla had the lowest affinity for BH_4 with a K_m of 2×10^{-5} M, followed by 6-MPH$_4$ (8×10^{-5} M), DMPH$_4$ (9×10^{-5} M), and finally tetrahydropterin (4×10^{-4} M) (Nagatsu et al., 1972a). These investigators also examined the inhibitory properties of tetrahydropteridines and found the following: (1) the structure corresponding to 2-amino-4-hydroxy-5,6,7,8-tetrahydropteridine, which is also the skeleton of the corresponding pterins, was crucial for inhibitory activity; (2) the H atom of N-8 may be necessary for inhibition since 8-substituted pteridines do not possess this hydrogen; (3) substitution of H at N-5 with -CH$_3$ or -CH$_2$C$_6$H$_5$ may produce inhibition; (4) replacement of the H atom at C-6 or C-7 with alkyl or phenyl groups was not essential for the inhibitory property of the pteridine.

An important observation was the feedback inhibition of tyrosine hydroxylase by norepinephrine (Spector et al., 1967) in vivo but not by DOPA. However, DOPA and other catechols were inhibitory to tyrosine hydroxylase in vitro (Udenfriend et al., 1965) and DOPA was found to be a "competitive inhibitor" of tetrahydropterin (Ikeda et al., 1966) though the "pattern of this inhibition" was characterized as "noncompetitive" (Kaufman, 1973). On phosphorylation of the enzyme with ATP, in presence of 3', 5'-cAMP and Mg^{2+}, the K_m of 6-MPH$_4$ dropped from 5×10^{-4} M to 1.6×10^{-4} M (Lovenberg et al., 1975).

Another pterin-dependent enzyme is tryptophan-5-hydroxylase (EC 1.14.16.4), which converts L-tryptophan and α-methyltryptophan to the corresponding 5-hydroxytryptophans. Tryptophan-5-hydroxylase from rabbit hind brain can also hydroxylate L-phenylalanine to L-tyrosine in presence of BH_4 (Tong and Kaufman, 1975). The dependence of this enzyme on the presence of reduced biopterin was soon recognized (Gál, 1965; Gál et al., 1966). Addition of NADPH$_2$ to DMPH$_4$ enhanced the activity of purified soluble tryptophan-5-hydroxylase (Nakamura et al., 1965) but did not affect the activity of the particulate-bound enzyme (Gál et al., 1966). Addition of mercaptoethanol, DMPH$_4$, and Fe^{2+} greatly enhanced enzymatic synthesis of L-5-hydroxytryptophan (5-HTP) (Lovenberg et al., 1967). The presence of Fe^{2+} was indirectly demonstrated through the inhibition of the enzyme by α,α'-dipyridyl and phenanthroline (Gál et al., 1966; Lovenberg et al., 1967). Similarly to other pterin-dependent monoozygenases, tryptophan-5-hydroxylase had a much lower apparent K_m for BH_4 than for its analogs. Also, at a concentration of 2×10^{-4} M of L-tryptophan, this substrate became inhibitory only in presence of the natural cofactor in vitro (Friedman et al., 1972) and in vivo (Gál, 1975; Gál et al., 1978c). Phospholipids did not stimulate this enzyme in presence of BH_4 (Tong and Kaufman, 1975). In search for a stimulating factor, a pteridinelike compound was found in the 30,000g supernatant of rat brain homogenates.

This factor would stimulate cerebral hydroxylation of L-tyrosine and L-tryptophan (Gál and Roggeveen, 1973). Unlike PHS, this factor is not a protein. It was found to be thermostable, alkali labile, dialyzable, light sensitive, and lost its activity after a few days of storage at -27 °C. The presence of BH_4 was an absolute requirement for its effect.

L-Erythro-5,6,7,8-BH_4 is the natural cofactor of the three hydroxylases discussed in this section. It is the natural cofactor by virtue of its demonstrated synthesis from GTP *in vivo* (Gál and Sherman, 1976) and by its unique role *in vivo* as the active hydrogen carrier for the enzymes it serves.

The natural cofactor, BH_4, of the three hydroxylases meets the criteria suggested (Kaufman, 1973): (1) it is specific; (2) it has catalytic functions; (3) it is utilized during a substrate-dependent enzymatic reaction of hydroxylation. The apparent affinity, K_m, of BH_4 for phenylalanine, tyrosine, and tryptophan hydroxylases is about the same order of magnitude for each enzyme (Table 14).

In a simplified manner, the overall catalyzing enzyme reactions are represented by two major steps, (1) and (2), starting with the L-erythro-q-BH_2 and can be thus written and balanced (3)

$$q\text{-}BH_2 + NADH + H^+ \xrightarrow{DHPR} BH_4 + NAD^+ \tag{1}$$

$$\underline{substrate + BH_4 + O_2 \xrightarrow{hydroxylase} product + q\text{-}BH_2 + H_2O} \tag{2}$$
$$NADH + H^+ + substrate + O_2 \rightarrow product + H_2O + NAD^+ \tag{3}$$

where q-$BH_2 \rightleftharpoons BH_4$ obviously represents the $2H^+ + 2e^-$ transfer through ratewise reduction of q-BH_2 by q-DHPR. A somewhat more detailed presentation is also given in Figure 4.

Some additional comments are in order as to the controlling factors of the

TABLE 14. Apparant K_m Values for Different Tetrahydropterins[a]

		Cofactors		
Monooxygenase	Source	BH_4	6-MPH_4	$DMPH_4$
Phenylalanine	Liver	0.6	4.5	7.0
Tyrosine	Brain	9.2	25.0	37.0
Tryptophan	Brain	3.5	9.7	43.0

[a] Data are from the reviewer's experiments and are expressed at $\times 10^{-5}$ M concentration for soluble enzymes without assessment of the extent of phosphorylation. Tissues from Sprague Dawley male rats. From Gál *et al.* (1974b) and E. M. Gál (unpublished data).

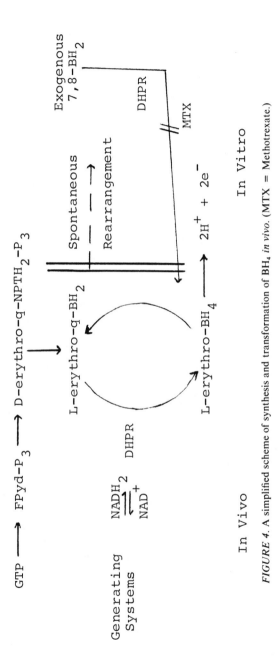

FIGURE 4. A simplified scheme of synthesis and transformation of BH_4 *in vivo.* (MTX = Methotrexate.)

reactions (1) and (2), particularly in relation to the role of dihydropteridine reductase, an enzyme over a thousand times in excess of its activity, in the reduction of q-BH$_2$. It was pointed out earlier that although, in the quantitative sense, the regional distribution of DHPR in brain varied, DHPR was ubiquitous and was present at levels sufficient to drive the continuous reduction of q-BH$_2$ to BH$_4$. It was demonstrated that the regional distribution of DHPR correlated well with that of tryptophan hydroxylase (Gál *et al.*, 1976) and of tyrosine hydroxylase (unpublished observations). Others did not find correlation between DHPR and tryptophan-5-hydroxylase (Bullard *et al.*, 1978). Yet these workers conceded that 25% of cerebral DHPR was associated with the synaptosomal enriched fractions. One may therefore deduce from their two observations that the synaptosomal DHPR must be exclusively localized in the adrenergic terminals. Of course, this was not borne out by experimental evidence, which revealed the presence of DHPR also in the serotonergic systems.

Another misconception pertains to the cerebral level of BH$_4$. By calculation of the actual cerebral or regional pool of BH$_4$ (Lloyd and Weiner, 1971; Gál *et al.*, 1976; Bullard *et al.*, 1978) there exists, in fact, an apparent state of unsaturation of the cofactor *vis á vis* tyrosine or tryptophan hydroxylase. This could therefore limit the activity of these hydroxylases. In reality complete arrest of the synthesis of q-BH$_2$ from GTP by dFPyd-P$_3$ in 3 hr and consequent reduction of the q-BH$_2$ and BH$_4$ pools by half did not bring about any change in the cerebral levels of 5-hydroxytryptamine (5-HT), dopamine (DA), and norepinephrine (NE) (Sherman and Gál, 1979). By extrapolation from the known cerebral turnover rates of q-BH$_2$ and BH$_4$ (Gál *et al.*, 1976) and from the rate of inhibition of their synthesis (Figure 5) a marked inhibition of the 5-HT, DA, and NE synthesis could not be attained even by the sixth hour following intraventricular injection of a third dose of 70 μg of FPyd-P$_3$ or DAO-Pyr (Gál and Whitacre, 1981). At this point, the cerebral cofactor pool was depleted to less than 10% of its original size.

A discussion of the role of BH$_4$ would be incomplete without mentioning the consequences of its deficiency in phenylketonuria (PKU). A recent review of the biochemical mechanism of PKU (Kaufman, 1977) has dealt with its complexities and semantics of terminology and definition. Therefore, a mere short overview will be given of the deficiencies in the level or synthesis of BH$_4$ as they relate to the function of phenylalanine hydroxylase.

Human liver phenylalanine hydroxylase was partially purified and studied for some of its properties (Friedman and Kaufman, 1973). Its instability and low activity, even with BH$_4$ in absence of lysolecithin, precluded accurate estimates of the K_m values. Nevertheless, these estimated values are the following: a K_m of 3×10^{-6} M for BH$_4$ (with lysolecithin added), and K_ms of 4×10^{-5} M and 5×10^{-5} M for 6-MPH$_4$ and DMPH$_4$ respectively. BH$_4$ and lysoleci-

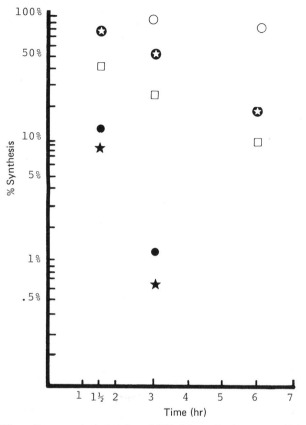

FIGURE 5. Effect of intraventricularly injected dFPyd-P_3 on the *de novo* synthesis of [^{14}C]-BH_2 (★) and [^{14}C]-BH_4 (●) from [U-^{14}C]-GTP; on the pool of BH_2 (□), BH_4 (✪), and levels of 5-HT (○) in rat brain. The 6 hr value by extrapolation.

thin failed to stimulate the synthesis of tyrosine by a sample of PKU liver beyond 0.27% of the normal liver (Friedman *et al.*, 1973).

A few years ago, PKU was reported in a male infant whose liver, brain, and skin fibroblast samples revealed the absence of dihydropterin reductase. The concentration of the sum of BH_2 and BH_4 in his liver sample was half that of normal subjects (6 nmol/g liver wet weight), less than one-sixth of the BH_4 content of the normal liver (Kaufman *et al.*, 1975). The brain biopsy of the frontal cortex from a DHPR-deficient patient revealed less than 1% activity of a control. Another case of DHPR deficiency was reported as a variant of phenylketonuria (Danks *et al.*, 1975). The patient was a severely retarded 17-

month-old girl excreting abnormally elevated amounts of 7,8-BH$_2$. Her serum level of biopterins in total was also high. Intravenous injection of BH$_4$ in graded doses from 1- to 100-mg quantities produced a transient decrease in the serum phenylalanine level of the patient. This experiment lent further support to the suggestion that BH$_4$ functions as a cofactor of phenylalanine hydroxylase *in vivo.* It also pinpointed the defect as being at the DHPR site. The level of phenylalanine hydroxylase in this deficiency did not seem to be affected when compared to cases of classic phenylketonuria, in which the enzyme levels were about 80 times lower (Friedman *et al.,* 1973).

It is well to note that though the human blood serum was found capable of effective binding of BH$_4$, possibly by α_2-macroglobulins (Rembold *et al.,* 1977), this binding, as well as the distribution and synthesis of BH$_4$, was greatly altered in diseases (Baker *et al.,* 1974).

Little is known of the effect of DHPR deficiency on tryptophan and tyrosine hydroxylases. Dihydrofolate reductase may have substituted to a limited extent for DHPR, though 7,8-BH$_2$ as a substrate for DHFR greatly decreases the rate of BH$_4$ synthesis. In some patients there was a total absence of BH$_4$ in spite of the presence of reducing substances, such as glutathione and ascorbic acid, which could have conceivably converted some 7,8-BH$_2$ to BH$_4$. A trial of ascorbate therapy in 5-g amounts daily for 19 days failed to be remedial in the patients with peripheral and neurological symptoms (Kaufman *et al.,* 1975). These observations, in the reviewer's estimate, strengthen the data discussed earlier (Gál and Sherman, 1978*a*; Gál *et al.,* 1979*a*) which indicated that (1) dihydrofolate has no significant functional role in the reduction of dihydropterin *in vivo* which is synthesized as q-BH$_2$, and (2) the cerebral levels of DHPR must fall below 10–5% before the synthesis of L-DOPA and 5-HTP becomes critically impaired. Such impairment might lead to the demise of the patient. DHPR-deficient patients revealed no observable defect in the biosynthetic route to 7,8-BH$_2$ as manifested by the excessive amounts of 7,8-BH$_2$. Appearance of urinary 7,8-dihydroxanthopterin and xanthopterin was also noted in these patients (Watson *et al.,* 1977). This defect might be construed as a mutation in the DHPR gene.

Another type of hyperphenylalaninemia was diagnosed as a result of low levels of reduced biopterins (Kaufman *et al.,* 1975; Milstien *et al.,* 1977; Rey *et al.,* 1977). The patient, a child, had normal phenylalanine DHPR, DFPR, and PHS protein as indicated by assays of his biopsied liver. However, reduced biopterins constituted only 5% of the normal level. Recently, additional reports appeared on patients with atypical phenylketonuria and with normal liver dihydropteridine reductase and phenylalanine-4-hydroxylase activities. These patients excreted neopterin and 3-hydroxysepiapterin but not biopterin or BH$_2$ in urine (Niederwieser *et al.,* 1979, 1980) and were treated with BH$_4$, BH$_2$, and sepiapterin, with promising results (Curtius *et al.,* 1979). The enzymatic block appears to be between the conversion of q-NPTH$_2$-P$_3$ to q-BH$_2$ along the biosynthetic pathway of q-BH$_2$ from GTP.

7.2. Oxygenases and Other Enzymes

Owing to their autooxidizable nature tetrahydropterins (Fisher and Kaufman, 1973a) were found to stimulate indoleamine 2:3 dioxygenase (Nishikimi, 1975), an enzyme found in the intestine (Yamamoto and Hayaishi, 1967) and in the brain (Gál *et al.*, 1966). This enzyme, like hepatic tryptophan dioxygenase, is a heme protein which oxidatively cleaves the pyrole ring of L-tryptophan to L-kynurenine, but unlike the liver enzyme, it also attacks D-tryptophan, D,L-5-HTP, 5-HT, tryptamine, and melatonin (Tsuda *et al.*, 1972; Hirata *et al.*, 1974). It is induced by tryptophan but not by cortisol (Gál, 1974a). Instead of oxygen, it requires superoxide O$_2^-$ for its catalysis. Tetrahydropterins generate superoxide during their autoxidation and together with catalase promote synthesis of L-kynurenine. The presence of catalase may prevent nonenzymatic oxidation of tetrahydropterins by H$_2$O$_2$ which is generated during their autoxidation. BH$_4$ was found to be the most effective among the tetrahydropterins in catalyzing the breakdown of tryptophan.

Although the indoleamine 2:3 dioxygenase preparation was not homogenous, it had no xanthine oxidase contamination. (Xanthine oxidase could have stimulated the ring cleavage of indoles.) The maximal activity of the enzyme was attained at a concentration of 2×10^{-4} M BH$_4$ and half maximal activity at 7×10^{-5} M which suggested to the author (Nishikimi, 1975) that BH$_4$ may serve as the natural cofactor of indoleamine 2:3 dioxygenase but could be inhibited by another enzyme, superoxide dismutase, which catalyzes the dissipation of O$_2^-$. At present there is no evidence that BH$_4$ is a cofactor of indoleamine 2:3 dioxygenase *in vivo*.

Recently, it was suggested that pteridines may participate in the light-dependent regulation of the hydroxyindole-O-methyltransferase (HIOMT) of the pineal gland and retina (Cremer-Bartels and Hollwich, 1978). The data on the effect of pteridines on the kinetics of HIOMT *in vitro* were supportive of such roles *in vivo*. The pineal gland was reported to contain biopterins (Have-Kirchberg *et al.*, 1977).

Another example of the participation of tetrahydropterins was revealed in the studies on the oxidation of glyceryl ethers by rat liver homogenates (Tietz *et al.*, 1964). An enzyme system of the liver which oxidized the long-chain alkyl ethers of glycerol to fatty acids and glycerol, with long-chain aldehydes as intermediates, was demonstrated to require oxygen and an unconjugated tetrahydropterin. L-erythro-NPTH$_4$ (BH$_4$ was not available to the experimenters) was six times as active as DMPH$_4$. Tetrahydrofolate (*l*-L-enantiomorph) at 5×10^{-5} M concentration was ten times less active than 6-MPH$_4$ in catalyzing the oxidation of glyceryl ethers to their hemiacetals which would spontaneously break down to glycerol and an aldehyde. The aldehyde is then oxidized by NAD^+ to the acid. The oxidative step could be accomplished by the use of well-washed microsomes, O_2, and a tetrahydropterin. In presence of *l*-L-tetrahydrofolate and DFPR, the reaction was inhibited by amethopterin (MTX).

The participation of tetrahydropterins was also implicated in the function of other oxygenases such as the one involved in the 17α-hydroxylation of progesterone (Hagerman, 1964). The synthesis of prostaglandine from 8,11,14-eicosatrienoic acid was stimulated by BH_4 *in vitro* (Samuelsson, 1972). Preliminary experiments *in vivo* did not show any change in the cerebral levels of prostaglandins $PGF_{1\alpha}$ and PGE_2 in rats whose cerebral synthesis of BH_2 and BH_4 was completely arrested and the pool sizes of reduced biopterins decreased by 50% (Sherman and Gál, 1979). Purified lipoyl dehydrogenase from pig brain was inhibited by pterins but its transhydrogenase and diaphorase activities were unaffected (Millard *et al.*, 1969).

7.3. Mitochondrial Respiration

It was noted that mitochondrial respiration, at the level of cytochrome C, was enhanced upon addition of tetrahydropterin without any effect on the ATP-generating system (Rembold and Buff, 1972). A more recent report has indicated that a 0.9 P:O ratio was obtained with rat liver mitochondria upon addition of $DMPH_4$. This implies phosphorylation at "site 3" of the electron transport system (Taylor and Hochstein, 1975). An interesting feature of this report was that the reduction of cytochrome C by the tetrahydropterin proceeded anaerobically and was not inhibited by superoxide dismutase. However, these experiments yielded no evidence for an enzymatic reduction of cytochrome C by $DMPH_4$ since this reduction did not increase when mitochondria or mitochondrial sonicate was added. The participation of tetrahydropterin as cofactor in the coupled oxidation of cytoplasmic reduced pyridine nucleotides by mitochondrial cytochrome C thus remains unresolved.

8. PHARMACOLOGICAL ASPECTS

The chemicals which inhibited the biosynthesis of biopterins *in vivo* have been considered in a previous section of this review.

Strictly speaking the effect of drugs on biopterins, as they regulate the affinity or rates of various enzymes, really belongs to the realm of quantitative biocatalysis. However, several drugs were reported to affect the kinetic parameters of various hydroxylases *in vivo* and *in vitro*. Examples like reserpine, haloperidol, and methiothepin are just a few of the drugs seen to exert their pharmacological actions on the brain either by altering the affinity of a hydroxylase toward its substrate, cofactor, or Ca^{2+}, or by altering corticosteroid levels. Intraperitoneal injection of reserpine (5 mg/kg) induced an increase in 5-HT synthesis *in vivo* (Tozer *et al.*, 1966), and a change in the K_m of $DMPH_4$ from 5.1×10^{-4} to 1.3×10^{-4} M for tyrosine hydroxylase of the striatum, which persisted in the experiments *in vitro*. Tyrosine hydroxylase of other cerebral areas, such as hypothalamus or brain stem, or of other organs, e.g., the adrenals, was not influenced by reserpine (Zivkovic *et al.*, 1975). Similar experiments with rats demonstrated that after intraperitoneal reserpine injection (5 mg/kg) the V_{max} of the substrate for brain stem tryptophan-5-hydroxylase increased without any change in the K_m (Hamon *et al.*, 1976). Injection of methiothepin (20 mg/kg) decreased the K_m for tryptophan but did not affect either the K_m or the V_{max} for $6-MPH_4$.

Changes in cerebral metabolism after administration of exogenous molecules such as drugs are manyfold. The mechanism of catalytic proteins could be altered by drugs. Their synthesis, catabolism, uptake, release from membrane surfaces, and, above all, their conformation through shifts of ionic charges and phosphorylation through appearance of stimulatory or inhibitory factors, could all be affected by drugs. In turn all these changes in mechanism may, to a varying degree, relate to the observed changes in the K_ms of BH_4 or the velocity maxima of the enzymes. No wonder, therefore, that this area of biochemical pharmacology is full of contradictions, controversies, redundancies, and very subjective interpretations (Mandell, 1978).

Another aspect that deserves some examination is the effect of pteridines as pharmacological agents. Studies in the late forties on the pharmacological actions of pteridines concentrated on three important fields of interest; namely (1) pteridines as anticarcinogenic agents, (2) pteridines as antifolates, and (3) pteridines as vitamin analogs. Between 1947 and 1950, a group of investigators at the University of California, Berkeley, noticed that of the five 4-amino-pteridines injected into rats, only the 2,4-diaminopteridines, but not the 2-thiol-4-aminopteridines, produced loss of weight. The weight loss could be correlated with the degree of crystalline deposits in the rat kidneys (La Du *et al.*, 1950). Crystalline deposits within the renal tubules were also observed after the administration of 2-amino-4,6-dihydroxypteridine (xanthopterin) and even after high doses of folic acid. Leukopenia was also reported, although no anemia, in weanling rats receiving 2,4-diamino-6,7-diphenyl pteridine (50 mg/100 kg) in their diet (Swenseid *et al.*, 1949). Subsequent biological assays with folate analogs in experimental animals and men unequivocally confirmed the need for 2,4-diamino substitutions of the pteridine ring for inhibitory and chemotherapeutic effectiveness. In 1958, it was reported that triamterene 2,4,7-triamino-6-phenylpteridine (SK&F 8542) was a good inhibitor (K_I 1.3×10^{-8} M) of dihydrofolate reductase (Doctor, 1958; Bertino *et al.*, 1965). Triamterene interfered with Na^+ reabsorption and simultaneous excretion of K^+ in the distal convoluted tubules of the nephron (Baba *et al.,* 1964). This is a direct action on transport processes in the tubular cells unrelated to competitive displacement of aldosterone. This drug is a moderately effective diuretic. After its oral administration in man, maximal diuresis was reached in about 2 hr (Baba *et al.,* 1964). Triamterene was excreted mainly as the sulfuric ester of its metabolite, 2,4,7-triamino-6-*p*-hydroxyphenylpteridine (Lehmann, 1965). It is of interest that pteridine diuretics displayed growth-inhibitory effects in *Crithidia* cultures, while pteridines, which were not diuretics, were not inhibitory (Dewey and Kidder, 1974). These authors have cautiously suggested that the diuretic activity might be related to the antagonism of these compounds to the natural cofactor since the growth inhibition of *Crithidia fasciculata* could be competitively reversed by L-erythroneopterin.

The reports on the therapeutic effectiveness of unconjugated pteridines are meager and may remain so. Yet a systematic search not only is justified but may be rewarding.

9. CONCLUSION

The reviewer attempted to convey the results of discoveries and explorations as well as the contentions of the biochemistry of pteridines. In general, the chemistry and biology of pteridines is an area of rapid growth; yet this growth, as it pertains to mammals, is still embryonic if not minuscule.

The biochemistry of pterins in mammals is ruled by similar mechanisms as those found in plant or other animal organisms. In some respects such as the biosynthesis of pterins the mammals appear to be strikingly different. The appearance of new enzymes in the mammalian tissue subserving this biosynthesis need not be viewed with skepticism through the distorting optics of scientific conservatism. Confirmation of new data by others, objectively interpreted, ought to reinforce facts and lead the skeptics out of their quandry. Confirmation of the work of others or discussion of differing results, be they ever so contrary to our own data, must never be glossed over. Nobody's work or priority should be ignored because of our antipathies or predilections or for reasons of self-aggrandizement. More and more, in this reviewer's opinion, one is given the impression that scientific achievements are born in a vacuum and that one does not owe anything to the work of others. This is scientific cannibalism, that devours the works of others. It forever assigns past achievements to oblivion at the mercy of the ignorant, the lazy, or the merely careless professionals and reviewers. It can safely be said, without fear of contradiction, that those who practice this art of cannibalism are perhaps skillful, competent professionals but lack the proper attitude, respect, and dignity of a philosophy which would rank them among scientists.

The above comments reveal not only this reviewer's disconcert but his attitude and earnest plea for respectful, balanced, and critical reviews. Hopefully, this chapter on the "Biosynthesis and Function of Unconjugated Pterins in Mammalian Tissues" will meet these objectives.

If there is anyone whose work in this area of narrow specialization has been overlooked, he/she should rest assured that the omission was unintentional and not due to disapprobation. If science is to flourish, and good research is to be stimulated, it must meet exacting requirements, and also it needs unbiased and generous encouragement. Thus it is incumbent upon all of us in science to exercise criticism without caprice and corrections without partisanship, for science thrives in its very essence and at its best through the toil, painstaking care, integrity, and, above all, through the expenditure of ideas and thoughts of its practitioners. Finally, the reviewer would like to thank his confreres of the present and past whose work he was privileged to review and cite. Their work has been an inexhaustible fountain of inspiration and an example of good science for the younger generation of scientists to emulate.

Goethe, in a quick but not too profound repartee, once said, "Everything has been thought of before, the difficulty is to think of it again." This certainly does not exemplify the scientist's daily encounter with refractory "Nature." A more correct appraisal of "Nature" which scientists can take to heart comes from P. Ehrlich, a great pundit of science, who thought that the basis of any discovery was to ask the "right questions" as "Nature" was ready with the "right answers."

ACKNOWLEDGMENTS

The reviewer is grateful to his colleagues, particularly Dr. A. D. Sherman, and also to Professors J. M. Musacchio and H. Rembold for permission to print Table 12 and Figure 3. The reviewer is indebted to his secretary, Ms. Linda Bair, for her conscientious work and her untiring review of the manuscript for corrections.

10. REFERENCES

Abelson, H. T., Spector, R., Gorka, C., and Fosburg, M., 1978, Kinetics of tetrahydrobiopterin synthesis by rabbit brain dihydrofolate reductase, *Biochem. J.* **171**:267–268.

Abita, J. P., Milstien, S., Chang, N., and Kaufman, S., 1976, *In vitro* activation of rat liver phenylalanine hydroxylase by phosphorylation, *J. Biol. Chem.* **251**:5310–5314.

Albert, A., 1957, Transformation of purines into pteridines, *Biochem. J.* **65**:124–127.

Andrews, K. J. M., Barber, W. E., and Tong, B. P., 1969, A new synthesis of biopterin, *J. Chem. Soc.* 928–930.

Archer, M.C., Vonderschmitt, D. J., and Scrimgeour, K. G., 1972, Mechanism of oxidation of tetrahydropterins, *Can. J. Biochem.* **50**:1174–1182.

Ayling, J. E., and Helfand, G. D., 1975, Effect of pteridine cofactor structure on the regulation of phenylalanine hydroxylase activity, in: *Chemistry and Biology of Pteridines* (W. Pfleiderer, ed.), pp. 305–318, W. de Gruyter, Berlin.

Baba, W. I., Tudhope, G. R., and Wilson, G. M., 1964, Site and mechanism of action of the diuretic, triamterene, *J. Clin. Sci.* **27**:181–193.

Bagnara, J. T., 1961, Chromatotrophic hormone, pteridines, and amphibian pigmentation, *Gen. Comp. Endocrinol.* **1**:124–133.

Bagnara, J. T., and Obika, M., 1965, Comparative aspects of integumental pteridine distribution among amphibians, *Comp. Biochem. Physiol.* **15**:33–49.

Bailey, S. W., and Ayling, J. E., 1975, High pressure liquid chromatography of substituted pteridines and tetrahydropteridines, in: *Chemistry and Biology of Pteridines* (W. Pfleiderer, ed.), pp. 633–643, W. de Gruyter, Berlin.

Bailey, S. W., and Ayling, J. E., 1978, Separation and properties of the 6 diastereoisomers of *l*-erythrotetrahydrobiopterin and their reactivities with phenylalanine hydroxylase, *J. Biol. Chem.* **253**:1598–1605.

Baker, H., Frank, O., Bacchi, D. J., and Hunter, S. H., 1974, Biopterin content of human and rat fluids and tissues determined protozoologically, *Am. J. Clin. Nutr.* **27**:1247–1253.

Bergmann, F., and Kwietney, H., 1959, Pteridines as substrates of mammalian xanthine oxidase. II. Pathways and rates of oxidation, *Biochem. Biophys. Acta* **33**:29–46.

Bertino, J. R., Perkins, J. P., and Johns, D. G., 1965, Purification and properties of dihydrofolate reductase from Ehrlich ascites carcinoma cells, *Biochemistry* **4**:839–846.

Blakley, R. L., 1957, The interconversion of serine and glycine: Preparation and properties of catalytic derivatives of pteroylglutamic acid, *Biochem. J.* **65**:331–342.

Blakley, R. L., 1969, *The Biochemistry of Folic Acid and Related Pteridines*, pp. 1–540, North-Holland Publishing, Amsterdam.

Boon, W. R., and Jones, W. G., 1951, Pteridines. Part II. The synthesis of some α-(5-nitro-4-pyrimidylamino)-ketones and their conversion into 7,8-dihydropterins and pteridines, *J. Chem. Soc.*, 591–596.

Brenneman, A. R., and Kaufman, S., 1964, The role of tetrahydropteridines in the enzymatic conversion of tyrosine to 3,4-dihydroxyphenylalanine, *Biochem. Biophys. Res. Commun.* **17**:177–183.

Broquist, H. P., and Albrecht, A. M., 1955, Pteridines and the nutrition of the protozoon *Crithidia fasciculata*, *Proc. Soc. Biol. Med.* **89**:178–180.

Brown, D. J., and Jacobsen, N. W., 1961, Pteridine studies. Part XIV. Methylation of 2-amino-4-hydroxypteridine and related compounds, *J. Chem. Soc.* 4413–4420.

Brown, G. M., 1971, The biosynthesis of pterins, in: *Advances in Enzymology* (A. Meister, ed.), Vol. 35, pp. 35–77, Wiley Interscience, New York.

Brown, G. M., Yim, J., Suzuki, Y., Heine, M. C., and Foor, F., 1975, The enzymic synthesis of pterins in *Escherichia Coli*, in: *Chemistry and Biology of Pteridines* (W. Pfleiderer, ed.), pp. 219–244, W. de Gruyter, Berlin.

Buff, K., and Dairman, W., 1975*a*, Biosynthesis of biopterin in the intact rat and in mouse neuroblastoma cells, in: *Chemistry and Biology of Pteridines* (W. Pfleiderer, ed.), pp. 273–284, W. de Gruyter, Berlin.

Buff, K., and Dairman, W., 1975*b*, Biosynthesis of biopterin by two clones of mouse neuroblastoma, *Mol. Pharmacol.* **11**:87–93.

Bullard, W. P., Guthrie, P. B., Russo, V., and Mandell, A. J., 1978, Regional and subcellular distribution and some factors in the regulation of reduced pterins in rat brain, *J. Pharmacol. Exp. Ther.* **206**:4–20.

Burchall, J. J., and Hitchings, G. H., 1965, Inhibitor binding analysis of dihydrofolate reductases from various species, *Mol. Pharmacol.* **1**:126–136.

Burg, A. W., and Brown, G. M., 1968, The biosynthesis of folic acid. VIII. Purification and properties of the enzyme that catalyzes the production of formate from carbon 8 of guanosine triphosphate, *J. Biol. Chem.* **243**:2349–2358.

Cheema, S., Soldin, S. J., Knapp, A., Hofmann, T., and Scrimgeour, K. G., 1973, Properties of purified quinonoid dihydropterin reductase, *Can. J. Biochem.* **51**:1229–1239.

Cone, J., and Guroff, G., 1971, Partial purification and properties of guanosine triphosphate cyclohydrolase, the first enzyme in pteridine biosynthesis from *Comamonas* sp. (ATCC 11299a), *J. Biol. Chem.* **246**:979–985.

Cotton, R. G. H., 1977, The primary molecular defects in phenylketonuria and its variants, *Int. J. Biochem.* **8**:333–341.

Craine, J. E., Hall, S. E., and Kaufman, S., 1972, The isolation and characterization of dihydropteridine reductase from sheep liver, *J. Biol. Chem.* **247**:6082–6091.

Cremer-Bartels, G., and Hollwich, F., 1978, Effects of pteridines on melatonin biosynthesis of pineal gland and retina, Abstract, 6th International Symposium on Chemistry and Biology of Pteridines, p. 24.

Curtius, H.-Ch., Niederwieser, A., Viscontini, M., Otten, A., Schaub, J., Scheibenreiter, S., and Schmidt, H., 1979, Atypical phenylketonuria due to tetrahydrobiopterin deficiency. Diagnosis and treatment with tetrahydrobiopterin, dihydrobiopterin and sepiapterin, *Clin. Chim. Acta* **93**:251–262.

Danks, D. M., Cotton, R. G., and Schlesinger, P., 1975, Tetrahydrobiopterin treatment of variant form of phenylketonuria, *Lancet* **2**:1043.

Descimon, H., and Barial, M., 1973, Correlation entre structure et proprietes chromatographiques des pterines, *Bull. Soc. Chim. France* **1**:87–92.

Dewey, V. C., and Kidder, G. W., 1967, The use of Sephadex for the concentration of pteridines, *J. Chromatogr.* **31**:326–336.

Dewey, V. C., and Kidder, G. W., 1971, Assay of unconjugated pteridines, in: *Methods of Enzymology* (D. B. McCormich, and L. D. Wright, eds.), Vol. 18B, pp. 618–624, Academic Press, New York.

Dewey, V. C., and Kidder, G. W., 1974, Pteridine diuretics as biopterin antagonists, *Biochem. Pharmacol.* **23**:773–779.

Dewey, V. C., Kidder, G. W., and Butler, F. P., 1959, Replacement of the biopterin requirement of *Crithidia*, *Biochem. Res. Commun.* **1**:25–28.

Doctor, V. M., 1958, Studies on the inhibitory nature of pteridines, *J. Biol. Chem.* **232**:617–626.

Donlon, J., and Kaufman, S., 1977, Modification of the multiple forms of rat hepatic phenylalanine hydroxylase by *in vitro* phosphorylation, *Biochem. Biophys. Res. Commun.* **78**:1011–1017.

Ehrenberg, A., Henmerich, P., Miller, F., Okada, T., and Viscontini, M., 1967, Uber pterinchemie. 18. Monohydro und trihydropterin-radikale, *Helv. Chim. Acta* **50**:411–416.

Elderfield, R. C., and Mehta, A. C., 1967, Heterocyclic compounds, in: *Heterocyclic Chemistry* (R. C. Elderfield, ed.), Vol. 9, pp. 45–107, J. Wiley and Sons, New York.

Ellenbogen, L., Taylor, R. J., and Brundage, G. B., 1965, On the role of pteridines as cofactors for tyrosine hydroxylase, *Biochem. Biophys. Res. Commun.* **19**:708–715.

Eto, L., Fukushima, K., and Shiota, T., 1976, Enzymatic synthesis of biopterin from D-erythro-dihydroneopterin triphosphate by extracts of kidney from Syrian golden hamsters, *J. Biol. Chem.* **251**:6505–6512.

Eugster, C. H., Frauenfelder, E. F., and Koch, H., 1970, Russulafarbstoff: Erkennung der roten Hautkomponenten als dimere Pteridineglykoside: Trennung von Pterinen durch isoelectrische Fokussierung in einem pH-Saccharose-Gradienten, *Helv. Chim. Acta* **53**:131–147.

Fisher, D. B., and Kaufman, S., 1972, The inhibition of phenylalanine and tyrosine hydroxylases by high oxygen levels, *J. Neurochem.* **19**:1359–1365.

Fisher, D. B., and Kaufman, S., 1973*a*, Tetrahydropterin oxidation without hydroxylation catalyzed by rat liver phenylalanine hydroxylase, *J. Biol. Chem.* **248**:4300–4304.

Fisher, D. B., and Kaufman, S., 1973*b*, The stimulation of rat liver phenylalanine hydroxylase by lysolecithin and α-chymotrypsin, *J. Biol. Chem.* **248**:4345–4353.

Fisher, D. B., Kirkwood, R., and Kaufman, S., 1972, Rat liver hydroxylase, an iron enzyme, *J. Biol. Chem.* **247**:5161–5167.

Fleming, A. F., and Broquist, H. P., 1967, Biopterin and folic acid deficiency, *Am. J. Clin. Nutr.* **20**:613–621.

Forrest, H. S., and Nawa, S., 1964, Recent work on the structures of isosepiapterin and the drosopterins and its relation to pteridine biosynthesis, in: *Pteridine Chemistry* (W. Pfleiderer and E. C. Taylor, eds.) pp. 281–289, Pergamon Press, Oxford.

Forrest, H. S., and Van Baalen, C., 1970, Microbiology of unconjugated pteridines, *Annu. Rev. Microbiol.* **24**:91–108.

Frank, O., Baker, H., and Sobotka, H., 1963, Blood- and serum-levels of water-soluble vitamins in man and animals, *Nature London* **197**:490–491.

Friedman, P. A., and Kaufman, S., 1973, Some characteristics of partially purified human liver phenylalanine hydroxylase, *Biochem. Biophys. Acta* **293**:56–61.

Friedman, P. A., Kappelman, A. H., and Kaufman, S., 1972, Partial purification and characterization of tryptophan hydroxylase from rabbit hind brain, *J. Biol. Chem.* **247**:4165–4173.

Friedman, P. A., Fisher, D. B., Kang, E. S., and Kaufman, S., 1973, Detection of hepatic phenylalanine-4-hydroxylase in classical phenylketonuria, *Proc. Natl. Acad. Sci. U.S.A.* **70**:552–556.

Fujimori, E., 1959, Interaction between pteridines and tryptophan, *Proc. Natl. Acad. Sci. U.S.A.* **45**:133–136.

Fukushima, T., 1970, Biosynthesis of pteridines in the tadpole of the bullfrog, *Rana catesbiana, Arch. Biochem. Biophys.* **139**:361–369.

Fukushima, T., and Akino, M., 1968, Nuclear magnetic resonance studies of some biologically active dihydropterins, *Arch. Biochem. Biophys.* **128**:1–5.

Fukushima, T., and Nixon, J. C., 1980, Analysis of reduced forms of biopterins in biological tissues and fluids, *Anal. Biochem.* **102**:176–188.

Fukushima, T., and Shiota, T., 1972, Pterins in human urine, *J. Biol. Chem.* **247**:4549–4556.

Fukushima, T., and Shiota, T., 1974, Biosynthesis of biopterin by Chinese hamster ovary (CHO K1) cell culture, *J. Biol. Chem.* **249**:4445–4451.

Fukushima, F., Eto, I., Saliba, D., and Shiota, T., 1975*a*, The enzymatic synthesis of Crithidia active substances(s) and a phosphorylated D-erythro-neopterin from GTP or GDP by liver preparations from Syrian golden hamsters, *Biochem. Biophys. Res. Commun.* **65**:644–651.

Fukushima, K., Eto, I., Mayumi, T., Richter, W., Goodson, S., and Shiota, T., 1975*b*, Biosynthesis of pterins in mammalian systems, in: *Chemistry and Biology of Pteridines* (W. Pfleiderer, ed.), pp. 247–263, W. de Gruyter, Berlin.

Fukushima, K., Richter, W. E., Jr., and Shiota, T., 1977, Partial purification of 6(D-erythro-1′,2′,3′-trihydroxypropyl)-7,8-dihydropterin triphosphate synthetase from chicken liver, *J. Biol. Chem.* **252**:5750–5755.

Fukushima, T., Kobayashi, K., Eto, I., and Shiota, T., 1978, A differential microdetermination for the various forms of biopterin. *Anal. Biochem.* **89**:71–79.

Gál, E. M., 1965, *In vitro* hydroxylation of tryptophan by brain tissue, *Fed. Proc. Fed. Am. Soc. Exp. Biol.* **24**:580.

Gál, E. M., 1974*a*, Cerebral tryptophan-2,3′-dioxygenase (pyrrolase) and its induction in rat brain, *J. Neurochem.* **22**:861–863.

Gál, E. M., 1974*b*, Tryptophan-5-hydroxylase: Function and control, in: *Advances in Biochemical Psychopharmacology* (E. Costa, G. L. Gessa, and M. Sandler, eds.,) Vol. 11, pp. 1–10, Raven Press, New York.

Gál, E. M., 1975, Hydroxylation of tryptophan and its control in brain, *Pavlovian J. Biol. Sci.* **10**:145–160.

Gál, E. M., and Roggeveen, A. E., 1973, Cerebral hydroxylases: Stimulation by a new factor, *Science* **179**:809–811.

Gál, E. M., and Sherman, A. D., 1976, Biopterin II: Evidence for cerebral synthesis of 7,8-dihydrobiopterin *in vivo* and *in vitro*, *Neurochem. Res.* **1**:627–639.

Gál, E. M., and Sherman, A. D., 1977a, Rapid isolation and quantitation of biopterin, neopterin, and their guanine ribotide precursor from biological samples, *Prep. Biochem.* **7**(2):155–164.

Gál, E. M., and Sherman, A. D., 1977b, Biosynthesis and control of pterins in the brain, in: *Structure and Function of Monoamine Enzymes* (E. Usdin, N. Weiner, and M. Youdim, eds.) pp. 23–42, Marcel Dekker, New York.

Gál, E. M., and Sherman, A. D., 1978a, Biosynthesis of reduced biopterins: Effect of methotrexate, *Fed. Proc. Fed. Am. Soc. Exp.* **37**:1346.

Gál, E. M., and Sherman, A. D., 1978b, Phosphorylation, a factor controlling the synthesis of L-erythro-dihydrobiopterin (BH$_2$), *Biochem. Biophys. Res. Commun.* **83**:593–598.

Gál, E. M., and Whitacre, D. H., 1981, Biopterin VII: Inhibition of synthesis of reduced biopterins and its bearing on the function of cerebral tryptophan-5 hydroxylase *in vivo, Neurochem. Res.* **6**:233–241.

Gál, E. M., Armstrong, J. C., and Ginsberg, B., 1966, The nature of *in vitro* hydroxylation of L-tryptophan by brain tissue, *J. Neurochem.* **13**:643–654.

Gál, E. M., Hanson, G., and Sherman, A. D., 1976, Biopterin I: Profile and quantitation in rat brain, *Neurochem. Res.* **1**:511–523.

Gál, E. M., Nelson, J. M., and Sherman, A. D., 1978a, Biopterin III: Purification and characterization of enzymes involved in the cerebral synthesis of 7,8-dihydrobiopterin, *Neurochem. Res.* **3**:69–88.

Gál, E. M., Henn, F. A., and Sherman, A. D., 1978b, Biopterin IV: Regional and subcellular aspects of L-erythro-7,8-dihydrobiopterin synthesis in brain, *Neurochem. Res.* **3**:493–499.

Gál, E. M., Young, R. B., and Sherman, A. D., 1978c, Tryptophan loading: Consequent effects on the synthesis of Kynurenine and 5-hydroxyindoles in rat brain, *J. Neurochem.* **31**:237–244.

Gál, E. M., Bybee, J. A., and Sherman, A. D., 1979a, Biopterin V: *De novo* synthesis of dihydrobiopterin: Evidence for its quinonoid structure and lack of dependence of its reduction to tetrahydrobiopterin on dihydrofolate reductase, *J. Neurochem.* **32**:179–186.

Gál, E. M., Dawson, M. R., Dudley, D. T., and Sherman, A. D., 1979b, Biopterin VI: Purification and sequence of the primary structure of mammalian D-erythro-7,8-dihydroneopterin triphosphate synthetase, *Neurochem. Res.* **4**:605–625.

Gerhart, J. D., and MacIntyre, R. J., 1970, Quantification of drosopterins in single eyes of *Drosophila melanogaster, Anal. Biochem.* **37**:21–25.

Guroff, G., and Strenkoski, C. A., 1966, Biosynthesis of pteridines and of phenylalanine hydroxylase cofactor in cell-free extracts of *Pseudomonas* species (ATCC 11299a), *J. Biol. Chem.* **241**:2220–2227.

Guroff, G., Rhoads, C. A., and Abramowitz, A., 1967, A simple radioisotope assay for phenylalanine hydroxylase cofactor, *Anal. Biochem.* **21**:273–278.

Hadorn, E., and Mitchell, H. K., 1951, Properties of mutants of *Drosophila melanogaster* and changes during development as revealed by paper chromatography, *Proc. Nat. Acad. Sci. U.S.A.* **37**:650–665.

Hagerman, D. D., 1964, Pteridine cofactors in enzymatic hydroxylation of steroids, *Fed. Proc. Fed. Am. Soc. Exp.* **23**:480.

Hama, T., 1953, Substances fluorescentes du type ptérinique dans la peau ou les yeux de la grenouille *(Rana nigromaculata)* et leurs transformation photochimiques, *Experientia* **8**:299–302.

Hama, T., 1963, The relation between the chromatophores and pterin compounds, *Ann. N.Y. Acad. Sci.* **100**:997–986.

Hamilton, G. A., 1974, Chemical models and mechanisms for oxygenases, in: *Molecular Mechanism of Oxygen Activation* (O. Hayaishi, ed.), pp. 405–451, Academic Press, New York.

Hamon, M., Bourgoin, S., Hery, F., Ternaux, J. P., and Glowinski, J., 1976, *In vivo* and *in vitro* activation of soluble tryptophan hydroxylase from rat brain stem, *Nature London* **260**:61–63.

Hamor, T. A., and Robertson, J. M., 1956, The crystal and molecular structure of pteridines, *J. Chem. Soc.,* 3586–3594.

Hasegawa, H., Matsura, S., Nagatsu, T., Ichiyama, A., and Imaizumi, 1978, Cofactor activity of diastereoisomers of tetrahydrobiopterin, Abstract, 6th International Symposium on the Chemistry and Biology of Pteridines, p. 44.

Haug, P., 1970, Mass spectral fragmentation of trimethylsilyl derivatives of 2-amino-4-hydroxypteridines, *Anal. Biochem.* **37**:285–292.

van der Have-Kirchberg, M. L. L., de Morée, A., van Laar, J. F., Gerwig, G. J., Versluis, C., Ebels, I., Haus-Citharel, A., L'Heritier, A., Roseau, S., Zurbrug, W., and Moszkowska, A., 1977, Separation of pineal extracts by gelfiltration. VI. Isolation and identification from sheep pineals of biopterin: comparison of the isolated compound with some synthetic pteridines and the biological activity in *in vitro* and *in vivo* bioassays, *J. Neural Transm.* **40**:205–220.

Hems, G., 1958, Effect of ionizing radiation on aqueous solutions of guanylic acid and guanosine, *Nature London* **181**:1721–1722.

Hillcoat, B. L., and Blakley, R. L., 1964, The reduction of folate by borohydride and dithionite, *Biochem. Biophys. Res. Commun.* **15**:303–307.

Hirata, F., Hayaishi, O., Tokuyama, T., and Senoh, S., 1974, *In vitro* and *in vivo* formation of two new metabolites of melatonin, *J. Biol. Chem.* **249**:1311–1313.

Hopkins, F. G., 1889, Note on a yellow pigment in butterflies, *Nature London* **40**:335.

Huang, C. Y., and Kaufman, S., 1973, Studies on the mechanism of action of phenylalanine hydroxylase and its protein stimulator. I. Enzyme concentration dependence of the specific activity of phenylalanine hydroxylase due to a non-enzymatic step, *J. Biol. Chem.* **248**:4242–4251.

Ikeda, M., Levitt, M., and Udenfriend, S., 1965, Hydroxylation of phenylalanine by purified preparations of adrenal and brain tyrosine hydroxylase, *Biochem. Biophys. Res. Commun.* **18**:482–488.

Ikeda, M., Fahien, L. A., and Udenfriend, S., 1966, A kinetic study of bovine adrenal tyrosine hydroxylase, *J. Biol. Chem.* **241**:4552–4456.

Iwai, K., Akino, M., Gota, M., and Iwanami, Y., 1970, *Chemistry and Biology of Pteridines,* pp. 1–473, International Academic Printing, Tokyo.

Iwanami, Y., and Akino, M., 1975, Evidence for enedial form of sepiapterin, *J. Nutr. Sci. Vitaminol.* **21**:143–145.

Jackson, R. J., and Shiota, T., 1971, Identification of the isomer of dihydroneopterin triphosphate synthesized by two enzyme fractions of Lactobacillus plantarum, *J. Biol. Chem.* **246**:7454–7459.

Jedlicki, E., Kaufman, S., and Milstien, S., 1977, Partial purification and characterization of rat liver phenylalanine hydroxylase phosphatase, *J. Biol. Chem.* **252**:7711–7714.

Jones, T. H. D., and Brown, G. M., 1967, The biosynthesis of folic acid. VII. Enzymatic synthesis of pteridines from guanosine triphosphate, *J. Biol. Chem.* **242**:3989–3997.

Katoh, S., 1971, Sepiapterin reductase from horse liver: Purification and properties of the enzyme, *Arch. Biochem. Biophys.* **146**:202–214.

Katoh, S., Nagai, M., Nagai, Y., Fukushima, T., and Akino, M., 1970, Some new biochemical aspects of sepiapterin and sepiapterin reductase, in: *Chemistry and Biology of Pteridines,*

(K. Iwai, M. Akino, M. Goto, and Y. Iwanami, eds.), pp. 225–234, International Academic Printing, Tokyo.

Kaufman, S., 1956, The enzymatic conversion of phenylalanine to tyrosine, *J. Biol. Chem.* **226**:511–524.

Kaufman, S., 1958, A new cofactor required for the enzymatic conversion of phenylalanine to tyrosine, *J. Biol. Chem.* **230**:931–939.

Kaufman, S., 1959, Studies on the mechanism of the enzymatic conversion of phenylalanine to tyrosine, *J. Biol. Chem.* **234**:2677–2682.

Kaufman, S., 1961, The nature of the primary oxidation product formed from tetrahydropteridines during phenylalanine hydroxylation, *J. Biol. Chem.* **236**:804–810.

Kaufman, S., 1962, On the structure of the phenylalanine hydroxylation cofactor, *J. Biol. Chem.* **237**:2712–2713.

Kaufman, S., 1963, The structure of phenylalanine hydroxylase cofactor, *Proc. Nat. Acad. Sci. U.S.A.* **50**:1085–1092.

Kaufman, S., 1964, Studies on the structure of the primary oxidation product formed from tetrahydropteridines during phenylalanine hydroxylation, *J. Biol. Chem.* **239**:332–338.

Kaufman, S., 1967*a*, Metabolism of phenylalanine hydroxylation cofactor, *J. Biol. Chem.* **242**:3934–3943.

Kaufman, S., 1967*b*, Pteridine cofactors, *Annu. Rev. Biochem.* **36**:171–184.

Kaufman, S., 1970, A protein that stimulates rat liver phenylalanine hydroxylase, *J. Biol. Chem.* **245**:4751–4759.

Kaufman, S., 1971, The phenylalanine hydroxylating system from mammalian liver, in: *Advances in Enzymology* (A. Meister, ed.), Vol. 35, pp. 245–319, Wiley Interscience, New York.

Kaufman, S., 1973, Cofactors of tyrosine hydroxylase, in: *Frontiers in Catecholanine Research* (E. Usdin and S. Snyder, eds.), pp. 53–60, Pergamon Press, Oxford.

Kaufman, S., 1975, Studies on the mechanism of phenylalanine hydroxylase: Detection of an intermediate, in: *Chemistry and Biology of Pteridines* (W. Pfleiderer, ed.), pp. 291–303, W. du Gruyter, Berlin.

Kaufman, S., 1977, Phenylketonuria: Biochemical aspects, in: *Advances in Neurochemistry* (B. W. Agranoff and M. H. Aprison, eds.), Vol. 2, pp. 1–116, Plenum Press, New York.

Kaufman, S., and Fisher, D. B., 1974, Pterin-requiring aromatic amino acid hydroxylases, in: *Molecular Mechanisms of Oxygen Activation* (O. Hayaishi, ed.), pp. 285–369, Academic Press, New York.

Kaufman, S., Holtzman, N. A., Milstien, S., Butler, L. J., Kurmholz, A., 1975, Phenylketonuria due to a deficiency of dihydropteridine reductase, *N. Engl. J. Med.* **293**:785–790.

Kidder, G. W., Dewey, V. C., and Rembold, H., 1964, Source of unconjugated pteridines in *Crithidia*, *Fed. Proc. Fed. Am. Soc. Exp.* **23**:529.

Koschara, W., 1936, Isolierung eines gelben Farbstoffs (Uropterin) aus Menschenharn, *Hoppe Seylers Z. Physiol. Chem.* **240**:127–151.

Kraut, H., Pabst, W., Rembold, H., and Wildemann, L., 1963, Uber das verhalten des biopterins im Saugetier-organismus. I. Bilanz- und wachstumsersuche an Ratten, *Z. Physiol. Chem.* **332**:101–108.

Krumdieck, C. L., Shaw, E., and Baugh, C. M., 1966, The biosynthesis of 2-amino-4-hydroxy-6-substituted pteridines, *J. Biol. Chem.* **241**:383–387.

Kuczenski, R., and Mandell, A. J., 1972, Regulatory properties of soluble and particulate rat brain tyrosine hydroxylase, *J. Biol. Chem.* **247**:3114–3122.

La Du, B. N., Jr., Fineberg, R. A., Gál, E. M., and Greenberg, D. M., 1950, Toxicity of some synthetic pteridines in rats, *Proc. Soc. Exp. Biol. Med.* **73**:107–109.

Lee, C., Fukushima, T., and Nixon, J. C., 1979, Biosynthesis of biopterin in rat brain, Abstract, 6th International Symposium on the Chemistry and Biology of Pteridines, p. 31.

Leeming, R. J., Blair, J. A., Melikian, V., and O'Gorman, D. J., 1976a, Biopterin derivatives in human body fluids and tissues, *J. Clin. Pathol.* **29**:444–451.

Leeming, R. J., Blair, J. A., Green, A., and Raine, D. N., 1976b, Biopterin derivatives in normal and phenylketonuric patients after oral loads of L-phenylalanine, L-tyrosine, and L-tryptophan, *Arch. Dis. Child.* **51**:771–777.

Lehmann, K. T., 1965, Isolierung und Identifizierung von Stoffwechsel-produkten des Triamterenes, *Arzneim. Forsch.* **15**:812–816.

Levy, C. C., 1964, Pteridine metabolism in the skin of the tadpole, *Rana catesbeiana, J. Biol. Chem.* **239**:560–566.

Lind, K. E., 1972, Dihydropteridine reductase—Investigation of the specificity of quinonoid dihydropteridine and the inhibition by 2,4-diaminopteridines, *Eur. J. Biochem.* **25**:560–562.

Lloyd, T., and Kaufman, S., 1974, The stimulation of partially purified bovine caudate tyrosine hydroxylase by phosphatidyl-L-serine, *Biochem. Biophys. Res. Commun.* **59**:1262–1269.

Lloyd, T., and Weiner, N., 1971, Isolation and characterization of tyrosine hydroxylase from bovine adrenal medulla, *Mol. Pharmacol.* **7**:569–580.

Lloyd, T., Markey, S., and Weiner, N., 1971, Identification of 2-amino-4-hydroxy-substituted pteridines by gas-liquid chromatography and mass spectrometry, *Anal. Biochem.* **42**:108–112.

Loo, T. L., and Adamson, R. H., 1965, The metabolite of 3′,5′-dichloro-4-amino-4-deoxy- N^{10}-methylpteroylglutamic acid (dichloromethotrexate) *J. Med. Chem.* **8**:513–515.

Lovenberg, W., Jequier, E., and Sjoerdsma, A., 1967, Tryptophan hydroxylation: Measurement in pineal gland, brain stem, and carcinoid tumor, *Science* **155**:217–219.

Lovenberg, W., Bruckwick, E. A., Hanbauer, I., 1975, ATP, cyclic AMP, and magnesium increase the affinity of rat striatal tyrosine hydroxylase for its cofactor, *Proc. Natl. Acad. Sci. U.S.A.* **72**:2955–2958.

Lund, H., 1975, Electrochemistry of pteridines, in: *Chemistry and Biology of Pteridines* (W. Pfleiderer, ed.), pp. 645–670, W. de Gruyter, Berlin.

Lynn, R., Rueter, M. E., and Guynn, R. W., 1977, Mammalian brain dihydrofolate reductase, *J. Neurochem.* **29**:1147–1149.

Mager, H. I. X., 1975, Autooxidative conversions of tetrahydropteridines and some related ring systems, in: *Chemistry and Biology of Pteridines* (W. Pfleiderer, ed.) pp. 753–771, W. de Gruyter, Berlin.

Mager, H. I. X., and Berends, W., 1965, Hydroperoxides of partially reduced quinoxalines, pteridines and (iso) alloxazines: Intermediates in oxidation processes, *Rev. Trav. Chim.* **84**:1329–1343.

Mandell, A. J., 1978, Redundant mechanisms regulating brain tyrosine and tryptophan hydroxylases, *Annu. Rev. Pharmacol. Toxicol.* **18**:461–493.

Matsubara, M., and Akino, M., 1964, On the presence of sepiapterin reductase different from folate and dihydrofolate reductase in chicken liver, *Experientia* **20**:574–575.

Matsubara, M., Katoh, S., Akino, M., and Kaufman, S., 1966, Sepiapterin reductase, *Biochem. Biophys. Acta* **122**:202–212.

McGeer, E. G., Gibson, S., and McGeer, P. L., 1967, Some characteristics of brain tyrosine hydroxylase, *Can. J. Biochem.* **45**:1557–1563.

McNutt, W. S., 1964, A spectrophotometric test for xanthopterin, *Anal. Chem.* **36**:912–914.

Millard, S. A., Kubose, A., and Gál, E. M., 1969, Brain lipoyl dehydrogenase. Purification, properties and inhibitors, *J. Biol. Chem.* **244**:2511–2515.

Milstien, S., Orloff, S., Spielberg, S., Berlow, S., Schulman, J. D., Kaufman, S., 1977, Hyperphenylalaninemia due to phenylalanine hydroxylase cofactor deficiency, *Ped. Res.* **11**:460.

Musacchio, J. M., Craviso, G. L., and Wurzburger, R., 1972, Dihydropteridine reductase in the rat brain, *Life Sci.* **11**:267–276.

Nagai, (Matsubara) M., 1968, Studies on sepiapterin reductase: Further characterization of the reaction product, *Arch. Biochem. Biophys.* **126**:426–435.

Nagatsu, T., Levitt, M., and Udenfriend, S., 1964, Tyrosine hydroxylase. The initial step in norepinephrine biosynthesis, *J. Biol. Chem.* **239**:2910–2917.

Nagatsu, T., Mizutani, K., Nagatsu, I., Matsuura, S., and Sugimoto, T., 1972*a*, Pteridines as cofactor or inhibitor of tyrosine hydroxylase, *Biochem. Pharmacol.* **21**:1945–1953.

Nagatsu, T., Mizutani, K., Sudo, Y., and Nagatsu, I., 1972*b*, Tyrosine hydroxylase in human adrenal glands and human pheochromocytoma, *Clin. Chim. Acta* **39**:417–424.

Nakamura, S., Ichiyama, A., and Hayaishi, O., 1965, Purification and properties of tryptophan hydroxylase in brain, *Fed. Proc. Fed. Am. Soc. Exp.* **24**:604.

Nathan, H. A., and Cowperthwaite, I., 1955, "Crithidia factor." A new member of the folic acid group of vitamins, *J. Protozool.* **2**:37–42.

Nawa, S., Matsuura, S., and Hirata, Y. J., 1953, Studies on pteridines. V. Reductive cleavage of pteridyl side chains, *J. Am. Chem. Soc.* **75**:4450–4451.

Nicolaus, B. J. R., 1960, Anwendung der Dünnschichtchromatographie auf Pteridine, *J. Chromatogr.* **4**:384–390.

Niederwieser, A., Curtius, H.-Ch., Bettoni, O., Bieri, J., Schircks, B., Viscontini, M., and Schaub, J., 1979, Atypical phenylketonuria caused by 7,8-dihydrobiopterin synthetase deficiency, *Lancet* 131–133.

Niiderwieser, A., Curtis, H.-Ch., Gitzelmann, R., Otten, A., Baerlocher, K., Blehova, B., Berlow, S., Grobe, H., Rey, F., Schaub, J., Scheibenreiter, S., Schmidt, H., and Viscontini, M., 1980, Excretion of pterins in phenylketonuria an phenylketonuria variants, *Helv. Paediatr. Acta* **35**:335–342.

Nielsen, K. H., 1969, Rat liver phenylalanine hydroxylase: A method for the measurement of activity, with particular reference to the distinctive features of the enzyme and the pteridine cofactor, *Eur. J. Biochem.* **7**:360–369.

Nishikimi, M., 1975, A function of tetrahydropteridines as cofactors for indolamine 2,3-dioxygenase, *Biochem. Biophys. Res. Commun.* **63**:92–98.

Numata (Sudo), Y., Kato, T., Nagatsu, T., Sugimoto, T., and Matsuura, S., 1977, Effects of stereochemical structures of tetrahydrobiopterin on tyrosine hydroxylase, *Biochim. Biophys. Acta* **480**:104–112.

Okada, T., and Goto, M., 1965, Syntheses of 2-amino-4-hydroxy-6-hydroxymethylpteridine-[10-^{14}C] and 2-amino-4-hydroxypteridine-[10-^{14}C] and their metabolism in *Drosophila melanogaster*, *J. Biochem. Tokyo* **58**:458–462.

Ortiz, E., Throckmorton, L. H., and Williams-Ashman, H. G., 1962, Drosopterins in the throatfans of some Puerto Rican lizards, *Nature London* **196**:595–596.

Pabst, W., and Rembold, H., 1966, Uber das Verhalten der Biopterins im Säugetierorganismus II. Einfluss vom Vitaminmangel und eines Antagonisten auf die Biopterin-ausscheidung und das Wachstum in der Ratte, *Z. Physiol. Chem.* **344**:107–112.

Patterson, E. L., Broquist, H. P., Albrecht, A. M., von Saltza, M. H., and Stokstad, E. K. R., 1955, A new pteridine in urine required for the growth of the protozoon *Crithidia fasciculata*, *J. Am. Chem. Soc.* **77**:3167–3168.

Pearson, A. J., and Blair, J. A., 1975, Autoxidation of tetrahydropterins, in: *Chemistry and Biology of Pteridines* (W. Pfleiderer, ed.), pp. 775–793, W. du Gruyter, Berlin.

Pfleiderer, W., 1957, Pteridine II. Uber 7-Hydroxy und 7-Hydroxy-6-methyl-2,4-dioxo-tetrahydropteridine, *Chem. Ber.* **90**:2588–2603.

Pfleiderer, W., 1964, Recent developments in the chemistry of pteridines, *Angew. Chem. Int. Ed. Engl.* **3**:114–132.

Pfleiderer, W., (ed.), 1975, *Chemistry and Biology of Pteridines*, 941 pp, W. de Gruyter, Berlin.

Pfleiderer, W., and Taylor, E. C., 1964, *Pteridine Chemistry,* Pergamon Press, Oxford.

Pfleiderer, W., Liedek, E., Lohrmann, R., and Rukwied, M., 1960, Pteridine X. Zur Struktur des Pterins, *Chem. Ber.* **93**:2015–2024.

Philipsborn, W. V., Stierlin, H., and Traber, W., 1964, Über die Protonen-resonanz-spektren von Pteridinen, in: *Pteridine Chemistry* (W. Pfleiderer and E. C. Taylor, eds.), pp. 169–179, Pergamon Press, Oxford.

Purrmann, R., 1940, Über die Flügelpigmente der Schmitterlinge. VII. Synthese des Leukopterins und Natur des Guanopterins, *Liebig's Ann. Chem.* **544**:182–190.

Purrmann, R., 1941, Konstitution und Synthese des sogenannten anhydroleucopterins. XII., *Liebig's Ann. Chem.* **548**:284–292.

Rembold, H., 1964, Untersuchungen über den Stoffwechsel des Biopterins und über die polarographishce Characterizierung von Pteridinen, in: *Pteridine Chemistry* (W. Pfleiderer and E. C. Taylor, eds.), pp. 465–484, Pergamon Press, Oxford.

Rembold, H., 1970, Catabolism of unconjugated pteridines, in: *Chemistry and Biology of Pteridines* (K. Iwai, M. Akino, M. Goto, and Y. Iwanami, eds.), pp. 163–178, International Academic Printing, Tokyo.

Rembold, H., and Buff, K., 1972, Tetrahydrobiopterin, a cofactor in mitochondrial electron transfer. Effect of tetrahydrobiopterin on intact rat liver mitochondria, *Eur. J. Biochem.* **28**:579–585.

Rembold, H., and Buschmann, L., 1962, Trennung von 2-amino-4-hydroxy pteridine durch Ionenaustauschen-chromatographie, *Hoppe Seylers Z. Physiol. Chem.* **330**:132–139.

Rembold, H., and Buschmann, L., 1963, Untersuchungen über die Pteridine der Bienenpuppe (Apis Mellifica), *Liebig's Ann. Chem.* **662**:72–82.

Rembold, H., and Gutensohn, W., 1968, 6-hydroxylation of the pteridine ring by xanthine oxidase, *Biochem. Biophys. Res. Commun.* **31**:837–841.

Rembold, H., and Gyure, W. L., 1972, Biochemistry of pteridines, *Angew. Chem. Int. Ed. Engl.* **11**:1061–1072.

Rembold, H., and Metzger, H., 1967*a*, Activierung von Biopterin in der Ratte, *Z. Naturforsch.* **22**:827–830.

Rembold, H., and Metzger, H., 1967*b*, On the behavior of biopterins in the mammalian organism. II. Effect of vitamin deficiency and of an antagonist on biopterin differentiation and on the growth of the rat, *Hoppe Seylers Z. Physiol. Chem.* **344**:107–112.

Rembold, H., Metzger, H., Sudershan, P., and Gutensohn, W., 1969, Catabolism of pteridine cofactors. I. Properties and metabolism in rat liver homogenates of tetrahydrobiopterin and tetrahydroneopterin, *Biochem. Biophys. Acta* **184**:386–396.

Rembold, H., and Simmersbach, F., 1969, Catabolism of pteridine cofactors. II. A specific pterin deaminase in rat liver, *Biochem. Biophys. Acta* **184**:589–596.

Rembold, H., Metzger, H., Sudershan, P., and Gutensohn, W., 1969, Catabolism of pteridine cofactors. I. Properties and metabolism in rat liver homogenates of tetrahydrobiopterin and tetrahydroneopterin, *Biochem. Biophys. Acta* **184**:386–396.

Rembold, H., Metzger, H., and Gutensohn, W., 1971*a*, Catabolism of pteridine cofactors. III. On the introduction of an oxygen function into position 6 of the pteridine ring, *Biochem. Biophys. Acta* **230**:117–126.

Rembold, H., Chandrashekar, V., and Sudershan, P., 1971*b*, Catabolism of pteridine cofactors. IV. *In vivo* catabolism of reduced pterins in rats, *Biochem. Biophys. Acta* **237**:365–368.

Rembold, H., Buff, K., and Hernings, G., 1977, Specificity and binding capacity of human blood serum for tetrahydropterins, *Clin. Chim. Acta* **76**:329–338.

Rey, F., Harpey, J. P., Leeming, R. J., Blair, J. A., Aicardi, J., and Rey, J., 1977, Les hyperphenylalaninemies avec acticité normale de la phenylalanine-hydroxylase, *Arch. Fr. Pediatr.*, **34**:109–120.

Röthler, F., and Karobath, M., 1976, Quantitative determination of unconjugated pterins in urine by gas chromatography/mass fragmentography, *Clin. Chim. Acta* **69**:457–462.

Samuelsson, B., 1972, Biosynthesis of prostaglandins, *Fed. Proc. Fed. Am. Soc. Exp. Biol.* **31**:1442–1450.

Scrimgeour, K. G., and Cheema, S., 1971, Discussion paper: Quinonoid dihydropterin reductase, *Ann. N.Y. Acad. Sci.* **186**:115–118.

Sherman, A. D., and Gál, E. M., 1979, Lack of dependence of amine or prostaglandin biosynthesis on absolute cerebral level of pteridine cofactor, *Life Sci.* **23**:1675–1680.

Shiota, T., 1971, The biosynthesis of folic acid and 6-substituted pteridine derivatives, in: *Comprehensive Biochemistry* (M. Florkin and E. H. Stotz, eds.), Vol. 21. Chapter 1, pp. 111–152.

Shiota, T., Palumbo, M. P., and Tsai, L., 1967, A chemically prepared formamidopyrimidine derivative of guanosine triphosphate as a possible intermediate in pteridine biosynthesis, *J. Biol. Chem.* **242**:1961–1969.

Shiota, T., Baugh, C. M., and Myrick, J., 1969, The assignment of structure to the formamidopyrimidine nucleotide triphosphate precursor of pteridines, *Biochem. Biophys. Acta* **192**:205–210.

Shiota, T., Jackson, R., and Baugh, C. M., 1970, The biosynthetic pathway of dehydrofolate, in: *Chemistry and Biology of Pterins* (K. Iwai, M. Akino, M. Goto, and Y. Iwanami, eds.), pp. 264–269, International Academic Printing, Tokyo.

Snady, H., and Musacchio, J. M., 1978a, Quinonoid dihydropterin reductase. I. Purification and characterization of the bovine brain enzyme, *Biochem. Pharmacol.* **27**:1939–1945.

Snady, H., and Musacchio, J. M., 1978b, Quinonoid dihydropterin reductase. II. Regional and subcellular distribution of rat brain enzyme, *Biochem. Pharmacol.* **27**:1947–1953.

Spector, R., Levy, P., and Abelson, H. T., 1977, Identification of dihydrofolate reductase in rabbit brain, *Biochem. Pharmacol.* **26**:1507–1511.

Spector, S., Gordon, R., Sjoersdma, R., and Udenfriend, S., 1967, End-product inhibition of tyrosine hydroxylase as a possible mechanism for regulation of norepinephrine synthesis, *Mol. Pharmacol.* **3**:549–555.

Stokstad, E. L. R., and Koch, J., 1967, Folic acid metabolism, *Physiol. Rev.* **47**:83–116.

Stone, K. J., 1976, The role of tetrahydrofolate dehydrogenase in the hepatic supply of tetrahydrobiopterin in rats, *Biochem. J.* **157**:105–109.

Storm, C. B., and Kaufman, S., 1968, The effect of variation of cofactor and substrate structure on the action of phenylalanine hydroxylase, *Biochem. Biophys. Res. Commun.* **32**:788–793.

Sugiura, K., and Goto, M., 1967, Biosynthesis of pteridines in *D. melanogaster, Biochem. Biophys. Res. Commun.* **28**:687–691.

Sugiura, K., and Goto, M., 1968, Biosynthesis of pteridines in the skin of the tadpole, *Rana catesbeiana, J. Biochem. Tokyo* **64**:657–666.

Sugiura, K., and Goto, M., 1973, Uber biosynthese von biopterin in säugetieren, *Experientia* **29**:1481–1482.

Swenseid, M. E., Wittle, E. L., Moersch, G. W., Bird, O. D., and Brown, R. A., 1949, Hematologic effect in rats of pterins structurally related to pteroylglutamic acid, *J. Biol. Chem.* **179**:1175–1182.

Taira, T., 1961, Enzymatic reduction of the yellow pigment of *Drosophila, Nature London* **189**:231–232.

Tauro, G. P., Danks, D. M., Rowe, P. B., van der Weyden, M. B., Schwartz, M. A., Collins, V. L., and Neal, B. W., 1976, Dihydrofolate reductase deficiency causing megaloblastic anaemia in two families, *New Engl. J. Med.* **294**:466–470.

Taylor, D., and Hochstein, P., 1975, Tetrahydrobiopterin: Reduction of cytochrome C and coupled phosphorylation at mitochondrial site 3, *Biochem. Biophys. Res. Commun.* **67**:156–162.

Taylor, E. C., and Jacobi, P. A., 1974, An unequivocal total synthesis of L-erythro-biopterin, *J. Am. Chem. Soc.* **96**:6781–6782.

Taylor, E. C., and Jacobi, P. A., 1977, Pteridines. XXXVII. A total synthesis of L-erythro-biopterin and some related 6-(polyhydroxyalkyl) pterins, *J. Am. Chem. Soc.* **98**:2301–2307.

Tietz, A., Lindberg, M., and Kennedy, E. P., 1964, A new pteridine-regin-ring enzyme system for the oxidation of glyceryl ethers, *J. Biol. Chem.* **239**:4081–4090.

Tong, J. H., and Kaufman, S., 1975, Tryptophan hydroxylase. Purification and some properties of the enzyme from rabbit hindbrain, *J. Biol. Chem.* **250**:4152–4158.

Tozer, T. N., Neff, N. H., and Brodie, B. B., 1966, Application of steady state kinetics to the synthesis rate and turnover time of serotonin in the brain of normal and reserpine treated rats, *J. Pharmacol. Exp. Ther.* **153**:177–182.

Tsuda, H., Noguchi, T., and Kido, R., 1972, 5-hydroxytryptophan pyrrolase in rat brain, *J. Neurochem.* **19**:887–890.

Turner, A. J., Ponzio, F., and Algeri, S., 1974, Dihydropteridine reductase in rat brain: Regional distribution and the effect of catecholamine-depleting drugs, *Brain Res.* **70**:553–558.

Turner, A. J., 1977, The roles of folate and pteridine derivatives in neurotransmitter metabolism, *Biochem. Pharmacol.* **26**:1009–1014.

Udenfriend, S., Zaltman-Nirenberg, P., and Nagatsu, T., 1965, Inhibitors of purified beef adrenal tyrosine hydroxylase, *Biochem. Pharmacol.* **14**:837–845.

Uyeda, K., and Rabinowitz, J. C., 1963, Fluorescence properties of tetrahydrofolate and related compounds, *Anal. Biochem.* **6**:100–108.

Valerino, D. M., and McCormack, J. J., 1969, Studies of the oxidation of some amino-pteridines by xanthine oxidase, *Biochim. Biophys. Acta* **184**:154–163.

Viscontini, M., and Schmidt, G. H. Z., 1965, Über die physiologische Bedeutung der Pteridine, *Z. Naturforsch. Teil B* **20**:327–331.

Viscontini, M., and Bobst, A., 1965, De la chimie des pterines sur la mécanisme d'oxydation des tetrahydroptérines en dihydroptérins á pH physiologique, *Helv. Chim. Acta* **48**:816–819.

Vonderschmitt, D. J., and Scrimgeour, K. G., 1967, Reaction of Cu^{2+} and Fe^{3+} with tetrahydropteridines, *Biochem. Biophys. Res. Commun.* **28**:302–308.

Vonderschmitt, D. J., Vitols, K. S., Huennekens, F. M., and Scrimgeour, K. G., 1967, Addition of bisulfite to folate and dihydrofolate, *Arch. Biochem. Biophys.* **122**:488–493.

Watson, B. M., Schlesinger, P., and Cotton, R. G. H., 1977, Dihydroxanthopterinuria in phenylketonuria and lethal hyperphenylalaninemia patients, *Clin. Chim. Acta* **78**:417–423.

Weygand, F., Simon, H., Dahms, G., Waldschmidt, M., Schliep, H. J., and Wacker, H., 1961, Über die Biogenese des Leucopterins, *Angew. Chem.* **73**:402–407.

Whiteley, J. M., and Huennekens, F. M., 1967, 2-amino-4-hydroxy-6-methyl-7,8-dihydropteridine as a model for dihydrofolate, *Biochemistry* **6**:2620–2625.

Wieland, H., and Schöpf, C., 1925, Über den gelben Flügelfarbstoff des Zitronenfalters (Gonepteryx rhamni), *Ber Dtsch. Chem. Ges.* **58**:2978–2183.

Yamamoto, S., and Hayaishi, O., 1967, Tryptophan pyrrolase of rabbit intestine D- and L-tryptophan cleaving enzyme or enzymes, *J. Biol. Chem.* **242**:5260–5266.

Yim, J. J., and Brown, G. M., 1976, Characteristics of guanosine triphosphate cyclohydrolase I purified from *Escherichia Coli, J. Biol Chem.* **251**:5087–5094.

Ziegler, I., 1964, Über natürlich vorkommende Tetrahydropteridinen, in: *Pteridine Chemistry* (W. Pfleiderer, and E. C. Taylor, eds.), pp. 295–305, Pergamon Press, Oxford.

Ziegler, I., and Harmsen, R., 1969, The biology of pteridines in insects, *Adv. Insect. Physiol.* **6**:139–203.

Zivkovic, B., Guidotti, A., and Costa, E., 1975, Effects of neuroleptics on striatal tyrosine hydroxylase: Changes in affinity for the pteridine cofactor, *Mol. Pharmacol.* **10**:727–735.

THE GANGLIOSIDES

HERBERT WIEGANDT

Physiologisch Chemisches Institut
Philipps Universität Marburg
Marburg, German Federal Republic

1. INTRODUCTION

Gangliosides are glycosphingolipids that contain sialic acid (N-acetyl- or N-glycolylneuraminic acid). They have elicited much interest since their discovery for a number of reasons. Gangliosides are typically found as membrane constituents in brain, a finding that suggests a specific functional role in the central nervous system (CNS). Furthermore, it has long been recognized that certain lipidoses that affect the nervous system, such as Tay Sachs disease, are characterized by ganglioside accumulation within cells of the brain. Further evidence for involvement of gangliosides in nervous system function is indicated by the behavior of the neurotoxin of *Clostridium tetani*. This toxin is specifically absorbed by the brain, and the property is believed to relate to the brain's ganglioside content (Wassermann and Takaki, 1898; W. E. van Heyningen, 1974). The elucidation of the chemical composition of sialic acid was accompanied by the recognition that it has specific biological properties and that the gangliosides are frequently the glycoconjugate carrier. More recently, it has become evident that gangliosides are ubiquitous, i.e., occurring not only in the nervous system, and should be considered important constituents of the surface membrane of most, perhaps all, animal cells of *Deuterostomia*.

In recent years a large number of detailed original reports as well as reviews have appeared dealing with various aspects of glycosphingolipids, including the gangliosides. This review is limited specifically to gangliosides and no attempt is made to cite recent surveys with broader scopes. The present review extends and updates a similar past effort of the author (Wiegandt, 1968).

2. CHEMISTRY AND ANALYSIS OF GANGLIOSIDES

2.1. Chemical Composition

The content of one or more sialic acid residues as a constituent carbohydrate distinguishes gangliosides from other glycosphingolipids. All consist of a long chain base, a "sphingoid," that is linked to fatty acid by an amide, thus forming the lipophilic "ceramide" portion. The sphingoid's primary hydroxyl carries the carbohydrate in a glycosidic linkage

$$CH_3 \cdot (CH_2)_{12} \cdot CH = CH \cdot CH(OH) \cdot CH \cdot CH_2 \cdot O \cdot glycosyl$$
$$\underset{\displaystyle acyl \cdot NH}{|}$$

Whereas the ceramide of glycosphingolipids shows microheterogeneity with regard to the sphingoid (Karlsson, 1970a,b) and the fatty acid, as do the lipophilic portion of other lipids, in most instances gangliosides have been isolated and characterized on the basis of their carbohydrate structures.

In general the glycosphingolipids may be classified in series according to their presumed biogenic relations, i.e., the sequential addition of monosaccharides to a ceramide and a growing sugar chain via glucosylceramide or galactosylceramide (Figure 1).

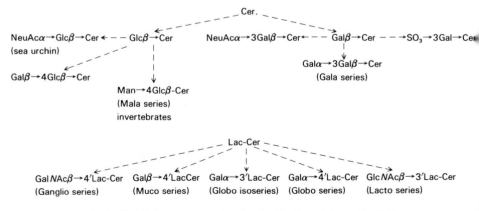

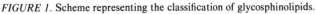
FIGURE 1. Scheme representing the classification of glycosphinolipids.

Glycosphingolipids that derive from one of the globoseries, the mucoseries, or from carbohydrate moieties containing mannose have so far not been reported to be substituted by sialic acid residues. Except for the sialocerebrosides, i.e., sialoglucosyl(or galactosyl)ceramide ($G_{Glc}1$ and $G_{Gal}1$) and the sialolactosylceramide, "hematoside" ($G_{Lac}1$), gangliosides carry sialo-oligosaccharides that belong to the ganglio or lacto series (see Figure 1). Though Seyama and Yamakawa (1974) found gangliotriaosylceramide as a major constituent of guinea pig erythrocytes and Matsumoto and Taki (1976) described a Fuc($\alpha1\rightarrow2$)Gal($\beta1\rightarrow3$)Gal $NAc(\beta1\rightarrow4$)Gal($\beta1\rightarrow4$)Glc$\beta\rightarrow$Cer from rat ascites hepatoma cells, glycolipids of the ganglioseries are usually found only as gangliosides, perhaps in consequence of their biosynthesis via sialolactosylceramide (see Section 3.2.1).*

The presence of sialic acid in gangliosides shows these lipids as typical cell surface constituents; for a sialic acid review, see Rosenberg and Schengrund (1976), and for isolation and characterization, see Schauer (1978). In aqueous solution free sialic acid is present as its β anomer (Holmquist and Ostman, 1975). In gangliosides, however, sialic acid is linked by an α-ketoside (Huang and Klenk, 1972; Sillerud et al., 1978). Sialic acid substitution of oligosaccharides usually takes place at branching or terminal positions.

Under acid conditions, sialic acids may form lactones that often give rise to a double spot formation of isolated gangliosides on thin layer chromatography (Cumar and Caputto, 1976) as well as in paper electrophoresis (Figure 2). Lactonization occurs with particular ease when two sialic acid molecules are linked to one another by an $\alpha2\rightarrow8$ glycoside bond. In this case, it is the terminal sialic acid residue that lactonizes preferentially (Wiegandt, 1973). It is tempting to speculate that lactonization of gangliosides, with a resultant alteration of electric charges at membrane sites, plays a role under in vivo conditions. Lipid-bound sialic acid isolated from human tissues was characterized in most cases as being exclusively N-acetylneuraminic acid or 9-O-acetyl-N-acetylneuraminic acid (Haverkamp et al., 1977b). However, in human HeLa cells† (Carubelli and Griffin, 1968) and human kidney (Mahieu and Winand, 1970) N-glycolylneuraminic acid was also identified. Therefore the possible presence of N-glycolylneuraminic acid in human gangliosides cannot be excluded entirely. The brain gangliosides of most other vertebrates, except for trace amounts of N-glycolylneuraminic acid (Tettamanti et al., 1965), also contain mostly N-acetylneuraminic acid or N,O-diacetylneuraminic acids (Ghidoni et al., 1979), the latter in high concentration in fish brain sialogly-

---

*Recently the presence of gangliotetraosylceramide was discovered in rat peritoneal exudate cells and nonimmunoglobulin bearing rat lymphocytes (Momoi et al., 1980; Young et al., 1980; Kasai et al 1980; Schwarting and Summers, 1980).

†N-glycolylneuraminic acid found in HeLa cells originated from calf serum constituents of the cell culture medium, according to Hof and Faillard (1973).

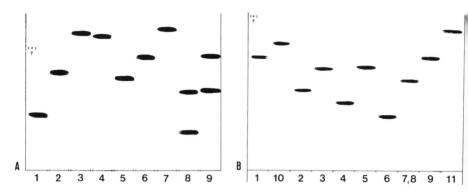

FIGURE 2. Paper electropherogram of N-acetylneuraminic acid, bis-N-acetylneuraminic acid, and free-reducing N-acetylneuraminyloligosaccharides derived from parent gangliosides, at pH 1.9 (A) and pH 6.4 (B). The slower-migrating component of 8 and 9 at pH 1.9 is due to lactone formation. (Paper from Schleicher and Schüll, Dassel, GFR; buffer at pH 1.9 comprised formic acid:acetic acid:H_2O = 50:150:800 v/v; buffer at pH 6.4 comprised pyridine:acetic acid:H_2O = 100:10:89 v/v.) Numerical code is as follows: 1, NeuAc; 2, II^{3}NeuAc-Lac; 3, II^3[NeuAc$\alpha\rightarrow$8NeuAcα]-Lac; 4, II^{3}NeuAc-GgOse$_3$; 5, II^3[NeuAc$\alpha\rightarrow$8NeuAcα]-GgOse$_3$; 6, II^{3}NeuAc-GgOse$_4$; 7, IV^{3}NeuAc-,II^{3}NeuAc-GgOse$_4$; 8, II^3[NeuAc$\alpha\rightarrow$8NeuAcα]-GgOse$_4$; 9, IV^{3}NeuAc-,II^3[NeuAc$\alpha\rightarrow$8NeuAcα]-GgOse$_4$; 10, NeuAc$\alpha\rightarrow$8NeuAc; and 11, IV^{3}NeuAc-, II^3[NeuAc$\alpha\rightarrow$8NeuAc$\alpha\rightarrow$8NeuAcα]-GgOse$_4$. from H. Wiegandt (unpublished results).

colipids (Ishizuka *et al.*, 1970). However, in gangliosides of bovine hypophysis (Clarke, 1975) and adrenal medulla (Ledeen *et al.*, 1968) more than 30% and 40%, respectively, of the sialic acid is N-glycolylneuraminic acid.

Extraneural gangliosides of nonhuman origin contain, besides N-acetylneuraminic acid, substantial amounts of the N-glycolyl derivative. Ganglioside $G_{Lac}1$ of horse erythrocytes contains N-glycolyl-4- O-acetylneuraminic acid.

Sugita and Hori (1976) discovered unusual types of sialic acids in the gangliosides of the starfish *Asterina pectinifora*. These gangliosides contained the following hematosides: sialolactosylceramides ($G_{Lac}1$), with the glycosylated sialic acid derivatives, Ara($\beta1\rightarrow$6)Gal($\beta1\rightarrow$4)NeuGl, Ara($\beta1\rightarrow$6) Gal($\beta1\rightarrow$4)[8-O-Mel] NeuGl or Ara($\beta1\rightarrow$6)Gal($\beta1\rightarrow$4)[Gal($\beta1\rightarrow$8)] NeuGl.

The gangliosides of lowest molecular weight that are derived from gluco- and galactocerebroside are NeuAc($\alpha2\rightarrow$6)Glc$\beta1\rightarrow$Cer ($G_{Glc}1$) and NeuAc($\alpha2\rightarrow$3)Gal$\beta1\rightarrow$Cer ($G_{Gal}1$).

Gangliosides of the class G_{Glc} containing only glucose as neutral sugar are characteristic of the gametes of sea urchin. Glucose was identified in its furanose form from gangliosides of the sea urchin by Zhukova and Smirnova (1969). The Russian authors also reported the composition of the ceramide of ganglioside $G_{Glc}1$ from sea urchin and identified 86% of its fatty acid as docosenoic acid ($C_{22:1}$) and sphing-4-enine ($C_{18:1}$) as the major long chain base constituent. Gangliosides NeuAc($\alpha2\rightarrow6$)Glc$\beta\rightarrow$Cer and NeuAc($\alpha2\rightarrow8$) NeuAc($\alpha2\rightarrow6$)Glc$\beta1\rightarrow$Cer($G_{Glc}2$) were isolated from spermatozoa of the sea urchin (*Pseudocentrotus depressus* and *Hemicentrotus pulcherrimus*) and structurally identified by Hoshi and Nagai (1975). Nagai and Hoshi (1975) also showed that the ganglioside composition in the gametes of sea urchin is characteristic for each species and gamete. By immunological localization using fluorescent-labeled antibody, Ohsawa and Nagai (1975) found the gangliosides are concentrated at the cell surface of the acrosomal region of the spermatozoa, where they may play a role in fertilization. A sialodiglucosylceramide was found in pig platelets by Heckers and Stoffel (1972).

Ganglioside $G_{Gal}1$ was isolated from human brain and its chemical structure elucidated by Kuhn and Wiegandt (1964). In contrast with other brain gangliosides, the majority of which are derived from gray matter, 2-hydroxy-fatty acids are present in ganglioside $G_{Gal}1$, as found in galactocerebroside of brain white matter (Klenk and Georgias, 1967; Siddiqui and McCluer, 1968). Indeed, $G_{Gal}1$ was identified as a typical and major ganglioside component of human CNS myelin (Ledeen *et al.*, 1973; Yu *et al.*, 1974), the myelin of human spinal cord (Ueno *et al.*, 1978), and oligodendroglia (Yu and Iqbal, 1977). Ganglioside $G_{Gal}1$, however, was not found in peripheral nerve myelin, including that of human sciatic nerve (Fong *et al.*, 1976). Apart from primate brain myelin, $G_{Gal}1$ also appears to be a major component of chicken brain white matter (Ando *et al.*, 1978) and chicken thymus (Narasimhan and Murray, 1978). In chicken egg yolk $G_{Gal}1$ was detected as a major ganglioside, in addition to gangliosides $G_{Lac}1$ and $G_{Lac}2$ (Li *et al.*, 1978).*

Gangliosides G_{Lac}, with one ($G_{Lac}1$) or two ($G_{Lac}2$) sialic acid residues, are the most abundant extraneural sialoglycolipids in vertebrates. They are, however, only minor constituents of the brain where higher hexosamine-containing gangliosides predominate. In a case of a hereditary disease, an accumulation of ganglioside $G_{Lac}1$ was reported to occur in the brain that was attributed to a deficiency in the transfer of N-acetylgalactosamine, i.e., $G_{Lac}1$:N-acetylgalactosamine transferase (Max *et al.*, 1974). Of the total ganglioside content $G_{Lac}1$ and $G_{Lac}2$ account for 74% and 19% in human kidney, 84% and 2.3% in human spleen (Wiegandt, 1973; Rauvala, 1976*b*); and 20% and 50% in buttermilk (Huang, 1973), respectively. In stomach and intestine $G_{Lac}1$ constitutes 68% and 44% of the total gangliosides, respectively (Keranen, 1975). $G_{Lac}2$ is the major component of mammalian retinal gangliosides (Handa and Burton, 1969; Holm *et al.*, 1972).

---

*Recently, $G_{Gal}1$ was characterized as a major ganglioside of mice erythrocytes (Hamanaka *et al.*, 1979).

In the group of lactose-derived gangliosides, one may also classify the sialoglycolipids that were isolated by Sugita (1979 a,b) from the invertebrate starfish *Asterina pectinifera* (see also Section 3.1.1).

The classical gangliosides, i.e., the predominant species in the brains of higher animals, contain carbohydrate moieties of the ganglio series:

Gangliotriaose	Gal$N$Ac(β1→4)Gal(β1→4)Glc
Gangliotetraose	Gal(β1→3)Gal$N$Ac(β1→4)Gal(β1→4)Glc
Gangliopentaose	Gal$N$Ac(β1→4)Gal(β1→3)Gal$N$Ac(β1→4)Gal(β1→4)Glc

All monosaccharide units of this series are linked by β-glycosides. Werries and Buddecke (1973) reported the occurrence of very small amounts of α-linked nonterminal galactose and glucose, although this suggestion has not yet been confirmed. Substitution with single or multiple α2→8-linked sialic acid occurs at the galactose residues of the gangliooligosaccharides at the 3-position (Table 1). Additional substitution by fucose occurs also (Wiegandt, 1973; Suzuki *et al.*, 1975; Ghidoni *et al.*, 1976; Sonnino *et al.*, 1978, 1979; Fredman *et al.*, 1980a,b).

A series of newly discovered gangliosides from the frog fat body was recently reported by Ohashi (1979 a,b). The structures of three of these gangliosides are derived from the monosialogangliotetraosylceramide by substitution of the terminal galactose residue in the 3-position by mono-, di-, and trigalactosyl units (Figure 1).

The most highly sialylated ganglioside identified thus far is a pentasialogangliotetraosylceramide, $G_{Gtet}5$, isolated from fish brain (Ishizuka and Wiegandt, 1972). In this species, the major tetrasialoganglioside has the structure of a IV³monosialo-II³trisialogangliotetraosylceramide. In contrast with fish brain, the major tetrasialoganglioside that is present in human and chicken brain is a IV³disialo-II³disialogangliotetraosylceramide (Ando and Yu, 1977a; Macher *et al.*, 1979).

Other brain gangliosides of the ganglio series are presented in Table 1. A ganglioside that was isolated from human erythrocyte membranes by Watanabe *et al.* (1979) has the unique structure of NeuAc(α2→3)Gal(β1→3)Gal$N$Ac(β1→4)Glcβ→Cer. Since it contains N-acetylgalactosamine substituted in the 3-position by galactose, it shows some similarity to gangliosides of the ganglio series.

Gangliosides that belong to the lacto series are more typical of those of extraneural origin. They contain the neutral oligosaccharide backbone of lactoneotetraosylceramide, i.e., Gal(β1→4)Glc$N$Ac(β1→3)Gal(β1→4)Glcβ1→ Cer. This structure may be extended with N-acetyllactosamine residues in the 3-position of the terminal galactose to lactoneohexaosylceramide, or in both 3-

and 6-positions of the terminal and nonterminal galactose (Watanabe *et al.*, 1975; Hakomori *et al.*, 1977; Yamashita *et al.*, 1977) to give the following:

$$\begin{array}{c}
\text{Gal}(\beta1\rightarrow4)\text{Glc}N\text{Ac}(\beta1\searrow_{6)} \\
\qquad\qquad\qquad \text{Gal}(\beta1\rightarrow4)\text{Glc}N\text{Ac}(\beta1\searrow_{6)} \\
\text{Gal}(\beta1\rightarrow4)\text{Glc}N\text{Ac}(\beta1\nearrow^{3)} \\
\qquad\qquad\qquad\qquad\qquad\qquad\qquad \text{Gal}(\beta1\rightarrow4)\text{Glc}N\text{Ac}(\beta1\rightarrow3)\text{Gal}(\beta1\rightarrow4)\text{Glc-Cer} \\
\qquad\text{Gal}(\beta1\rightarrow4)\text{Glc}N\text{Ac}(\beta1\nearrow^{3)}
\end{array}$$

It has long been recognized that a conspicuous parallelism exists between the oligosaccharide structures of gangliosides, or other neutral glycosphingolipids of the lacto series, and the sugars secreted in milk (for review, see Wiegandt and Egge, 1970).

In analogy to gangliosides of the ganglio series, those of the lacto series may carry fucose residues in branching or terminal positions, e.g., as shown in a human kidney ganglioside, IV³NeuAc-,III³Fuc-nLcOse₄-Cer by Rauvala (1976*b*). Another fucoganglioside with blood group H activity was identified in human erythrocytes. It has a branched sialooligosaccharide chain with the following structure: VI³NeuAc-,IV⁶[Fuc(α1→2)Gal(β1→4)Glc$N$Acβ] nLcOse₆-Cer (Watanabe *et al.*, 1978).

A ganglioside of the lacto series that contains a β-N-acetylgalactosaminide, i.e., NeuAcα2→3Gal$N$Acβ1→3Galβ1→4Glc$N$Acβ1→3Galβ→4Glcβ1 →Cer, was discovered in human erythrocytes (Watanabe and Hakomori, 1979).

The ceramide moiety of gangliosides generally reflects the fatty acid and sphingoid composition of other neutral glycosphingolipids that are derived from the same cellular material (for review, see Karlsson, 1970*a,b*; Wiegandt, 1971). Frequently, however, it has been observed that the ceramide composition of glycosphingolipids deviates from that expected on the basis of the biogenic relations of their carbohydrate portion. Thus, ganglioside $G_{Lac}1$ may show a fatty acid content quite dissimilar to that of the lactosylceramide from the same tissue (Henning and Stoffel, 1973). Similarly, an increase of eicosasphing-4-enine ($C_{20:1}$) over sphing-4-enine ($C_{18:1}$) is found in brain gangliosides with increasing sialic acid content (Schengrund and Garrigan, 1969; Iwamori and Nagai, 1978*b*). Yohe *et al.* (1976) believe that the ganglioside content of eicosasphing-4-enine relative to the degree of sialylation is a decisive factor for physicochemical homogeneity of ganglioside domains functioning to prevent phase separations.

The mechanisms that regulate the balance between the composition of the ceramide of gangliosides compared to that of their carbohydrate portion are not yet understood.

2.2. Nomenclature

In 1967, the Commission on Biochemical Nomenclature proposed rules for the designation and short notation of the long chain base or "sphingoid" (IUPAC-IUB, 1967). Examples are

4-sphingenine (sphingosine, 2-D-amino-octadec-4-ene-1,2-diol)
$CH_3 \cdot (CH_2)_{12} \cdot CH = CH \cdot CH(OH) \cdot CH(NH_2) \cdot CH_2 \cdot OH$

sphinganine (dihydrosphingosine)
$CH_3 \cdot (CH_2)_{14} \cdot CH(OH) \cdot CH(NH_2) \cdot CH_2 \cdot OH$

4-D-hydroxysphinganine (phytosphingosine)
$CH_3 \cdot (CH_2)_{13} \cdot CH(OH) \cdot CH(OH) \cdot CH(NH_2) \cdot CH_2 \cdot OH$

4-eicosasphingenine
$CH_3 \cdot (CH_2)_{14} \cdot CH = CH \cdot CH(OH) \cdot CH(NH_2) \cdot CH_2 \cdot OH$

These proposals were extended by the "Recommendations" (IUPAC-IUB, 1978) including a semisystematic nomenclature for higher glycosphingolipids. It is based on trivial names for specific oligosaccharides. Accordingly, the sialoglycolipids, i.e., gangliosides, are named *N*-acetyl(or *N*-glycolyl-)neuraminosyl(x)osylceramide, where (x) stands for the root name of the neutral oligosaccharide to which the sialosyl residue is attached. The position of the sialic acid group may be indicated by a Roman numeral, for the number of the monosaccharide residues to which the sialic acid is linked; this is accompanied by an Arabic numeral superscript indicating the position, within that residue, to which the sialic acid is attached. The neutral oligosaccharides are represented by specific symbols in which the number of monosaccharide units (-oses) is indicated by Ose_n, preceded by two letters giving the trivial name of the oligosaccharide. To conserve space, Ose can be omitted:

ganglio-	"Gg"	Globo-	"Gb"
lacto-	"Lc"	globoiso	"*i*Gb"
lactoneo-	"*n*Lc"	muco-	"Mc"

For other short notations of gangliosides in this review the abbreviations suggested earlier are used (Wiegandt, 1973). Gangliosides are thereby designated according to their neutral oligosaccharide moiety and the number and nature of sialic acid constitutents, i.e., G stands for ganglioside therefore the index, e.g., G_{Gal}, is an abbreviation for its neutral sugar moiety. To this index is added the number and nature of the sialic acid residues, using arabic numerals and lower case letters, to distinguish between positional sialoisomers, e.g.,

$G_{Gtet}2aNeuAc$. Abbreviations for neutral oligosaccharides are the following: Lac represents lactose; Gtri represents gangliotriaose ($GgOse_3$); Gtet represents gangliotetraose ($GgOse_4$); Gpt represents gangliopentaose ($GgOse_5$); Gfpt represents gangliofucopentaose ($IV^2Fuc-GgOse_4$); Ltri represents lactotriaose ($LcOse_3$); L$n$tet represents lactoneotetraose ($nLOse_4$); L$n$fpt represents lactoneofucopentaose ($III^3Fuc-nLcOse_4$); L$n$hex represents lactoneohexaose ($nLcOse_6$). A comparison of ganglioside nomenclature is given in Table 1.

2.3. Chemical Synthesis

Work on the complete chemical synthesis of gangliosides was performed almost exclusively in the laboratory of David Shapiro at the Weizmann Institute (for list of publications, see *Chem. Phys. Lipids,* 1974). In 1957 Shapiro *et al.* reported the first successful synthesis of sphing-4-enine. Only very recently, Shoyama *et al.* (1978) succeeded in synthesizing all four sphingosine stereoisomers and their corresponding ceramides.

As a key intermediate for the synthesis of higher sphingolipids, Shapiro employed sphingosine with its secondary hydroxyl and the amino group protected by formation of an oxazoline:

$$CH_3 \cdot (CH_2)_{12} \cdot CH = CH \cdot CH - CH \cdot CH_2 \cdot OH$$

$$\begin{array}{cc} | & | \\ O & N \\ \diagdown & \diagup \\ & C \\ & | \\ & C_6H_5 \end{array}$$

Using this intermediate, Shapiro and Rachaman (1964) achieved the total synthesis of lactosylceramide and in 1973 the synthesis of gangliotriaosylceramide (Shapiro *et al.*, 1973).

2.4. Chemical and Enzymatic Alterations

In recent years a variety of useful chemical and enzymatic reactions were applied to gangliosides that yielded products which were instrumental in studies of the biological function of these sialoglycolipids.

2.4.1. Alteration of the Ceramide Moiety

Cleavage of the sphingoid-*N*-acyl group of gangliosides by mild alkaline degradation in butanol yields the corresponding psychosine-type sialoglycolipid

TABLE 1. Gangliosides, Chemical Structure and Abbreviation

Structure	Designation according to IUPAC-IUB recommendations	Short notations according to:		Reference[a]
		Wiegandt	Svennerholm	
GANGLIOSIDES OF THE GANGLIO SERIES				
Gal(β1→4)Glcβ1→Cer, $\left(\begin{smallmatrix}3\\\uparrow\\2\alpha\end{smallmatrix}\right)$NeuAc	II³NeuAc-Lac-Cer	$G_{Lac}1$	G_{M3}	
Gal(β1→4)Glcβ1→Cer, $\left(\begin{smallmatrix}3\\\uparrow\\2\alpha\end{smallmatrix}\right)$NeuAc(8←2$\alpha$)NeuAc	II³NeuAc$_2$-Lac-Cer	$G_{Lac}2$	G_{D3}	
Gal(β1→4)Glcβ1→Cer, $\left(\begin{smallmatrix}3\\\uparrow\\2\alpha\end{smallmatrix}\right)$NeuAc(8←2$\alpha$)NeuAc NeuAc	II³NeuAc$_3$-Lac-Cer	$G_{Lac}3$	G_{T3}	
Gal$N$Ac(β1→4)Gal(β1→4)Glcβ1→Cer, $\left(\begin{smallmatrix}3\\\uparrow\\2\alpha\end{smallmatrix}\right)$NeuAc	II³NeuAc-GgOse$_3$-Cer	$G_{Gtn}1$	G_{M2}	
Gal$N$Ac(β1→4)Gal(β1→4)Glcβ1→Cer, $\left(\begin{smallmatrix}3\\\uparrow\\2\alpha\end{smallmatrix}\right)$NeuAc($\beta$←2$\alpha$)NeuAc	II³NeuAc$_2$-GgOse$_3$-Cer	$G_{Gtn}2$	G_{D2}	1
Gal$N$Acβ1→4Gal(β1→4)Glcβ1→Cer, $\left(\begin{smallmatrix}3\\\uparrow\\2\alpha\end{smallmatrix}\right)$NeuAc(8←2$\alpha$)NeuAc (8	II³NeuAc$_3$-GgOse$_3$-Cer	$G_{Gtn}3$	G_{T2}	2

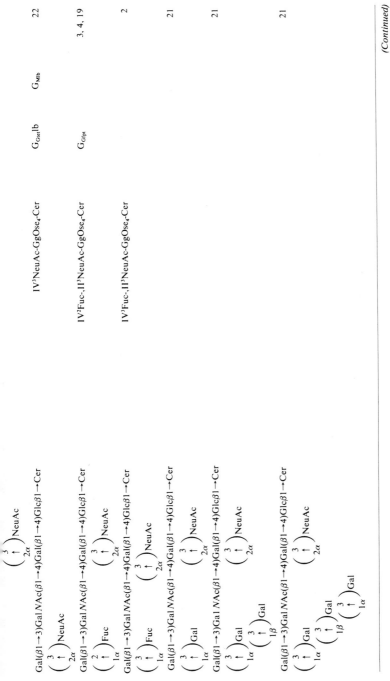

IV³NeuAc-GgOse₄-Cer	G_Giel1b	G_M1b	22
IV²Fuc-,II³NeuAc-GgOse₄-Cer	G_Gfpt		3, 4, 19
IV³Fuc-,II³NeuAc-GgOse₄-Cer			2
			21
			21
			21

(Continued)

TABLE 1. (Continued)

Structure	Designation according to IUPAC-IUB recommendations	Short notations according to:		Reference[a]
		Wiegandt	Svennerholm	
Gal($\beta1\rightarrow3$)GalNAc($\beta1\rightarrow4$)Gal($\beta1\rightarrow4$)Glc$\beta1\rightarrow$Cer, ($\overset{3}{\underset{2\alpha}{\uparrow}}$) NeuAc($8\leftarrow2\alpha$)NeuAc	II³NeuAc₂-GgOse₄-Cer	$G_{Glet}2b$	G_{Dlb}	
Gal($\beta1\rightarrow3$)GalNAc($\beta1\rightarrow4$)Gal($\beta1\rightarrow4$)Glc$\beta1\rightarrow$Cer, ($\overset{2}{\underset{1\alpha}{\uparrow}}$) Fuc, ($\overset{3}{\underset{2\alpha}{\uparrow}}$) NeuAc($8\leftarrow2\alpha$)NeuAc	IV²Fuc-,II³NeuAc₂-GgOse₄-Cer	$G_{Glpt}2$		5
Gal($\beta1\rightarrow3$)GalNAc($\beta i\rightarrow4$)Gal($\beta1\rightarrow4$)Glc$\beta1\rightarrow$Cer, ($\overset{3}{\underset{2\alpha}{\uparrow}}$) NeuAc, ($\overset{3}{\underset{2\alpha}{\uparrow}}$) NeuAc	IV³NeuAc-,II³NeuAc-GbOse₄-Cer	$G_{Glet}2a$	G_{Dla}	
Gal($\beta1\rightarrow3$)GalNAc($\beta1\rightarrow4$)Gal($\beta1\rightarrow4$)Glc$\beta1\rightarrow$Cer, ($\overset{3}{\underset{2\alpha}{\uparrow}}$) NeuAc($\beta\leftarrow2\alpha$)NeuAc, ($\overset{8}{\underset{2\alpha}{\uparrow}}$) NeuAc	II³NeuAc₃-GgOse₄-Cer	$G_{Glet}3c$	G_{Tlc}	6
Gal($\beta1\rightarrow3$)GalNAc($\beta1\rightarrow4$)Gal($\beta1\rightarrow4$)Glc$\beta1\rightarrow$Cer, ($\overset{3}{\underset{2\alpha}{\uparrow}}$) NeuAc, ($\overset{3}{\underset{2\alpha}{\uparrow}}$) NeuAc($8\leftarrow2\alpha$)NeuAc	IV³NeuAc-,II³NeuAc₂-GgOse₄-Cer	$G_{Glet}3b$	G_{Tlb}	7
Gal($\beta1\rightarrow3$)GalNAc($\beta1\rightarrow4$)Gal($\beta1\rightarrow4$)Glc$\beta1\rightarrow$Cer, ($\overset{3}{\underset{2\alpha}{\uparrow}}$) NeuAc($8\leftarrow2\alpha$)NeuAc, ($\overset{3}{\underset{2\alpha}{\uparrow}}$) NeuAc	IV³NeuAc₂-,II³NeuAc-GgOse₄-Cer	$G_{Glet}3a$	G_{Tla}	8
Gal($\beta1\rightarrow3$)GalNAc($\beta1\rightarrow4$)Gal($\beta1\rightarrow4$)Glc$\beta1\rightarrow$Cer, ($\overset{3}{\uparrow}$) NeuAc($8\leftarrow2\alpha$)NeuAc, ($\overset{3}{\uparrow}$) NeuAc($8\leftarrow2\alpha$)NeuAc	IV³NeuAc₂-,II³NeuAc₂-GgOse₄-Cer	$G_{Glet}4b$	G_{Qlb}	

Structure	Abbreviation	Ref.
	G_{Plc}	
$$\begin{array}{l}\left(\overset{3}{\underset{2\alpha}{\uparrow}}\right)\!NeuAc \qquad \left(\overset{3}{\underset{2\alpha}{\uparrow}}\right)\!NeuAc(8{\leftarrow}2\alpha)NeuAc \\ \hspace{4.5cm}\left(\overset{8}{\underset{2\alpha}{\uparrow}}\right)\!NeuAc \\[4pt] Gal(\beta1{\rightarrow}3)Gal\mathit{N}Ac(\beta1{\rightarrow}4)Gal(\beta1{\rightarrow}4)Glc\beta1{\rightarrow}Cer \\ \left(\overset{3}{\underset{2\alpha}{\uparrow}}\right)\!NeuAc(8{\leftarrow}2\alpha)NeuAc \end{array}$$	$G_{Get}5c$	6
$$\begin{array}{l}Gal\mathit{N}Ac(\beta1{\rightarrow}4)Gal\mathit{N}Ac(8{\leftarrow}2\alpha)NeuAc \\ \hspace{3.2cm}\left(\overset{8}{\underset{2\alpha}{\uparrow}}\right)\!NeuAc \\[4pt] Gal\mathit{N}Ac(\beta1{\rightarrow}3)Gal\mathit{N}Ac(\beta1{\rightarrow}4)Gal(\beta1{\rightarrow}4)Glc\beta1{\rightarrow}Cer \\ \hspace{4cm}\left(\overset{3}{\underset{2\alpha}{\uparrow}}\right)\!NeuAc \end{array}$$	$G_{Gpt}1a$	9
$$\begin{array}{l}Gal\mathit{N}Ac(\beta1{\rightarrow}4)Gal\mathit{N}Ac(\beta1{\rightarrow}3)Gal\mathit{N}Ac(\beta1{\rightarrow}4)Gal(\beta1{\rightarrow}4)Glc\beta1{\rightarrow}Cer \\ \hspace{2.6cm}\left(\overset{3}{\underset{2\alpha}{\uparrow}}\right)\!NeuAc \hspace{2.8cm}\left(\overset{3}{\underset{2\alpha}{\uparrow}}\right)\!NeuAc \end{array}$$	$G_{Gpt}2a$	10

GANGLIOSIDES OF THE LACTO SERIES

Structure	Abbreviation	Ref.
$$\begin{array}{l}Gal(\beta1{\rightarrow}4)GlcNAc(\beta1{\rightarrow}3)Gal(\beta1{\rightarrow}4)Glc\beta1{\rightarrow}Cer \\ \left(\overset{3}{\underset{2\alpha}{\uparrow}}\right)\!NeuAc \end{array}$$	$G_{Lntet}1a$	11,12,13
$$\begin{array}{l}Gal(\beta1{\rightarrow}4)GlcNAc(\beta1{\rightarrow}3)Gal(\beta1{\rightarrow}4)Glc\beta1{\rightarrow}Cer \\ \left(\overset{6}{\underset{2\alpha}{\uparrow}}\right)\!NeuAc \end{array}$$	$G_{Lntet}1b$	3,20
$$\begin{array}{l}Gal(\beta1{\rightarrow}4)GlcNAc(\beta1{\rightarrow}3)Gal(\beta1{\rightarrow}4)Glc\beta1{\rightarrow}Cer \\ NeuAc(8{\leftarrow}2\alpha)NeuAc? \end{array}$$	$G_{Lntet}2$	16,20
$$\begin{array}{l}Gal(\beta1{\rightarrow}4)GlcNAc(\beta1{\rightarrow}3)Gal(\beta1{\rightarrow}4)Glc\beta1{\rightarrow}Cer \\ \left(\overset{3}{\underset{2\alpha}{\uparrow}}\right)\!NeuAc \left(\overset{3}{\underset{1\alpha}{\uparrow}}\right)\!Fuc \end{array}$$	$G_{Lrpt}1$	4

Structural‐name designations:
$IV^3NeuAc_2{-},II^3NeuAc_3{-}GgOse_4{-}Cer$ — $G_{Get}5c$ — 6
$II^3NeuAc{-}GgOse_5{-}Cer$ — $G_{Gpt}1a$ — 9
$IV^3NeuAc{-},II^3NeuAc{-}GgOse_5{-}Cer$ — $G_{Gpt}2a$ — 10
$IV^3NeuAc{-}nLcOse_4{-}Cer$ — $G_{Lntet}1a$ — 11,12,13
$IV^6NeuAc{-}nLcOse_4{-}Cer$ — $G_{Lntet}1b$ — 3,20
$IV^3NeuAc_2{-}nLOse_4{-}Cer$ — $G_{Lntet}2$ — 16,20
$IV^3NeuAc{-},III^3Fuc{-}nLcOse_4{-}Cer$ — $G_{Lrpt}1$ — 4

(Continued)

TABLE 1. (Continued)

Structure	Designation according to IUPAC-IUB recommendations	Short notations according to: Wiegandt	Svennerholm	Reference[a]
Gal(β1→4)GlcNAc(β1→3)Gal(β1→4)Glcβ1→Cer $\;\;\left(\begin{smallmatrix}3\\\uparrow\\1\beta\end{smallmatrix}\right)$ Gal1(3←2α)NeuAc	IV³[NeuAcα2→3Galβ1→]-nLcOse₄-Cer			18
Gal(β1→4)GlcNAC(β1→3)Gal(β1→4)Glcβ1→Cer $\;\;\left(\begin{smallmatrix}3\\\uparrow\\1\beta\end{smallmatrix}\right)$ GalNAc(3←2α)NeuAc	IV³[NeuAcα2→3GalNAcβ1→]-nLcOse₄-Cer			20
Gal(β1→4)GlcNAc(β1→3)Gal(β1→4)Glcβ1→Cer $\;\;\left(\begin{smallmatrix}3\\\uparrow\\2\alpha\end{smallmatrix}\right)$ NeuAc	VI³NeuAc-nLcOse₆-Cer	$G_{Lnhex}1a$		15,20
Gal(β1→4)GlcNAc(β1→3)Gal(β1→4)Glcβ1→Cer $\;\;\left(\begin{smallmatrix}6\\\uparrow\\2\alpha\end{smallmatrix}\right)$ NeuAc	VI⁶NeuAc-nLcOse₆-Cer	$G_{Lnhex}1b$		20
Gal(β1→4)GlcNAc(β1→3)Gal(β1→4)GlcNAc(β1→3)Gal(β1→4)Glcβ1→Cer $\;\;\left(\begin{smallmatrix}\beta1\\\downarrow\\6\end{smallmatrix}\right)$ Fuc$\left(\begin{smallmatrix}\alpha1\\\downarrow\\2\end{smallmatrix}\right)$ Gal(β1→4)GlcNAc $\;\;\left(\begin{smallmatrix}3\\\uparrow\\2\alpha\end{smallmatrix}\right)$ NeuAc	VI³NeuAc-,IV⁶[Fucα→2Galβ→4GlcNAcβ]-nLcOse₆Cer			117

[a] Literature references: (1) L. Kobata and Ginsburg (1972); (2) Ohashi and Yamakawa (1977); (3) Wiegandt (1973); (4) Ghidoni et al. (1976); (5) Sonnino et al. (1978); (6) Ishizuka and Wiegandt (1972); (7) Kuhn and Wiegandt (1963); (8) Ando and Yu (1977); (9) Iwamori and Nagai (1978a); (10) Svennerholm et al. (1973); (11) Wiegandt and Schulze (1969); (12) Uemura et al. (1978); (13) Li et al. (1973); (14) Rauvala (1976b); (15) Wiegandt (1976b); (16) Keranen (1976); (17) Watanabe (1978); (18) Watanabe et al. (1974); (19) Suzuki et al. (1975); (20) Watanabe et al. (1979); (21) Ohashi (1979b); (22) Hirabayashi et al. (1979).

(Taketomi and Kawamura, 1970). With this method, Taketomi *et al.* (1975) obtained sialosyllactosylsphingosine from ganglioside $G_{Lac}1$. By *N*-deacylation and re-*N*-acetylation, Holmgren *et al.* (1974) prepared the *N*-acetyl derivative of ganglioside $G_{Gtet}1$. Glycolipids with only one aliphatic long carbon chain have physicochemical properties typical of "lyso" lipids (Taketomi and Kawamura, 1970).

A different approach to "lyso" glycolipids is by removal of part of the aliphatic long carbon chain of the sphingoid. This may be achieved by cleavage of the sphingoid carbon–carbon double bond with ozone followed by reduction with sodium borohydride (Taketomi *et al.*, 1975; Wiegandt *et al.*, 1976):

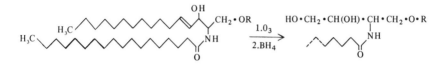

Alternatively, the product that is obtained by cleavage of gangliosides or other glycosphingolipids by ozone can be further oxidized to contain a carboxyl function which allows for a coupling of the fragment glycolipid to matrices such as aminoalkylagarose. Prior to coupling, the carboxyl group of sialic acid must be protected, e.g., by esterification (Laine *et al.*, 1974; Young *et al.*, 1979):

$$uAc[Me\text{-}ester](\alpha2\rightarrow3')Lac\text{-}Cer \xrightarrow[\text{AcOH}]{O_3 \quad H_2O_2}$$

$$uAc[Me\text{-}ester](\alpha2\rightarrow3')Lac\text{-}O \cdot CH_2 \cdot CH \cdot CH(OH) \cdot CO_2H \xrightarrow[\text{2. NaOCH}_3]{\substack{\text{1. } H_2N \cdot CH_2CH_2 \cdot NH\text{-agarose} \\ \text{(carbodiimide)}}}$$

$$NH \cdot CO \cdot R$$

$$uAc(\alpha2\rightarrow3')Lac\text{-}O \cdot CH_2 \cdot CH \cdot CH(OH) \cdot CO \cdot NH \cdot CH_2 \cdot CH_2NH \cdot agarose$$

$$NH \cdot CO \cdot R$$

C-3 of the sphingoid of glycosphingolipids carrying a secondary hydroxyl group may selectively be oxidized by 2,3-dichloro-5,6-dicyanobenzoquinone (Kishimoto and Mitry, 1974; Iwamori *et al.*, 1975b). The 3-keto derivative thereby obtained may be used for the specific tritium labeling of the ceramide moiety by borotritiide with retention of the sphingoid carbon double bond (Iwamori *et al.*, 1975a). Oxidation of gangliosides by dichlorodicyanobenzoquinone has not been as satisfactory, because of the formation of side products of sialic acid oxidation (unpublished observation).

Radioactive labeling of components of the ceramide moiety of gangliosides by catalytic hydrogenation with tritium gas has been described (Seyama *et al.*, 1968; Dicesare and Rapport, 1974). Borotritiide in the presence of palladium can be used more conveniently and with no apparent hydrogenolytic decomposition for the reduction of the carbon double bonds (Schwarzmann *et al.*, 1978).

Gangliosides that bear a lipophilic substitute for ceramide, "gangliosidoides" were synthesized by Wiegandt and Ziegler (1974). The isolated, free reducing sialooligosaccharides of gangliosides, obtained by oxidative cleavage of the sphingoid carbon double bond by either ozonolysis (Wiegandt and Bücking, 1970) or osmium tetroxide–periodate oxidation (Hakomori and Siddiqui, 1972) followed by alkaline fragmentation, were used. After treatment of the sialosugar with cyanoborohydride in the presence of ammonia, the reductaminated oligosaccharide is coupled to a fatty acid by an amide. A sialoglycolipid is directly obtained, when the reductamination is performed with a long aliphatic carbon chain amine*:

$$R \cdot CH = O\text{-} \quad \begin{array}{l} \xrightarrow{\text{NH}_4^+} R \cdot CH_2 \cdot NH_2 \xrightarrow{R'' \cdot CO_2H} R \cdot CH_2 \cdot NH \cdot CO \cdot R'' \\ \text{NaCNBH}_3 \\ \xrightarrow[R' \cdot NH_3^+]{} R \cdot Ch_2 \cdot NH \cdot R' \xrightarrow{R'' \cdot CO_2H} R \cdot CH_2 \cdot NR'' \cdot CO \cdot R' \end{array}$$

Gangliosidoides with two long aliphatic carbon chain residues have also been obtained by the following reaction sequence (Mraz *et al.*, 1980)*:

$$R \cdot CH_2 \cdot NH_2 + O_2N \cdot C_6H_4 \cdot O_2C \cdot CHN_3 \cdot (CH_2)_n \cdot CH_3 \rightarrow$$

$$R \cdot CH_2 \cdot NH \cdot CO \cdot CHN_3 \cdot (CH_2)_n \cdot CH_3 \xrightarrow{H_2/Pt}$$

$$R \cdot CH_2 \cdot NH \cdot CO \cdot \underset{\underset{NH_2}{|}}{CH} \cdot (CH_2)_n \cdot CH_3 \xrightarrow{+ R' \cdot CO_2 \cdot C_6H_4 \cdot NO_2}$$

$$R \cdot CH_2 \cdot NH \cdot CO \cdot \underset{\underset{NH \cdot CO \cdot R'}{|}}{CH} \cdot (CH_2)_n \cdot CH_3$$

---

*Where R represents oligosaccharide residue, R' represents aliphatic carbon chain, and R'' represents long aliphatic carbon chain.

2.4.2. Alteration of the Carbohydrate Moiety

Chemical as well as enzymatic reactions involving the sialooligosaccharide moiety of gangliosides in many instances are aimed at an introduction of some label that would allow for the detection of minute quantities of compounds or serve as probes for neighboring groups. In addition, the specific degradation of gangliosides by enzymes proved to be a powerful tool in the elucidation of their chemical constitution.

Gangliosides with free terminal galactose can be tritiated as described by Hajra *et al.* (1966). The galactose residue is oxidized by galactose oxidase from *Polyporus circinatus* (EC 1.1.3.9) and subsequently reduced with borotritiide (Radin *et al.*, 1969; Ghidoni *et al.*, 1974). This method also allows labeling of terminal N-acetylgalactosamine, as in ganglioside $G_{Gtri}1$, by tritium (Suzuki and Suzuki, 1972).

Another convenient way to introduce tritium label into the sialooligosaccharide of some gangliosides is to oxidize terminal sialic acid residues by treatment with low concentrations of periodate, followed by reduction with borotritiide. By choosing appropriate conditions, only the C-7 to C-9 side chain of sialic acid is affected with negligible destruction of other monosaccharide residues. Model studies showed that sialic acid is converted mainly to the C-8-analog by this procedure (Veh *et al.*, 1977).

Both labeling methods (galactose oxidase and periodate oxidation) have successfully been applied to the examination of gangliosides in intact cell cultures (Moss *et al.*, 1977*a*).

Recently described was an endo-β-galactosidase from *Escherichia freundii* that cleaves ganglioside $G_{Lntet}1a$ or ganglioside VI^{3}NeuAc-,IV^6 [Fuc($\alpha\rightarrow$2)Gal($\beta\rightarrow$4)Glc NAcβ]-nLcOse$_6$-Cer at the nonterminal galactose residue, e.g., IV^{3}NeuAc-nLcOse$_4$-Cer$\rightarrow$NeuAc(α2$\rightarrow$3)Gal($\beta\rightarrow$4)Galc NAc ($\beta\rightarrow$3)Gal + Glc-Cer (Fukuda *et al.*, 1978; Watanabe *et al.*, 1978).

Sequential and selective removal of sialic acid residues from brain gangliosides by neuraminidase (N-acetylneuraminate glycohydrolase, EC 3.2.1.18) has provided a first clue in the understanding of their structural relationship. It was fortunate that neuraminidases of various bacterial and viral origins have different substrate specificities with regard to the nature of the sialic acid and its linkage to the aglycon (Table 2). Ketosides of sialic acids substituted at the 4-hydroxyl site are not cleaved by such sialidases.

It was recognized early that the sialic acid residue of ganglioside $G_{Gtri}1$ and $G_{Gtet}1$, which is linked by an α2$\rightarrow$3 ketoside to a C-4-substituted galactose, proved characteristically resistant to the neuraminidases of viral and bacterial origin. There are now five gangliosides known to contain "neuraminidase-resistant" sialic acid residues: the monosialocompounds II^{3}NeuAc-GgOse$_3$-Cer ($G_{Gtri}1$), II^{3}NeuAc-GgOse$_4$-Cer ($G_{Gtet}1$), II^{3}NeuAc-GgOse$_5$-Cer ($G_{Gpt}1$),

TABLE 2.   Specificities of Viral and Bacterial Neuraminidases[a]

	Literature references[b]				
	1,2,3,4,5	11,12,13	2,6,7,10		8,9
Linkage type	Vibrio cholerae	Clostridium perfringens	FPV[c]	NDV[d]	Arthrobacter ureafaciens
NeuAc(α2→3)Gal<	+	+	+	+	+
NeuAc(α2→3)Gal[4←GalNAc]<	−	−[e]	−	−	+
NeuAc(α2→3)Gal[4←GalNAc]< (in gangliosides)	−	+	−	−	+
NeuAc(α2→3)Gal[4←βGalNAc3←βGal2←αFuc]< (in gangliosides)	−			−	− (trace +)
NeuAc(α2→6)Gal<	+	−			+
NeuAc(α2→6)GlcNAc[3←]<	+	+	−		+
NeuAc(α2→8)NeuAc<	+	+	−		+

[a] +, Neuraminidase-labile; −, neuraminidase-resistant.
[b] Literature References: (1) Kuhn et al. (1961); (2) Drzeniek and Gauhe (1970); (3) Suttajit and Winzler (1971); (4) Isizuka and Wiegandt (1972); Cassidy et al. (1965); (6) Drzeniek et al., (1966); (7) Drzeniek (1967); (8) Uchida et al. (1976); (9) Sugano et al. (1978); (10) Huang and Orlich (1972); (11) Wenger and Wardell (1973); (12) Rauval (1976b); (13) Schauer et al. (1970).
[c] FPV, chicken fowl plague virus.
[d] NDV, newcastle disease virus.
[e] NeuAc is cleaved by C. perfringens neuraminidase from reductaminated monosialogangliotetraose, i.e. Gal(β1→3)GalNAc(β1→4)Gal[3←2αNeuAc](β1→3)[1-aminosorbitol] (R. Schauer and M. Wiegandt, unpublished results).

IV²Fuc-,II³NeuAc-GgOse₄-Cer   ($G_{Gfpt}1$)   and   the   disialoganglioside IV³NeuAc-,II³NeuAc-GgOse₅-Cer ($G_{Gpt}2a$). The "neuraminidase-resistance" in such cases was attributed to steric hindrance at the vicinally cis-substituted galactose (Kuhn and Wiegandt, 1963a). Indeed, ^{13}C-NMR resonance data of a sialic acid in such sialidase-resistant positions suggest an anisotropy effect caused by the steric hindrance due to the neighboring groups (Harris and Thornton, 1978). A steric arrest of this sialic acid residue, as in ganglioside $G_{Gtet}1$, by the adjacent N-acetylcarbonyl group of N-acetylgalactosamine may also be the reason that its vertical dipole moment, contributing to the surface potential at air–water interfaces as measured by Maggio et al. (1978b), is opposite that of the terminal sialic acid residues in gangliosides $G_{Gtet}2a$ and $G_{Gtet}3b$. It was also suggested that a tight packing of the hydrophilic head groups of gangliosides in their micelles made sialic acid residues that otherwise are labile to the enzyme inaccessible to neuraminidase (Huang and Orlich, 1972). In support of this concept, it was shown that a marked hydrolysis of ganglioside $G_{Gtri}1$ or $G_{Gtet}1$ by Clostridium perfringens neuraminidase occurred below the "critical micellar concentration" (CMC) of these lipids (Lipovac et al., 1971; Rauvala, 1976c) or in the presence of bile salt (Wenger and Wardell, 1973a,b). Marginal splitting of ganglioside $G_{Gtet}1$ was also reported for Arthro-

bacter ureafaciens neuraminidase (Sugano *et al.*, 1978). An enlargement of the hydrophobic matrix by addition of sodium cholate below the CMC leads to a more effective splitting of otherwise resistant sialic acid residues. Thus far unexplained, however, is the fact that in contrast to the respective ganglioside $G_{Gtet}1$, its sialogangliotetraose residue is not (or is much less effectively) cleaved by *Clostridium perfringens* neuraminidase (R. Schauer, personal communication). In this case cholate shows no effect on the action of the enzyme towards the free sialo-oligosaccharide (Sugano *et al.*, 1978).

Sialidases from mammalian tissue that effectively cleave sialic acid from ganglioside $G_{Gtri}1$ have been described, such as rat intestine (Kolodny *et al.*, 1971) and heart muscle (Tallman and Brady, 1973).

The accessibility of neuraminidase-labile gangliosides to the action of exogeneous enzyme has been used to probe the localization of the glycolipid in biological membranes. However, reports in the literature are not yet unequivocal. Almost complete conversion of polysialogangliosides in rat brain microsomes by *Clostridium perfringens* neuraminidase was shown by Maccioni *et al.* (1974), whereas DiCesare and Rapport (1973) reported that gangliosides in neuronal membranes were not readily accessible to this enzyme preparation. In mouse fibroblasts (L cells) Weinstein *et al.* (1970) also found ganglioside resistance to *Clostridium perfringens* sialidase, while *Vibrio cholera* neuraminidase did not cleave sialic acid from small intestinal mucosa (Holmgren *et al.*, 1975) or from the hematoside present in dog erythrocytes (Keenan *et al.*, 1974*a*). On the other hand, Wherrett (1973) reported release of 80% of the lipid-bound sialic acid from human erythrocyte by the *Vibrio cholera* enzyme.

2.5. Preparation of Gangliosides

2.5.1. Isolation

Homogeneity here refers to the sialo sugar portion rather than to constituents of the ceramide of gangliosides. Recent improvements in techniques for ganglioside isolation and characterization have contributed to the field.

Gangliosides are usually extracted from biological material with aqueous chloroform–methanol and partitioned against an aqueous phase (Folch *et al.*, 1957; Suzuki, 1965). In a different procedure, aimed at quantitative isolation and separation from glycoproteins, tetrahydrofuran was used for extraction followed by addition of ether and partitioned against aqueous buffer (Tettamanti *et al.*, 1973). The extraction of gangliosides from tissues appears to necessitate the prior breaking of noncovalent association with protein. Therefore, the presence of salt (e.g., sodium acetate or potassium chloride) in the extraction medium is necessary. Weinstein *et al.* (1970) have reported that higher gangliosides ($G_{Gtet}2$) could be extracted from cell membranes only after tryptic digestion.

Instead of the partition of gangliosides into an aqueous phase, direct isolation from an extract is achieved by sequential elution from anion-exchange matrices such as DEAE-cellulose (Saito and Hakomori, 1971; Winterbourn, 1971), DEAE-Sephadex (Ledeen *et al.*, 1973; Momoi *et al.*, 1976; Ueno *et al.*, 1978), DEAE-Sepharose (Iwamori and Nagai, 1978*b*), DEAE-silica gel (Kundu and Roy, 1978), or porous glass beads covered with crosslinked DEAE-Dextran (Fredman *et al.*, 1980*b*). The gangliosides can thereby be separated into groups according to their number of sialic acid residues. Resolution of glycosphingolipids into single component species is achieved by chromatography on silica gel (Ando *et al.*, 1976) or silica gel–Kieselguhr (Kawamura and Taketomi, 1977). An effective method for the mapping of gangliosides was elaborated based on these techniques by Iwamori and Nagai (1978*b*). These authors showed that mammalian and chicken brain gangliosides contain, in addition to the thirteen structurally known sialoglycolipid species, some twenty-five as yet unidentified components.

2.5.2. Characterization

Separation of small quantities of gangliosides for preliminary identification is best achieved by thin layer chromatography (TLC) on silica gel; it may be combined with colorimetric determination of single components (Smid and Reinisova, 1973; Yates and Thompson, 1977; Harth *et al.*, 1978). Ando *et al.* (1978) used high-performance TLC and direct densitometric evaluation of the resorcinol–HCl developed plates with high sensitivity and reproducibility. A microquantitation of glycosphingolipids following ^{14}C-acetylation was described by Blomberg (1978).

The structural elucidation of gangliosides has been greatly advanced in recent years by introduction of newly developed gas chromatographic techniques, particularly in combination with mass spectrometry (for review, see Egge, 1978; Rickert and Sweeley, 1978).

The long chain base sphingoid composition (for review, see Karlsson, 1970*a,b*) can be analyzed after hydrolysis of the glycosphingolipid (Gaver and Sweeley, 1965) by direct gas-liquid chromatography of the trimethylsilyl derivatives (Carter and Gaver, 1967).

In another approach, the oxidation products of sphingoids are studied by gas chromatography. The aldehydes, obtained either by periodate oxidation of the free sphingoids or ozonolysis of the intact glycosphingolipids, are identified directly (Evans and McCluer, 1969) or after borohydride reduction as the trimethylsilyl derivatives of the fatty alcohols (Kawamura and Taketomi, 1977).

Ceramide composition was studied by Samuelsson and Samuelsson (1970) using combined gas chromatography–mass spectrometry. Information was obtained regarding not only the overall constitution of a ceramide mixture, but also the distribution of molecular species. Mass spectrometry by chemical ionization of the ceramide moiety of glycosphingolipids was reported by Markey and Wenger (1974).

The early studies on the mass spectrometry of glycosphingolipids yielded information on the ceramide composition and the constituent sugars other than sialic acids (Sweeley and Dawson, 1969; Dawson and Sweeley, 1971; Yogeeswaran et al., 1972). Karlsson (1973) first obtained a mass peak as high as m/e 1854 for the methylated reduced trimethylsilylated derivative of ganglioside $G_{Gtet}1$ with specific information on type and ratio of sugars including their sequence. Gradually with time, gangliosides of increasing size and complexity were analyzed by mass spectrometry; some examples are the following: $G_{Lac}1$ (Karlsson, 1973), $G_{Gtet}1$ (Karlsson et al., 1974b), $G_{Gtet}2a$ (Karlsson, 1974a) and $G_{Gtet}4b$ (Freeman et al., 1980a). Data for intact gangliosides obtained with electron impact mass spectrometry are often complicated by the presence of small fragment ion species arising from both the carbohydrate and aliphatic moieties. This difficulty is overcome by chemical ionization which favors the appearance of fragments in the high mass range. Complications can further be reduced by analysis of the separated sialo-oligosaccharide moiety by chemical ionization mass spectrometry (Ando et al., 1977).

The identification of partially methylated alditol acetates derived from glycolipids by gas chromatography–mass spectrometry was described by Bjorndahl et al. (1970). Permethylation of glycosphingolipids by dimethylsulfoxide methylsulfinylcarbanion methyliodide (Hakomori, 1964; Sandford and Conrad, 1966) leads to N-methylated acetamido groups of constituent hexosamines inducing a high resistance of adjacent glycosidic bonds towards acid hydrolysis. It was therefore an important improvement in the gas chromatographic analysis of partially methylated 2-deoxy-2- N-methylacetamidohexitol acetates when Stellner et al. (1973) suggested the use of acetolysis to cleave hexosamine-glycosidic bonds. Methylation analysis by gas chromatography–mass spectrometry of the major gangliosides of human intestinal mucosa was recently described by Keranen (1976) and led to the structure determination of the ganglioside $G_{Lntet}2b$ (IV^3NeuAc_2-$nLcOse_4$-Cer).

In a recent development in the methylation analysis of sialo-oligosaccharides, Haverkamp et al. (1977a) included the detection of neuraminic acid derivatives. These authors confirmed the structure of ganglioside $G_{Gtet}3b$ as previously established by Kuhn and Wiegandt (1963b) using periodate–Smith-degradation analysis.

2.6. Physicochemical Characteristics of Gangliosides

2.6.1. Gangliosides in Solution

The molecular combination of two heterophilic regions of comparable volume, the lipophilic ceramide and the hydrophilic carbohydrate carrying a negative charge under physiological conditions, makes gangliosides highly polar lipids with rather complex physicochemical properties. Their extreme amphipathic nature is very responsive to the environment provided by the solvent and additional complexing molecules. Depending in a complex way on the number of sialic acid residues, as well as the presence of mono- or divalent cations and protein, gangliosides have drastically different solubility characteristics. This is shown by the partitioning behavior of gangliosides between solvent phases of different polarities (Hayashi and Katagiri, 1974).

Pascher (1976) has shown that the ceramide portion of glycosphingolipids adopts a preferential conformation that stems primarily from the rigidity of its planar amide group, resulting in a parallel orientation of the axes of the two hydrocarbon tails. The carbon–carbon trans-double bond in sphing-4-enine promotes condensation of ceramides in a closely packed arrangement. Condensation is further promoted by hydroxyl groups on the sphingoid and D-hydroxy fatty acids, if present, in the ceramide. Löfgren and Pascher (1977) propose that this effect is brought about by lateral interactions via hydrogen bond formation, partaking in a general hydrogen-bond belt located in biomembranes at the level of ester carbonyl groups of phospholipids.

Chemical shift data of ^{13}C-NMR resonance of C-3 and C-4 of the sphing-4-enine of gangliosides in different solvents also point to solvation effects on the conformation in this region of the long chain base (Harris and Thornton, 1978). NMR data showed that ganglioside–ceramide in mixture with phospholipids intercalates with the lipid portion of the latter (Harris and Thornton, 1978).

As compared with ceramide, less information is available regarding the conformation of the ganglioside sugar portion. A model based on ^{13}C-NMR spin lattice relaxation data was proposed for sialic acid by Czarniecki and Thornton (1977a). These authors suggested (Czarniecki and Thornton, 1977b) that gangliosides embedded with ceramide in the membrane lipid bilayer have carbohydrate structures stabilized by solvation and "anchoring" in the solution by sialic acid residues. The sialic acid thereby exerts a stabilizing influence on the conformation of the ganglioside carbohydrate in water solutions. As a result of a network of intermolecular hydrogen bondings in aqueous media, sialic acid was shown to be the least mobile constituent in a ganglioside–sialo-oligosaccharide chain (Czarniecki and Thornton, 1977a,b).

In the ganglioside $G_{Gtet}1$, the sialic acid is very likely to adopt a preferred position of its ring perpendicular to that of the neighboring N-acetylgalactosamine (Harris and Thornton, 1978).

The ionic properties of sialic acid appear to be strongly influenced by the presence and the nature of an aglycon. This was tentatively deduced from the mobility of free sialic acid and ganglioside-derived sialo-oligosaccharides in paper electrophoresis at low pH values. As shown in Figure 2, at pH 1.9 monosialolactose migrates faster than free sialic acid. Further elongation of the sialo sugar by N-acetylgalactosamine to monosialogangliotriaose again shows an increase in mobility as compared to monosialolactose. Moreover, as demonstrated by the comparative electrophoretic migration of disialooligosaccharides at pH 1.9, the terminal sialic acid residues in a NeuAc($\alpha2\rightarrow8$)NeuAc-linkage, does not enhance the mobility when N-acetylgalactosamine is a second neighbor (Wiegandt, unpublished results).

It was discovered early that gangliosides exist as monomers in organic solvents such as dimethylformamide, dimethylsulfoxide, or tetrahydrofuran and form higher ordered structures in aqueous systems. Such properties will be strongly influenced by the conformation of both ceramide and sialo-oligosaccharide moieties.

Over the hydration range of 18–56% water, gangliosides exist as hexagonally packed rodlike structures (Curatolo et al., 1977). With higher percentage water, gangliosides form isotropic micellar solutions. The presence of micelles explains the macromolecular behavior of gangliosides in polyacrylamide gel electrophoresis (Dutton and Barondes, 1972). Electrophoresis also showed that ganglioside aggregates are rather stable in aqueous media, with little detectable monomer exhange, within 12 hr at 20 °C (Heuser et al., 1974). Upon dilution, however, Howard and Burton (1964) found a breakdown of ganglioside micelles within 30 min. Addition of phosphatidylcholine to ganglioside results in an increasing size of mixed micelles (Hill and Lester, 1972; Harris and Thornton, 1978). At higher lecithin to ganglioside ratios, cylindrical and lamellar structures are obtained that can be pelleted in the ultracentrifuge (Hill and Lester, 1972). A similar association between ganglioside and cholesterol has been shown by McCabe and Green (1977).

The aggregation properties of gangliosides in aqueous systems are determined in a subtle way by the ratio of C_{20}- to C_{18}-sphingoid fatty acids as well as the sialo-oligosaccharide (Yohe et al., 1976). The apparent micellar size is also sharply influenced by the presence of metal counter ions (Paglini and Zapata, 1975). Typical values for brain ganglioside micelles range from 300,000 M_r, with 220 monomers, and an apparent CMC of 7.5×10^{-5} M for ganglioside $G_{Gtet}1$ to 250,000 M_r, with 120 monomers, and apparent CMC of 1×10^{-4} M for ganglioside $G_{Gtet}3b$ (Yohe and Rosenberg, 1972; Yohe et al., 1976). The micellar shape is globular and in the form of an oblate ellipsoid. The inner part of the ganglioside micelle in aqueous solution may be partly permeable and house penetrating molecules as was suggested, e.g., for the triiodide ion, by Yohe and Rosenberg (1972).

Apart from the described micellar properties, several unrelated observations suggest that at levels below these CMC gangliosides may still exist in similar aggregate forms. Indications for this notion include conductivity measurements that show no well-defined break (Gammack, 1963; Howard and

Burton, 1964), alinearity of the absorbancy of the triiodide ion with change in ganglioside concentrations (Yohe and Rosenberg, 1972), and very low rate of dialysis of gangliosides below their apparent CMC. Additional evidence for the existence of ganglioside aggregate structures at very low concentrations (10^{-9} to 10^{-10} M) comes from ultracentrifugal sedimentation analysis of ganglioside $G_{Gtet}1$ in the presence and absence of the multivalently binding B protomer of cholera toxin (Schwarzmann *et al.*, 1978) as well as other gangliosides (Formisano *et al.*, 1979; Mraz *et al.*, 1979, 1980). In view of these more recent results, a reevaluation of all earlier data that report phase transition concentrations at much higher concentrations appears necessary.

2.6.2. Gangliosides in Membranes

The surface behavior of different gangliosides at the water–air interface was studied by Maggio *et al.* (1978*b*). It was reported that owing to electrostatic repulsion, the area requirement of the ganglioside predominantly depends on the charge of the molecule, with approximately 38–45 Å^2 in the uncharged state (44 Å^2 for dipalmitoylphosphatidylcholine). Gangliosides $G_{Lac}1$, $G_{Gtri}1$, and $G_{Gtet}1$ or $G_{Lac}2$ have similar area requirements within 10 Å^2. The authors suggest that electric charges in ganglioside molecules induce an increase in the fluidity of films that also is typical of lytically active lysolipids. And indeed, di- and trisialogangliosides were found capable of inducing membrane fusion in erythrocytes (Maggio *et al.*, 1978*a*). Perturbations of membranes by gangliosides may also be reflected by the release of dopamine from synaptosomal preparations upon addition of gangliosides (Cumar *et al.*, 1978) or the release of glucose from ganglioside-containing liposomes by biogenic amines (Maggio *et al.*, 1977). Another instance of lytic properties is seen in the disruption of the Sendai virus envelope caused by 10^{-6} M ganglioside (Tiffany, 1973). The role of ganglioside in liposome fusion by Sendai virus, however, may depend on their receptor properties towards the hemagglutinin-neuraminidase part of the spike glycoprotein, the fusion itself being effected by the fusogenic portion of the virus spike (Haywood, 1974*a,b*; Holmgren *et al.*, 1980).

According to studies by Sharom and Grant (1978), who employed electron spin resonance spectroscopy, gangliosides in membranes tend to cooperate via hydrogen bonding by clustering, particularly in the presence of physiological concentrations of Mg^{2+} and Ca^{2+} ions. An aggregation of gangliosides around glycoprotein in the membrane was also postulated.

2.6.3. Cation Binding to Gangliosides

Early hypotheses on the possible function of gangliosides implicated these lipids in special cation binding and transport or release mechanisms in biological membranes, particularly in the CNS (Triggle, 1971; Caputto *et al.*, 1977). Gangliosides have an affinity for divalent cations of approximately 1.5×10^3 M^{-1}. Abrahamson *et al.* (1972) showed that in a beef brain ganglioside mixture, the sialic acids can be titrated to roughly 50% at pH 4. In the presence of divalent cations, some of the carboxyl groups complex with the metal Ca^{2+}, being 20 times more effective than Mg^{2+}. The authors concluded that Ca^{2+} binds more strongly to ganglioside than to phospholipid because of the formation of chelate structures. Behr and Lehn (1973) showed with purified gangliosides that as the Ca^{2+} concentration increases a change in the binding stoichiometry occurs. This phenomenon is explained by the invariant tendency of ganglioside micelles to complex as much Ca^{2+} from the environment as possible; at high Ca^{2+} concentrations this is achieved in micellar structural configurations that allow for a correspondingly lower sialic acid to Ca^{2+} ratio. From solvent partition experiments by Hayashi and Katagiri (1974) it can be seen that Ca^{2+} may complex ganglioside to protein. Potassium chloride as well as acetylcholine inhibit such complex formation. ^{13}C Nuclear magnetic resonance spin lattice relaxation data yielded more precise information on the metal complexation site of ganglioside molecules, i.e., the atoms involved in the cation coordination sphere (Jacques *et al.*, 1977; Czarniecki and Thornton, 1977*b,c*). With this technique, Czarniecki and Thornton (1977*c*) discovered that the β-anomer of sialic acid complexes Ca^{2+} much more strongly than the naturally occurring α-anomer in ketosidic linkage [see also Jacques *et al.* (1977)]. Nevertheless, gangliosides are able to complex Ca^{2+} more strongly than free sialic acid alone. Sillerud *et al.* (1978) found that metal ion binding to ganglioside $G_{Gtet}1$ occurs via the carboxyl and the glycerol side chain of sialic acid. Additional ligands are donated by the *N*-acetylgalactosaminylpyranoside and the terminal galactose residue.

3. BIOCHEMICAL PROPERTIES OF GANGLIOSIDES

3.1. Occurrence in Nature

3.1.1. *Animal Species*

The available data on the phylogenetic occurrence and distribution of gangliosides allow some general conclusions to be drawn. Gangliosides are found in phyla of the *Deuterostomia*. They have not even been detected in the most highly developed protostomia. Since the cells of the nervous system are those most highly enriched with gangliosides, comparisons show that the level of higher brain organization correlates to a higher ganglioside content. Whereas mammals, birds, and reptiles have similar brain ganglioside content and component profile with only minor species peculiarities (Iwamori and Nagai,

1978*b*), teleost fish brain contains two to three times less ganglioside. An evolutionary trend is perhaps reflected in a shortening of the average neutral oligosaccharide chain length of gangliosides. Thus, the sialoglycolipids of the brain of mammals, birds, amphibians, and teleost fish contain predominantly gangliotetraose, though with a different degree of sialylation. In ray and bony fish, *Chondroichthies*, a high proportion of the brain gangliosides show shorter carbohydrates derived from lactose and gangliotriaose, respectively. The gangliosides from starfish *Asterina pectinifera*, contain ceramide-linked lactose substituted by *N*-glycolylneuraminosylresidues (Sugita and Hori, 1976), i.e., Ara($\beta 1 \rightarrow 6$)Gal($\beta 1 \rightarrow 4$)[8-OMe] NeuGl($\alpha 2 \rightarrow 3$)Gal($\beta 1 \rightarrow 4$)Glc$\beta 1 \rightarrow$Cer, Ara ($\beta 1 \rightarrow 6$)Gal($\beta 1 \rightarrow 4$)NeuGl($\alpha 2 \rightarrow 3$)Gal($\beta 1 \rightarrow 4$)Glc$\beta 1 \rightarrow$Cer and Ara($\beta 1 \rightarrow 6$) Gal($\beta 1 \rightarrow 4$) [Gal($\beta 1 \rightarrow 8$)] NeuGl($\alpha 2 \rightarrow 3$)Gal($\beta 1 \rightarrow 4$)Glc$\beta 1 \rightarrow$Cer.

Sea urchins have gangliosides derived only from glucose to which sialic acid is linked. The comparison of echinodermata gangliosides in this context may, however, be of less interest, since no comparable organ structures exist.

The ceramides of brain gangliosides in various animal species were studied by Avrova (1971) and Avrova and Zabelinski (1971). Whereas stearic acid is the predominant fatty acid in the major mammalian brain gangliosides, cold-blooded animals contain comparably more palmitic and monoenoic acids. In addition, the high amount of eicosasphingoid in major mammalian brain gangliosides typically found (23–48%) compares with only 3–12% of C_{20}-sphingoid in cold-blooded animals. The eicosasphingoid content and the generally higher degree of sialylation of gangliosides of poikilotherm (also promoting fluidization), may be interpreted as an adaption of membrane fluidity to heterotherm environmental conditions. In a similar direction, Breer (1975) and Breer and Rahmann (1976) observed that the brain ganglioside component profile of fish depends on the ambient temperature with a higher contribution of polysialylated compounds in the cold. This, as well as the varying degree of sialylation found in brain gangliosides of different vertebrate species, was believed to originate from a temperature adaption of the Ca^{2+}-complexing capacity of the sialoglycolipids in neuronal elements of the CNS (for review, see Rahmann, 1978).

3.1.2. Organ Distribution

Gangliosides are present in most, if not all, mammalian tissues (Table 3). The highest concentration and the highest degree of complexity is seen in cells of the CNS. In the CNS gangliosides are derived mostly from the ganglio series (see Section 2.1). Gangliosides in peripheral nerve and extraneural sites usually contain a high proportion of complex gangliosides derived from the lacto series (Wiegandt and Bücking, 1970; Svennerholm *et al.*, 1972). It has not yet been shown whether gangliosides of the ganglio and the lacto series may actually occur in one and the same cell.

TABLE 3. Ganglioside Content of Tissues[a]

Tissue of origin	Animal species	Ganglioside content	Reference[b]
Brain			
Whole	Man	321	1
Forebrain	Man	309	1
Cerebellum	Man	121	1
Stem	Man	297	1
Cerebrum	Rat	822	2
Cerebellum	Rat	406	2
Gray matter	Man	875	2
White matter	Man	275	2
Gray matter	Chimpanzee	374	2
	Monkey	300	2
	Chick	620	2
	Cattle	326	2
	Sheep	342	2
	Pig	406	2
Myelin			
Peripheral	Cattle	67–88	5
Spinal root	Cattle	218–287	5
Sciatic nerve, human	Cattle	218–287	5
Nerve			
Sciatic	Rabbit	83	6
Femoral	Man	33	4
Neurohypophysis	Cattle	453	3
Adenohypophysis	Cattle	71	3
Adrenal gland			
Medulla	Cattle	223	8
Mammary gland	Cattle	27	7
Retina	Man	113	10
	Cattle	126	10
	Rabbit	178	10
	Chick	123	11
	Rat	149	11
	Calf	179	11
Plasma	Man, cattle	3.7	9
	Rabbit	0.87	9
	Man	3.8	13
Erythrocytes	Man	7.7	13
	Man	2.9	14
Intestine, small, mucosa	Man	0.03	12
	Pig	0.6	12
	Cattle	13.3	12

[a] Units used throughout table are μg lipid-bound sialic acid/g fresh weight.

[b] Key to references: (1) Yusuf *et al.* (1977); (2) Ando *et al.* (1978); (3) Clarke (1975); (4) Svennerholm *et al.* (1972); (5) Fong *et al.* (1976); (6) Yates and Wherret (1974); (7) Keenan (1974b); (8) Ledeen *et al.* (1968); (9) Yu and Ledeen (1972); (10) Holm *et al.* (1972); (11) Edel-Harth *et al.* (1973); (12) Holmgren *et al.* (1975); (13) Portoukalian *et al.* (1978); (14) Wherret (1973); (15) Rösner *et al.* (1973).

3.1.2.1. Central Nervous System. In representative analyses on sphingoid bases, Kawamura and Taketomi (1977) estimated in mammalian brain a ganglioside content of 1.3–1.7 μmol in gray matter and 0.5–0.7 μmol in white matter, expressed per gram fresh tissue weight. In fish (carp) and frog total brain, lower values of gangliosides occur with 0.39 and 0.36 μ/mol sphingoid per gram wet weight, respectively. A detailed quantitative analysis of the ganglioside component distribution in brain of various animal species was reported by Ando *et al.* (1978). These authors confirmed the report of Ledeen *et al.* (1973) that ganglioside $G_{Gtet}1$ and $G_{Gal}1$ are the predominant sialolipids of brain white matter in primates and chicken, with other species having a much lower content of the latter compound.

Myelin of human or bovine peripheral nerve contains only some 50% of the ganglioside content of the myelin of the central nervous tissue. It does not show the presence of ganglioside $G_{Gal}1$ (Fong *et al.*, 1976). Gangliosides $G_{Gal}1$ and $G_{Gtet}1$ of central white matter are constituents of differentiated mature oligodendroglial myelin. Neuronal axons (bovine) derived from myelinated brain tissue have a different ganglioside profile with $G_{Gtet}1$, 2a, 2b, and 3, and an enrichment of the gangliosides $G_{Lac}2$ and $G_{Gtri}1$. The latter two components account for 40% of the total sialolipid (DeVries and Norton, 1974). Bovine oligodendrocytes from white matter (Poduslo and Norton, 1973) and hamster glial cells in culture (Robert *et al.*, 1975) also have $G_{Lac}2$ and $G_{Gtri}1$ as major gangliosides. Astroblasts in primary culture (96% $G_{Lac}1$ and 4% $G_{Lac}2$) or other glial tumor cells (Dawson *et al.*, 1971; Stoolmiller *et al.*, 1975), show only $G_{Lac}1$ and $G_{Lac}2$. No hexosamine-containing gangliosides have been discovered in glial tumors by Stoolmiller *et al.* (1975).

Two other neuronal elements have been isolated in fair purity and studied for their gangliosides, i.e., perikarya and nerve ending particles (for review, see Ledeen, 1978).

Neuronal cell bodies have a ganglioside content that is lower than that of whole brain (Norton and Poduslo, 1971; Hamberger and Svennerholm, 1971). On the other hand, synaptosomal fractions show enriched levels of gangliosides (Morgan *et al.*, 1972, 1973; Breckenridge *et al.*, 1972, 1973; Avrova *et al.*, 1973). The sialolipids appear to be concentrated among elements of the nerve ending plasma membrane. Synaptic vesicles and mitochondria contain no ganglioside (Wiegandt, 1967). Synaptic junctions have been isolated that are almost devoid of gangliosides (Morgan *et al.*, 1976).

There are obvious constraints on conclusions drawn from the observed occurrence of gangliosides in cultured cells concerning the distribution in the tissue of origin (for review, see Sato, 1973). Thus, established cells of neuronal origin derived from the mouse C-1300 tumor, that indeed retain many of the characteristics of neurons, show a general glycosphingolipid profile not very typical of fresh brain tissue-derived cells, especially in their having a tetrahexaosylceramide and a lack in higher oligosialogangliosides (Yogeeswaran *et al.*, 1973; Dawson and Stoolmiller, 1976). The glycolipid pattern of these cells does not change on neurite outgrowth, which is believed to represent some state of differentiation (Dawson, 1979).

3.1.2.2. *Peripheral Nerve.* Gangliosides have been identified in peripheral nerve tissue, including the neuro- and adenohypophysis, the adrenal medulla, and the visual tract.

The ganglioside distributions were reported by Svennerholm *et al.* (1972) for human femoral nerve, by Yates and Wherret (1974) for rabbit sciatic nerve, and by Klein and Mandel (1975) for rat sciatic nerve. All three groups showed thin layer chromatographic data for the peripheral nerve gangliosides, which were, however, not well-characterized or consistent.

Clarke (1975) showed that the bovine neurohypophysis contains a high concentration of gangliosides similar to those of cerebral cortex, consisting of more than 50% ganglioside $G_{Gtet}2a$, in addition to $G_{Gtet}2b$, and small amounts of $G_{Gtet}1$. However, unlike brain, a high proportion of ganglioside sialic acid is *N*-glycolylneuraminic acid.

The adenohypophysis on the other hand showed a drastically different distribution of gangliosides, with more than 43% of the total lipid-bound sialic acid in $G_{Lac}1NeuGl$ and $G_{Gtri}1NeuAc$.

Adrenal medulla, a component of the autonomic peripheral nervous system, is rich in gangliosides, with some 50% of the molar concentration present in brain gray matter (Ledeen *et al.*, 1968). Similar to the adenohypophysis, the ganglioside pattern more closely resembles that of extraneural sources in its low content of C_{20}-sphingoids and hexosamine-containing constituents. More than 90% of bovine adrenal medulla ganglioside consists of $G_{Lac}1$ (Price *et al.*, 1975). In this case, notably the membrane of an intracellular structure, the adrenal chromaffin granules were shown to contain ganglioside, predominantly G_{Lac} (Dreyfus *et al.*, 1977).

Several groups reported detailed analyses of the distribution of gangliosides in various parts of the visual system. The optic pathway, considered to be a part of the CNS, provided an attractive system for study. Reasons for this were, among others, easy accessibility and comparable structural simplicity. Elements of the retina, the optic nerve, and tectum can be isolated in purified form. Furthermore, the system is specifically excitable by light (Dreyfus *et al.*, 1974).

In the lens (Windeler and Feldman, 1970) and iris (Windeler and Feldman, 1969) the major ganglioside, representing more than 90% of the total sialo lipid, is $G_{Lac}1$. In contrast, ganglioside of mammalian retina consists mostly of $G_{Lac}2$ (35–46% of the total sialo lipids). There are minor species variations among mammals (Handa and Burton, 1969; Holm *et al.*, 1972). Other gangliosides of the retina are those found in brain with the exception of $G_{Gtri}1$.

Chicken retina gangliosides have a different component distribution than mammalian retinal sialolipids. They show, in addition to ganglioside $G_{Gtri}1$, predominantly $G_{Gtet}2a$, contributing more than 30% of the total gangliosides (Dreyfus *et al.*, 1974; Harth *et al.*, 1978). In frog photoreceptors, Hess *et al.* (1971) found only two gangliosides, tentatively identified as $G_{Gtet}2b$ and $G_{Gtet}3$.

The ganglioside $G_{Lac}2$ of mammalian whole retina appears localized in the outer segments of rod photoreceptor cells. Isolated rod outer segments have a ganglioside composition similar to whole retina. They show, however, a some-what higher content of $G_{Lac}1$ and $G_{Lac}2$ and a relative decrease of $G_{Gtet}2a$ com-pared to whole retina (Edel-Harth *et al.*, 1973). This suggests that hexosa-mine-containing gangliosides of the retina may be positioned in other retinal structural elements. Analyses of the ceramides derived from retinal ganglio-sides support this view. Whereas the ceramide of retinal $G_{Lac}2$ consists of mostly sphing-4-enine and $C_{20:0}–C_{22:0}$ fatty acids, retinal G_{Gtet} series ganglio-sides resemble brain gangliosides, with most of the fatty acid as $C_{18:0}$ and a high proportion of eicosasphingoid (Holm *et al.*, 1972; Holm and Mansson, 1974*a*). In addition, retinal $G_{Lac}2$ differs sharply in its metabolism from the other retinal gangliosides (Holm and Mansson, 1974*c*). The hexosamine-con-taining gangliosides may be characteristic constituents of retinal ganglion cells. In mammalian optic nerve, which contains the axons of retinal ganglion cells, no ganglioside $G_{Lac}2$ was detected (Holm and Mansson, 1974*b*). Instead, the four major brain gangliosides $G_{Gtet}1$, $G_{Gtet}2a$, $G_{Gtet}2b$, and $G_{Gtet}3$ constitute more than 90% of the sialolipid.

3.1.3. Cellular Localization

There is general agreement that gangliosides are most highly enriched in the outer cell surface membrane (Renkonen *et al.*, 1970; Weinstein *et al.*, 1970; Dnistrian *et al.*, 1975). However, Keenan *et al.* (1972*a*) and Critchley *et al.* (1973) pointed out the possibility of a more complex distribution, with localization not restricted to the plasma membrane. Keenan *et al.* (1972*b*) showed that besides Golgi membranes and plasma membranes gangliosides are indigenous to liver endoplasmic reticulum. Low levels of gangliosides may even occur as soluble constituents of the cytoplasm (Sonnino *et al.*, 1979). Tamai *et al.* (1974) found an absence of glycolipid in the rough-surfaced microsomal membranes from rat brain.

If indeed a precursor–product relationship is reflected in glycosphingolipid localization, the findings of Weinstein *et al.* (1970) may represent such a sit-uation. These authors report localization of gangliosides G_{Lac} and $G_{Gtet}2a$ in the plasma membrane of L-cells, whereas ceramide dihexoside and ganglioside $G_{Gtet}1$ were localized intracellularly.

An intracellular localization of gangliosides was also clearly demonstrated in rabbit muscle, where they are constituents of the sarcoplasmic reticulum

(Narasimhan *et al.*, 1974). In other studies, ganglioside was detected in smooth and rough endoplasmic reticulum (Cheema *et al.*, 1970), Golgi membranes (Keenan *et al.*, 1972*a*), primary and secondary lysosomal membranes (Huterer and Wherret, 1974; Henning and Stoffel, 1973), and membranes of adrenal medullary chromaffin granules (Dreyfus *et al.*, 1977).

Localization of ganglioside at the cell surface of sea urchin spermatozoa was reported by Ohsawa and Nagai (1975).

Viruses may contain ganglioside in their envelope derived from the host cell; this was demonstrated in the case of Sindbis virus. Stoffel and Sorgo (1976) found all of the sialolipid in the outer leaflet of its membrane. This strongly suggests that in uninfected cells as well, ganglioside is restricted to the outer leaflet of the membrane lipid bilayer.

Localization of gangliosides in brain tissue by histochemical methods using antibodies was reported by Baecque *et al.* (1976). Cholera toxin labeled with ^{125}I or peroxidase was employed for the electron microscopic visualization of ganglioside $G_{Gtet}1$ (Manuelidis and Manuelidis, 1976*a,b*; Hansson *et al.*, 1977). These studies showed ganglioside evenly distributed on the external side of the outer membranes of isolated neuronal, as well as glial cells. Little labeling, owing to the presence of ganglioside $G_{Gtet}1$, was seen in intracellular vesicles.

Ultrastructural localization of ganglioside $G_{Gtet}1$ by labeling with antibody to cholera toxin in extraneural tissue was previously demonstrated in the gastrointestinal epithelium (Peterson *et al.*, 1972). These studies are in agreement with the findings of Tamai *et al.* (1974) on an isolated central nerve perikaryal preparation and autoradiographic studies by Rösner *et al.* (1973). Both studies reveal that gangliosides, in contrast to cerebrosides and sulfatides, show a diffuse distribution over the entire cell surface.

Cholera toxin could also be used to divide C-1300 neuroblastoma cells into subpopulations on the basis of a cell surface receptor believed to be ganglioside $G_{Gtet}1$. Separation was achieved magnetophoretically with cholera toxin-conjugated magnetic microspheres that attach themselves to the cells (Kronick *et al.*, 1979).

Gangliosides positioned at the cell surface may not be accessible to nonpenetrating probes. Thus gangliosides were frequently reported not to be susceptible to neuraminidase degradation *in situ* (see Section 2.4.2).

3.2. Metabolism

3.2.1. Biosynthesis

Numerous reviews in recent years have summarized the published information on the biosynthesis of gangliosides (Ohman, 1970; Fishman, 1974;

Brady and Fishman, 1974; Richardson et al., 1975; Fishman and Brady, 1976).

The available evidence suggests that glycosyltransferases primarily control the transfer of nucleotide-activated monosaccharides onto the growing carbohydrate chain in ganglioside biosynthesis. To ensure a regulated sequential transfer, the existence of ordered multienzyme complexes were postulated by Roseman (1970) and Caputto's group (Maccioni et al., 1971; Arce et al., 1971). The precise cellular localization of all glycosyltransferases is not yet clear, particularly for ganglioside synthesis where the assembly of neutral or oligosialylated precursors may be at one locus, and final sialylation at another. Work from Keenan's laboratory (Keenan et al., 1972a,b, 1974b; Keenan, 1974) shows glycosyltransferases of glycosphingolipid biosynthesis located in the Golgi membranes. In fact it appears that much of the ganglioside that is found intracellularly resides in membranes for biosynthesis or lysosomal degradation. Several earlier reports, however, claim that glycosyltransferases (Patt and Grimes, 1974) and sialyltransferases (Pricer and Ashwell, 1971) could also be found at the cell surface, where they were thought to be involved in cis or trans (cell to cell) glycosylation reactions (Bosman, 1971, 1972; Roth and White, 1971). But more recent, careful studies with intact, viable cells under conditions that minimize extracellular hydrolysis of nucleotide-activated sugar precursors have cast considerable doubt on the existence of a glycosyltransferase activity on the surface of the cell (for reviews, see Keenan and Morré, 1975; Deppert and Walter, 1978).

In the brain, it was reported that nerve endings contain all necessary glycosyltransferases for incorporation of hexosamines and sialic acid into gangliosides (Den and Kaufman, 1968; Bosman and Hemsworth, 1970; Festoff et al., 1971).

In the chick tectum opticum the main site of ganglioside biosynthesis, however, was found to be in the neurona pericarya from where they may be translocated to the nerve endings (Landa et al., 1979).

The major route of ganglioside biosynthesis in the brain is outlined in Figure 3.

Kemp and Stoolmiller (1976) showed that neither the conversion of lactosylceramide to gangliotriaosylceramide nor the synthesis of $G_{Gtri}1$ from the latter trihexosylceramide takes place to any significant degree in rat neuroblastoma cells. This makes the transfer of N-acetylgalactosamine in the reac-

---

$\longrightarrow$

FIGURE 3. Pathway of brain ganglioside biosynthesis. Numbers in parentheses indicate references cited. Key to references: 1, Basu et al. (1973); 2, Yu and Lee (1976); 3, Yu and Ando (1977); 4, DiCesare and Dain (1971); 5, Kemp and Stoolmiller (1976); 6, Steigerwald et al. (1975); 7, Yip and Dain (1970); 8, Yip (1972); 9, Cumar et al. (1971); 10, Cumar et al. (1972); 11, Arce et al. (1971); 12, Moskal et al. (1974); 13, Duffard and Caputto (1972); 14, Mestrallet et al. (1974); 15, Yohe and Yu (1980).

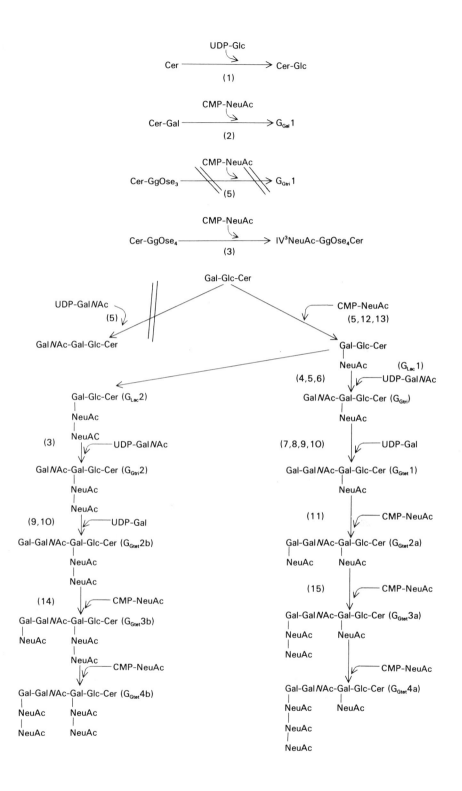

tion the key step in the main biosynthetic pathway of gangliosides of the ganglio series:

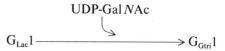

At this point ganglioside anabolism perhaps differs from catabolism. As reported by Tallman and Brady (1972), lysosomal brain neuraminidase and hexosaminidase may both act on ganglioside $G_{Gtri}1$:

$$-NeuAc \qquad GalNAc\text{-}Gal\text{-}Glc\text{-}Cer$$

$$GalNAc\text{-}GalNeuAc\text{-}Glc\text{-}Cer$$

$$NeuAc \qquad -GalNAc \qquad NeuAc\text{-}Gal\text{-}Glc\text{-}Cer$$

The presence of gangliotriaosylceramide, which is found in neuroblastoma NB41A cells by Dawson *et al.* (1971), and similarly that of ganglioside $G_{Gpt}1$ ($II^3NeuAc\text{-}GgOse_5\text{-}Cer$) in brain (Iwamori and Nagai, 1978a) may therefore possibly represent products of ganglioside catabolism rather than of biosynthesis. Transfer of *N*-acetylgalactosamine to lactosylceramide could, however, represent a prominent route of biosynthesis in other, perhaps nonneuronal, cell types, e.g., the neutral gangliotriaosylceramide found as the major glycosphingolipid in guinea pig erythrocytes, the gangliotetraosylceramide of rat T-lymphocytes and macrophages (Momoi *et al.*, 1980), the *Vibrio cholera* neuraminidase-labile ganglioside $G_{Gtet}1b$ ($IVNeuAc\text{-}GgOse_4\text{-}Cer$) occurring in rat hepatoma cells (Hirabayashi *et al.*, 1979), human erythrocytes (Watanabe *et al.*, 1979b), and tumors derived from Kirstern virus-transformed 3T3 mouse fibroblasts.

Glycosyltransferase (Yip and Dain, 1970) and sialyltransferase (Duffard and Caputto, 1972) activities are inhibited by added ganglioside. This, however, contrasts with the observation of Langenbach and Kennedy (1978) of an increased formation of higher gangliosides after addition of gangliosides to cells.

3.2.2. Biodegradation and Storage Diseases

Enzymes and enzyme activators involved in ganglioside biodegradation received particular attention because of their implications in hereditary storage diseases (for review, see O'Brian *et al.*, 1971; van Hoof, 1973; Baker *et al.*, 1976; Sandhoff, 1977; Brady, 1978).

With the possible exception of a ganglioside $G_{Lac}1$ storage disease, apparently all gangliosidoses are caused by deficiencies in the activity of degrading hydrolases. The basis may be a missing or faulty enzyme, or activator protein of such enzymes. Gangliosidoses can be classified according to the defects as listed in Table 4.

In "G_{MI}-gangliosidosis," near-normal levels of β-galactosidase could be demonstrated immunologically (Norden and O'Brien, 1975). The enzyme shows, however, a much decreased activity, believed to result from a structural gene mutation.

In the B and O variants of classical Tay Sachs disease, the deficiency in ganglioside hexosaminidase activity is caused by a reduction or absence of this enzyme. An explanation for the interrelationship between the gangliosidosis variants, based on β-hexosaminidase deficiencies, was derived from the structural constitution of the enzymes. According to the work of Geiger and Arnon (1976), hexosaminidase A consists of subunits α_2 and β_2, each containing two peptide chains linked by a disulfide. Hexosaminidase B, with a $\beta_2\beta_2$ configuration, has only one type of peptide. Another enzyme found in trace amounts, hexosaminidase S, consists of the corresponding $\alpha_2\alpha_2$ subunits only (Geiger et al., 1977). This may explain why hexosaminidase A never occurs without concomitant expression of hexosaminidase B (Lalley et al., 1974). It is concluded that in variant B of Tay Sachs disease, the α chain, and in variant O, the β chain of the hexosaminidase are inactive or missing.

The breakdown of gangliosides by degrading enzymes is greatly enhanced by glycoprotein activators first isolated from human liver (Li et al., 1974; Li and Li, 1976). Two such activators have been isolated, one specific for the conversion of $G_{Gtet}1$ to $G_{Gtri}1$ by human hepatic β-galactosidase (Li and Li, 1976), and the other for the degradation of $G_{Gtri}1$ to $G_{Lac}1$ by β-hexosaminidase (Hechtman and LeBlanc, 1977). The mechanism of action of these two separate protein activators (Li et al., 1979), although not yet known, may be dif-

TABLE 4.   Gangliosidoses

Ganglioside stored	Enzyme deficiency	Variant
II³NeuAc-GgOse₄-Cer	β-Galactosidase	G_{MI}-gangliosidosis
II³NeuAc-GgOse₃-Cer	Hexosaminidase A,S	Variant B (defect α-chain)
II³NeuAc-GgOse₃-Cer, GgOse₃-Cer,GbOse₄-Cer	Hexosaminidase A,B	Variant O (defect β-chain)
II³NeuAc-GgOse₃-Cer	Activator protein for hexosaminidase	Variant AB
	Acid neuraminidase	Mucolipidosis II (I-cell disease)

ferent from the nonspecific stimulation of enzymatic degradation *in vitro* caused by detergents such as taurocholate (Li and Li, 1979).

Sandhoff *et al.* (1977) reported that the enzymatic activity of human hexosaminidase, A or B, could be increased by detergents or by a natural activator protein preparation. Under such conditions, hexosaminidase B was more active towards GgOse$_3$-Cer than hexosaminidase A, whereas only the hexosaminidase A activity against substrate ganglioside $G_{Gtri}1$, and not that of the B enzyme, could be enhanced by activator or detergent. This may explain the method of storage of this ganglioside in the B variant of Tay Sachs disease. Recently Conzelmann and Sandhoff (1978), in a case of Tay Sachs AB variant, were able to demonstrate a deficiency of an activator for hexosaminidase A. Gangliosidoses also occur in animals (Handa and Yamakawa, 1971). An O variant Tay Sachs disease was detected in cats (Cork *et al.*, 1977). Storage of ganglioside $G_{Gtet}1$ due to reduced β-galactosidase activity was observed in a calf fibroblast cell line (Sheahan *et al.*, 1977).

Another group of "mucolipidoses" is caused by a deficiency in the action of lysosomal neuraminidases, i.e., mucolipidosis of type I (sialidosis) and type II (I-cell disease). Systematic studies by Cantz and collaborators employing fibroblast cultures obtained from patients with these respective mucolipidoses revealed characteristic differences of the endogenous sialidase activities towards sialic acid-containing substrates. Whereas in the case of mucopolidosis type I no sialidase activity was detected for sialo-oligosaccharide added to the cell culture, a normal activity was found for the substrate gangliosides $G_{Lac}1$, $G_{Lac}2$, and $G_{Gtet}2$, as well as endogenous sialoglycoconjugates (Cantz *et al.*, 1977; Michalski *et al.*, 1977; Spranger *et al.*,1977; Spranger and Cantz, 1978). Mucolipidosis type II fibroblasts are also unable to cleave sialic acid from sialo-oligosaccharide substrates. In addition, in this case a much reduced sialidase activity (20–40% of normal) with substrate gangliosides $G_{Lac}1$, $G_{Lac}2$, and $G_{Gtet}2$, as well as with endogenous sialoconjugates, was observed by Cantz and Messer (1979). These authors postulate that mucolipidosis type II is caused by a multiple hydrolase deficiency that is probably "secondary to an as yet unknown genetic lesion." In this respect it may be relevant that the neuraminidase of brain is believed to be localized preferentially in the neuronal plasma membrane, whereas the other ganglioside hydrolases, including extraneural sialidases, are of predominantly lysosomal origin (Schengrund and Rosenberg, 1970; Tettamanti *et al.*, 1972).

Storage of ganglioside $G_{Lac}1$ in the brain of a patient was reported by Max *et al.* (1974) and Fishman *et al.* (1975). Since in this case all higher gangliosides were missing, it was thought likely that the disease was caused by a deficiency in ganglioside biosynthesis. A marked increase of ganglioside $G_{Lac}1$ and $G_{Lac}2$ beyond the normal levels was also observed in cultured skin fibroblasts of a patient with mucolipidosis IV (Bach *et al.*, 1975).

In a recent study, Constantino-Ceccarini and Suzuki (1978) extracted a protease-sensitive factor from rat brain that inhibited the transfer of glucose or galactose to ceramide. It may therefore be assumed that activators of glycohydrolases as well as inhibitors of the glycosyltransferases may represent decisive factors that influence the ganglioside profile of tissues.

Other genetic disorders that affect the CNS but are not primarily caused by an error in ganglioside metabolism may nevertheless cause a derangement of the normal ganglioside pattern. In adrenoleukodystrophy the presence of extremely long chain fatty acid was reported by Igarashi *et al.* (1976). Also alterations of gangliosides were found in multiple sclerosis but they were not well characterized (Yu *et al.*, 1974).

3.3. Changes *in Vivo* in Ganglioside Composition

3.3.1. Developmental Changes in Brain

The gangliosides of the CNS undergo characteristic local changes in their component profile and composition of the ceramide moiety (for review, see Svennerholm, 1974). From these observations it was hoped that functional aspects of gangliosides might be revealed. At fetal stages of mammalian brain development, gangliosides are already prominent constituents of the CNS. Gangliosides increase in quantity, particularly during periods that parallel the rapid outgrowth of dendrites and axons, and the establishment of neuronal connections. The compositional pattern of gangliosides thereby changes, as has been shown in mammals (Yusuf *et al.*, 1977; Merat and Dickerson, 1973; Rösner, 1977), birds (Schengrund and Rosenberg, 1971; Irwin *et al.*, 1976), and fish (Breer and Rahmann, 1977).

During fetal development in mammals the relative quantities, as well as the absolute content, of monosialogangliosides $G_{Lac}1$, $G_{Gtri}1$, and $G_{Gtet}1$ decrease. Perinatally, particularly in the forebrain, ganglioside $G_{Gtet}2a$ content increases rapidly, whereas ganglioside $G_{Gtet}3a$, which is more abundant in human brain at the early fetal stage, shows a relative decrease in concentration (Svennerholm, 1974). The developmental changes in ganglioside patterns in human cerebellum and brain stem are different from forebrain and rather less pronounced (Yusuf *et al.*, 1977). At all times, ganglioside $G_{Gtet}2a$ is the major ganglioside in the cerebellum of man and rat.

Developmental ganglioside changes may be interpreted variously and it must be considered that they not only represent alterations in morphology, but also reflect differentiation and maturation of membrane structures. Therefore, if sialylation were a measure of the establishment of structural cell–cell connections and differentiation, the ganglioside $G_{Gtet}3b$ could be expected to arise in early completed connections of fetal brain. Ganglioside $G_{Gtet}2a$ might then reflect a later stage of development and newly completed structures that are dormant after a rapid division.

It was shown in humans by Manson *et al.* (1978) that individual gangliosides change their ceramide composition with increasing age. The ratio of C_{20} to C_{18} sphingoid increases rapidly until 10 yr of age. It then levels off with 60–70% C_{20} sphingoid after 30 yr of age. In addition, the fatty acids of ganglioside ceramide, which are comprised of 93% stearic acid at birth, have at the age of 98 yr a content of only 78% of this $C_{18:0}$ fatty acid, whereas the C_{20} fatty acids increase from 3 to 9%.

This change in ceramide composition with age is interpreted to reflect a physicochemical balancing of the hydro- and lipophilic portion of the ganglioside secondary to a general increase in the degree of sialylation.

3.3.2. Changes Related to Nerve Stimulation

Several groups have examined effects of physiological stimulation on ganglioside composition. Stimulating rats with light and sound, Maccioni *et al.* (1971 *b*) observed a redistribution of gangliosides within different subcellular compartments of brain tissue, with an increased content in the mitochondrial fraction and a decrease in synaptosomes and microsomes. This finding may, in some way, be compared to the observations made by Dreyfus *et al.* (1974), who reported that the rod outer segments in calf retina showed a 40% increase in the content of ganglioside after stimulation with light, with no change in their component distribution.

In other studies, behavioral stimulation was correlated with alteration of ganglioside metabolism. Irwin and Samson (1971) observed an increase in ganglioside $G_{Gtet}3$ with concomitant decrease in $G_{Gtet}2b$ in rats that were forced to swim in a deep water tank.

3.3.3. Changes at the Cellular Level

3.3.3.1.   Changes under Normal in Vitro Growth Conditions. The nature of a cell's gangliosides (e.g., ganglio or lacto series) results from a primary genetic expression. It is not clear at present whether quantitative alterations of ganglioside profiles, as observed, e.g., in clonal isolates of normal or transformed cells (Yogeeswaran *et al.*, 1972; Yogeeswaran and Murray, 1973; Moskal *et al.*, 1974) or upon chemical or viral transformation, are due to epigenetic variations in the regulation of gene expression.

The glycosphingolipid composition of cells, including gangliosides, is significantly and sensitively dependent on the physiological state of the cell. Biosynthesis and biodegradation vary with phases of the cell cycle. Using human epidermoid carcinoma KB cells in galactose incorporation studies, Chatterjee *et al.* (1973, 1975*a*) reported that glycosphingolipid and ganglioside were synthesized mainly during mitosis and the G_1-phase, with some biosynthesis also during S and G_2 phases. The chemical quantities of penta- and tetrahexosylceramides during the various phases of hamster NIL-cell cycle were found to be nearly constant, whereas tri- and dihexosylceramides were significantly increased during mitosis and in G_1 phase (Gahmberg and Hakomori, 1974). In a similar system of synchronized NIL-cells, Wolfe and Robbins (1974) showed that galactose incorporation into tetra- and trihexosylceramides occurred only during G_1 and S phase. Chatterjee *et al.* (1975*b*) deduced that glycosyltransferases with peak activity during the S phase, and glycosylhydrolases are synthesized at alternate times in cells with careful regulation. From this it can be expected that arrest of cells in G_1 phase is paralleled by an increase in glycosphingolipids. Indeed, certain agents that reduce cell growth or arrest cells in G_1, or a similar phase which at present can not yet precisely be defined (usually with a parallel change in cell morphology), cause alterations in glycosphingolipid profiles.

Inasmuch as the cell cycle is affected by cellular growth conditions, perhaps via cell–cell contact or adhesion, the metabolism of the cellular glycosphingolipids can limit their chemical quantity. The mode of growth in monolayer, as compared to suspension culture, appears to influence the profile of glycolipids, including the gangliosides, in a direction similar to that observed in resting versus rapidly dividing cells (Chatterjee *et al.*, 1975*a*).

Cells arrested in growth by cell–cell contact show a dramatic increase in chemical quantity and metabolic activity of the glycosphingolipids (Hakomori, 1970; Robbins and MacPherson, 1971). Whereas, in NIL 2 cells, predominantly neutral glycolipids are enhanced at confluence (Robbins and MacPherson, 1971), a cell line lacking in these lipids (NIL 1c1) shows an increase of ganglioside $G_{Lac}1$ upon cell–cell contact (Sakiyama *et al.*, 1972).

In contrast to hamster cell lines, such as BHK and NIL, which contain more neutral glycolipids, fibroblasts of murine origin have principally hexosamine-containing gangliosides (Yogeeswaran *et al.*, 1972). In BALB/c3T3 mouse fibroblasts, the synthesis and quantity of ganglioside $G_{Gtet}1$ and $G_{Gtet}2a$ is particularly high at early stages of cell contact, when still no growth inhibition occurs. The basis of this increase was related to a decrease in sialidase activity at touching phase of the cells (Yogeeswaran and Hakomori, 1975).* Recently, Patt *et al.* (1978) showed that the cell density-dependent inhibition of cell growth that can be reinduced in chemically or virally transformed cells

---

*An increase in sialidase activity in plasma membranes obtained from transformed cells in contrast to normal, untransformed cells was reported by Schengrund *et al.* (1973) and Visser and Emmelot (1973).

by retinol or retinoic acid was associated with changes in the ganglioside complement of the cells, with a particular increase in ganglioside $G_{Lac}1$ and promotion of the cell contact-dependent enhancement of $G_{Gtet}1$ and $G_{Gtet}2a$ synthesis.

An instance where stimulation of cell division is accompanied by increased glycolipid biosynthesis is seen in the lectin-induced changes in lymphocytes. Peripheral blood lymphocytes stimulated by phytohaemagglutinin M (Inouye *et al.*, 1974) or concanavalin A (Narasimhan *et al.*, 1976) change their compositional profile of glycolipids, including gangliosides.

Rosenfelder *et al.* (1978) showed an enhanced biosynthesis of neutral glycosphingolipids, as well as gangliosides, in concanavalin A-stimulated mouse thymocytes. In a more detailed study, Rosenfelder *et al.* (1979) also followed the effects of mitogens that are specific for T or B lymphocytes on glycolipid biosynthesis. The two cell types thereby showed an increased labeling of their specific ganglioside patterns.

A change in concentration of $G_{Lac}1$ (twofold in 10 min) in human platelets after treatment with thrombin was discovered by Chatterjee and Sweeley (1973). There is a concomitant reduction in the amount of free ceramide and lactosylceramide in these cells.

3.3.3.2. Changes Related to Cell Transformation. Transformation of cells either spontaneously or induced by virus (Fishman *et al.*, 1972), X rays (Coleman *et al.*, 1975), or chemical agents (Brady *et al.*, 1969) results in the loss of growth regulation mechanisms such as cell–cell contact-dependent growth inhibition. This loss is paralleled by a similar reduction in the levels of more complex neutral glycosphingolipids and gangliosides (Langenbach and Kennedy, 1978) similar to that seen in cells that are in a state of rapid division as compared to the resting state (for review, see Hakomori, 1973; Murray *et al.*, 1973; Brady and Fishman, 1974; Richardson *et al.*, 1975; Morré *et al.*, 1978). In Table 5, instances are listed where the change in ganglioside biosynthesis in cells undergoing transformation could be correlated to a block in the activity of corresponding glycosyltransferases, thus explaining increases in neutral precursor glycosphingolipid observed upon transformation (Lingwood *et al.*, 1978).

Transformation, induced chemically or by x-irradiation effects, effects changes in cellular ganglioside patterns that resemble those produced by oncogenic DNA viruses. Most studies of the glycosphingolipid changes that follow transformation of cells were performed with oncogenic viruses (Brady *et al.*, 1969; Coleman *et al.*, 1975). Infectious processes or drugs that inhibit cell protein biosynthesis also interfere with the production of enzymes involved in glycosphingolipid biosynthesis (Fishman *et al.*, 1974*b*; Simmons *et al.*, 1975; Vakirtzi-Lemonias and Evangelatos, 1978).

After viral transformation cells do not necessarily change their glyco-

TABLE 5. Enzymatic Block in Biosynthesis of Gangliosides in Transformed Cells

Depressed glycosylation reaction	Reference
$G_{Lac}1 \xrightarrow{+ GalNAc} G_{Gtri}1$	Keenan and Dodak (1973) Itaya and Hakomori (1976)
$G_{Gtri}1 \xrightarrow{+ Gal} G_{Gtet}1$	Keenan and Dodak (1973) Coleman et al. (1975) Fishman et al. (1974a)
$G_{Gtet}1 \xrightarrow{+ NeuAc} G_{Gtet}2$	Keenan and Morré (1973)
$G_{Gtet}2 \xrightarrow{+ NeuAc} G_{Gtet}3$	Siddiqui and Hakomori (1970) Cheema et al. (1970)

sphingolipid pattern; nor do they share the cell density-dependent glycolipid alteration response of the normal parent cells (Sakiyama et al., 1972).

3T3-cell revertants of DNA-virus transformation regain their normal ganglioside complement to a great extent (Mora et al., 1971). Similarly, the ganglioside status (i.e., the chemical quantity of ganglioside components) of cell lines that show temperature-dependent expression of transformed phenotype parallels the changes in growth regulation at permissive versus nonpermissive temperatures (Itaya and Hakomori, 1976; Lingwood et al., 1978).

Apart from ad hoc transformation of cells, changes in the ganglioside profile (generally with simplification of pattern) will also be a consequence of the slow dedifferentiation seen in cell cultures with increasing passages and aging (Stoker and MacPherson, 1961; Hakomori, 1970; Sakiyama et al., 1972; Manuelidis and Manuelidis, 1976b).

When cells grown as a solid tumor or in cell culture are compared, the tissue shows a pattern similar to that of single cells, but with increased amounts of gangliosides. A well-studied example of this type is the rat hepatoma (Cheema et al., 1970; Siddiqui and Hakomori, 1970; Dyatlovitskaya et al., 1974; Dnistrian et al., 1975; Leblond-Larouch et al., 1975; Skipski et al., 1975). During tumor growth a high increase in ganglioside-biosynthesizing enzymes is observed in the tumor itself and the surrounding tissue. Perhaps as a result of shedding of tumor enzyme, the increase is reflected in the serum; not only the ganglioside level increased (Skipski et al., 1975; Portoukalian et al., 1978), but also the concentration of sialic acid transferase (Bernacki and Kim, 1977). Similar observations were made in mammary tumor-bearing animals (Kloppel et al., 1977).

3.3.3.3. Drug-Induced Ganglioside Changes. Rather little is known about the factors mediating signals received by cells that result in regulation of ganglioside biosynthesis. Observations in which drugs induce alterations of cellular glycosphingolipids may therefore be useful in elucidating regulating events.

The possibility that the cellular cAMP level, via activation of enzymes, may directly influence glycoprotein and glycolipid biosynthesis is often proposed, but as yet has not been unequivocally demonstrated. Dibutyryl-cAMP has been used to increase the intracellular cAMP level, but its possible action on glycolipid biosynthesis is still uncertain. No effect of dibutyryl-cAMP on glycolipid synthesis was seen by Sakiyama *et al.* (1972). Dawson (1979) reported that "no profound" changes of gangliosides could be induced with dibutyryl-cAMP or with cholera toxin in mouse oligodendroglioma cells. In other reports, however, different results were presented. Dawson *et al.* (1979) mentioned an overall stimulation of ganglioside biosynthesis in mouse neuroblastoma cells. In mouse adrenal tumor cells, Yeung *et al.* (1974) showed that a shift in the ratio of different glycolipids, including ganglioside $G_{Lac}1$, occurred upon treatment with with dibutyryl-cAMP, with an increase in the higher glycosylated components. An increase in the biosynthesis of glycosphingolipids paralleled by an elevation in activity of galactosyl- and sialyltransferase was shown by Stoolmiller *et al.* (1974) in neuroblastoma cells after treatment with dibutyryl-cAMP. In all of the cases, it still needs to be clarified whether the effects of dibutyryl-cAMP are due to the product of hydrolysis (i.e., cAMP) or to the presence of butyrate.

Short chain fatty acids, including propionate, butyrate, and pentanoate may cause distinct morphological changes in cells. These changes are paralleled by an increase in ganglioside biosynthesis. The effect of butyrate can be related to an induction of a CMP-sialic acid:lactosylceramide sialyltransferase, while other glycotransferases remain unaffected (Fishman *et al.*, 1974*b*, 1976*b*; Simmons *et al.*, 1975). The drug norepinephrine increases the cAMP level in cells and also stimulates the incorporation of glucosamine into gangliosides of C1300 mouse neuroblastoma cells owing to an increased specific activity of UDP-Gal$N$Ac:$G_{Lac}1$-GalNAc-transferase (Stoolmiller *et al.*, 1974). On the other hand, when mouse neuroblastoma cells were cultured in the presence of opiates, as well as an enkephalin analogue, [D-Ala^2, D-Leu^5], an inhibition of [^{3}H]glucosamine and [^{14}C]galactose incorporation into gangliosides and glycoproteins was observed by Dawson *et al.* (1979).

A parallel effect on the metabolism of gangliosides and glycoproteins is also seen in the almost complete inhibition of ganglioside biosynthesis in the liver after administration of high doses of galactosamine (Rupprecht *et al.*, 1976).

3.3.4. Uptake of Exogenous Gangliosides

It is still an open question as to what extent *in vivo* alterations of endogenous gangliosides are directly related to any of the observed biological properties of cells. In order to approach this problem from a different angle, attempts have been made to incorporate exogenous gangliosides into cells artificially.

In vitro incubation of cells in the presence of exogenous gangliosides (except for $G_{Lac}1$) results in a saturable uptake of these lipids (Keenan *et al.*, 1974*a*; Moss *et al.*, 1976*a*). The cell accumulation of ganglioside thereby causes an inhibition of cell growth (Keenan *et al.*, 1975) and an increase in the biosynthesis of more complex gangliosides (Langenbach and Kennedy, 1978). Such an effect of ganglioside on cells may be related to the observation that ganglioside inhibits the recognition of cell surface receptors, as shown in the case of peripheral lymphocytes (Seiler *et al.*, 1976). The exact location of cell-incorporated exogenous ganglioside is unknown. Sharom and Grant (1978) used electron spin resonance-labeled ganglioside to probe the vicinity of cell-associated exogenous ganglioside. A considerable portion of cell-associated exogenous ganglioside was found in neuraminidase- and trypsin-labile positions and thus differed from endogenous glycolipid (Keenan *et al.*, 1974*a*; Callies *et al.*, 1977; Radsak *et al.*, 1979). Therefore, there is still doubt whether or not gangliosides, with a CMC of about 10^{-10} M, can be inserted into the lipid bilayer of the outer cell surface membrane. On the other hand, ganglioside analogs that contain a single, electron spin-labeled aliphatic hydrocarbon chain instead of the ceramide moiety (CMC $\simeq 10^{-4}$) are irreversibly incorporated into liposomes as well as erythrocytes, as shown by the change in ESR signal, indicating immobilization of the probe (Kanda *et al.*, 1979). Gangliosides are taken up poorly by cells in the presence of serum-containing media (Barkai and DiCesare, 1975; Fishman *et al.*, 1977). In addition, it is known that some, but not all, glycolipid components present in plasma may be transferred to erythrocytes (Dawson and Sweeley, 1970; Koscielak *et al.*, 1978). These findings indicate that competing structures in serum bind gangliosides very tightly. In addition, it was shown by Filipovic *et al.* (1978) that ganglioside is taken up by serum lipoprotein, causing an inhibition of the high affinity binding that otherwise leads to internalization of the lipoprotein by cultured cells.

3.4. Immunologic Properties of Gangliosides

The immunogenicity of glycosphingolipids, including gangliosides, was reviewed comprehensively by Rapport and Graf (1969) and Marcus and Schwarting (1976).

Gangliosides contribute to the immunologic expression of cells. Reports of Esselman and Miller (1974 *a,b*) and Miller and Esselman (1975 *a,b*) of the ganglioside nature of the murine Thy-1 (theta) allo-antigen, a surface marker present on T lymphocytes in brain and epidermal cells, could not be confirmed by Stein-Douglas *et al.* (1976).

In a more recent investigation, Wang *et al.* (1978) isolated Thy-1 active glycolipid from mouse brain. This compound demonstrated chromatographic properties similar to ganglioside $G_{Gtet}1$. It could, however, be separated from the latter by thin layer chromatography. The nonidentity of ganglioside $G_{Gtet}1$ and Thy-1 antigen was also stressed by de Cicco and Greaves (1978), who showed the Thy-1 antigen to have a mobility at the cell surface different from this ganglioside. Since certain membrane proteins with Thy-1 antigenicity have also been isolated (Williams *et al.*, 1977), it appears that Thy-1 specific carbohydrate residues may exist in glycolipids as well as in glycoproteins.

Ganglioside $G_{Lnhex}1a$ (VI^3NeuAc-$nLcOse_6$-Cer) from human erythrocytes showed the immunocharacteristics of iI blood group (Nieman *et al.*, 1978). The sialic acid of this ganglioside, however, is not required for expression of the i and I activities.

The induction of ganglioside antibodies by injection of lipid micelles and methylated bovine serum albumin was described by Nagai and Ohsawa (1974); for methodology, see Hakomori (1972) and Marcus (1976). Using this immunization procedure, high titer antisera could be raised against gangliosides $G_{Gtet}1$ and $G_{Gtet}2b$, whereas gangliosides with terminal sialic acid residues produced only low or negligible levels of ganglioside antibodies (Nagai *et al.*, 1976). Naiki *et al.* (1974) gave a comparative description of the properties of antisera prepared by a single injection of ganglioside $G_{Gtet}1$ or gangliotetraosylceramide. It was shown that antibodies exist that specifically recognize ganglioside $G_{Gtet}1$ and are inhibited by monosialogangliotetraose.

The production of antibodies and their Fab fragments for ganglioside $G_{Lac}1NeuGl$ was reported by Laine *et al.* (1974). The specificity of these antibodies, which were purified by affinity chromatography on $G_{Lac}1$-coupled to agarose, is mainly directed against the *N*-glycolylneuraminic acid residue of this ganglioside.

Antisera to gangliosides exhibit a number of biological actions in cellular systems that reflect the involvement of gangliosides in cell surface membrane-mediated processes of cell regulation. Thus, spleen lymphocytes coated with ganglioside were able to trigger a "mixed lymphocyte reaction" in autologous thymus-derived lymphocytes (Sela, 1980). Furthermore, ganglioside $G_{Gtet}1$ antibodies in rat thymocytes stimulate mitosis and induce cap formation (Sela *et al.*, 1978). Recently, Lingwood *et al.* (1978) showed that monovalent Fab fragments of ganglioside $G_{Lac}1$ and $G_{Gtet}1$ antibodies effectively inhibit the expression of transformed phenotypes in virus transformed cells. This property of antiganglioside is shared by Fab fragment of LETS protein antibodies.

Various reports describe the application of ganglioside antisera to nervous tissue. Injection of ganglioside antisera into the cat sensorimotor cortex induced spiking in the electroencephalogram and led to seizures (Karpiak *et al.*, 1976*a*,*b*; Rapport and Karpiak, 1976). These authors also observed an effect of antisera to brain gangliosides on learning, memory, and behavior of rats (Karpiak *et al.*, 1976*a*–*c*; Rapport and Karpiak, 1976). These observations may relate to the induction of an epileptiform status by the ganglioside G_{Gtet}1-binding B protomer of cholera toxin (Karpiak *et al.*, 1978). Gangliosides also appear involved in immunopathologies observed in humans such as "serum sickness." Higashi and Naiki (1977) presented evidence that the heterophile antibodies found in patients that have received animal sera are directed against ganglioside with terminal N-glycolylneuraminyl($\alpha2\rightarrow3$)galactosyl residues, as found in ganglioside G_{Lac}1NeuGl and G_{Lmet}1aNeuGl.

3.5. Biological Effects of Gangliosides on Nerve Tissue

Several reports show that gangliosides can influence nervous tissue with pathological consequences that may occur partly as a result of immunologic events. Immunodamage, likely to be caused by ganglioside antibodies and sensitized lymphocytes, and closely resembling experimental encephalomyelitis with concomitant extensive degeneration of peripheral nerves, was experimentally induced with brain ganglioside (Nagai *et al.*, 1976).

Whereas in the CNS the encephalitogenic peptide of basic myelin protein can alone induce demyelination, in peripheral nervous tissue the corresponding myelin P2 protein has full capacity to induce experimental allergic peripheral neuritis only in the presence of glycosphingolipids, such as ganglioside (Nagai *et al.*, 1978) or cerebroside (Saida *et al.*, 1979). From their studies, Nagai *et al.* (1978) suggest the possibility that the immunologic properties of ganglioside are directly responsible for the peripheral myelitis-inducing activity of the complex.

A very different effect of ganglioside on nerve tissue was reported by Ceccarelli *et al.* (1976). These authors point out that ganglioside may offer "substantial protection against damage caused by different types of experimental polyneuritis." According to their findings, an intraperitoneal injection of gangliosides in cats following anastomosis greatly influences peripheral sympathetic nerve regeneration and reinnervation by promotion of outgrowth of axons. It may be relevant that denervation of muscle itself causes a change in the ganglioside pattern in this tissue (Max, 1970).

A remarkable property of gangliosides was proposed by Micelli *et al.*

(1977), who introduced these lipids for the therapy of mental deterioration. The authors report that patients who had received a dose of 10 mg of mixed bovine brain gangliosides by intramuscular injection twice daily (!) showed a significant lessening in the degree of dementia.

4. BINDING PROPERTIES OF GANGLIOSIDES

4.1. Interaction of Gangliosides with Toxins, Hormones, and Interferon

Perhaps one of the most exciting recent developments in ganglioside research was initiated by the pioneering work of W. E. van Heyningen. Van Heyningen was first to show the remarkable binding properties of gangliosides to the exotoxins of *Clostridium tetani* and *Vibrio cholerae*. Numerous articles and reviews have since dealt with this subject; for review, see W. E. van Heyningen (1974), Fishman and Brady (1976), Bennett *et al.* (1976), and Wiegandt (1979).

The study of the interaction between these bacterial toxins and gangliosides appeared particularly attractive since a more general function of sialolipid in cell surface receptors might emerge. Indeed, the interactions of gangliosides with toxins bear many of the characteristics of the binding of hormones to receptors.

The following toxins were reported to bind to ganglioside*: *Clostridia* neurotoxins, tetanus toxin (W. E. van Heyningen, 1959*a,b,c*); botulinus toxin (Simpson and Rapport, 1971); exoenterotoxins, cholera toxin (W. E. van Heyningen *et al.*, 1971); *Escherichia coli* toxin (Donta and Viner, 1975); staphylococcus α toxin (Kato and Naiki, 1976); and hemolysins of *Streptococcus parahemolyticus* (Takeda *et al.*, 1976), and that of the sea wasp (Crone, 1976).

Tetanus toxin in its extracellular form consists of two peptide chains of approximately 100,000 and 40,000 M_r, linked by a disulfide bond. Only the heavy chain contains the intact ganglioside binding site of the toxin (S. van Heyningen, 1976; Helting *et al.*, 1977). The structural requirements of ganglioside for fixation by the toxin were first studied by W. E. van Heyningen (1963, 1974). He showed, with ganglioside insolubilized by cerebroside, that optimal fixation was achieved only with gangliosides of the ganglio series that carried two sialic acid residues at the nonterminal galactose of the gangliotetraose, i.e., $G_{Gtet}2b$ and $G_{Gtet}3b$ (W. E. van Heyningen and Mellanby, 1968). Gangliosides $G_{Gtet}1$ and $G_{Gtet}2a$ could fix tetanus toxin some 7–12 times less, whereas with ganglioside $G_{Gtri}1$ the binding amounted to only 0.02% of that of

---

*References are to initial reports.

$G_{Gtet}2b$. These data agree well with those obtained by Lee *et al.* (1978), who used binding of [^{125}I]-tetanus toxin to ganglioside-containing liposomes. In a different assay system employing Sephadex-adsorbed tetanus toxin and radio-labeled sialoglycolipids, Helting *et al.* (1977) showed that ganglioside binds to the toxin in a 1:1 molar ratio with half saturation at 10^{-8} M for the ligand. All the gangliosides tested in this assay system, including $G_{Lac}1$, $G_{Gtri}1$, $G_{Gtet}1$, $G_{Gtet}2b$, and $G_{Gtet}3b$, as well as structurally unrelated synthetic sialoglycolipid, bound to the toxin to a comparable extent (Helting *et al.*, 1977; Wiegandt, 1979). Besides the presence of sialic acid, a lipid moiety of the ligand was required for binding to tetanus toxin.

The results obtained with the Sephadex matrix procedure are in contrast to the ganglioside selectivity, i.e., $G_{Gtet}2b \approx G_{Gtet}3 \gg G_{Gtet}1 \approx G_{Gtet}2a \gg G_{Gtri}1$, shown in other test systems. This discrepancy may perhaps be explained by an influence of the Sephadex matrix on the ganglioside-ligand interaction.

Tetanus toxin is fixed by isolated brain nerve ending preparations known to contain gangliosides in high concentration (Mellanby and Whittaker, 1968; Habermann, 1976). However, in experiments showing tetanus toxin binding by direct immunofluorescence, Zimmermann and Gifferetti (1977) claimed that differentiating mouse neuroblastoma C1300 cells pretreated with neuraminidase and β-galactosidase still fixed toxin by a mechanism unrelated to ganglioside.

According to Stoeckel *et al.* (1975), tetanus toxin is internalized at peripheral nerve terminals and transported retrogradely. Ganglioside $G_{Gtet}3b$ reduced this axonal transport by only 50% (Stoeckel *et al.*, 1977).

A conspicuous parallelism appears to exist for the binding of tetanus toxin and the thyroid stimulating hormone, thyrotropin, to membranes of the thyroid gland (Habig *et al.*, 1978). The two effector molecules could replace each other specifically at these membranes and it was postulated that gangliosides are involved as receptors for both the hormone and the toxin (Mullin *et al.*, 1976*a,b*; Meldolesi *et al.*, 1976). Gangliosides added to thyrotropin inhibit its binding to thyroid membranes with a similar sequence of efficiency as observed for tetanus toxin, i.e., $G_{Gtet}2b \geqslant G_{Gtet}3b > G_{Gtet}1 > G_{Gtri} = G_{Lac}1 > G_{Gtet}2a$ (Mullin *et al.*, 1976*a*). The specific binding of thyrotropin was also shown with ganglioside-containing lipid bilayer systems (Aloj *et al.*, 1977; Poss *et al.*, 1978).

Thyrotropin prevents and reverses the binding of tetanus toxin to thyroid membranes in a similar way to that observed with cholera toxin, which also binds to ganglioside (Mullin *et al.*, 1976*b*; Ledley *et al.*, 1977).

Speculations that gangliosides act solely as tetanus toxin or thyrotropin receptors were, however, contradicted by the finding of Lee *et al.* (1978) that both effectors may also specifically interact with a glycoprotein component from thyroid gland. Therefore, ganglioside (or possibly other acidic lipids) and a specifically binding glycoprotein may both be involved in the reception of the tetanus toxin, or thyrotropin, and the mediation of effector information at the plasma membrane.

The discovery of the specific and multivalent binding of cholera toxin to ganglioside was made by W. E. van Heyningen et al. (1971); for review, see Gill (1977). Later studies of this phenomenon emanated mainly from the laboratories of Cuatrecasas (Bennett et al., 1976), Svennerholm (1976), and Wiegandt (1979).

Of the two cholera toxin protomer subunits, the A protein, carrying an ADP-ribosyltransferase activity, and the pentamer B protein, only the latter binds to ganglioside (Sattler et al., 1975; Bennett et al., 1976). The interaction is cooperative in nature and highly specific for ganglioside $G_{Gtet}1$ (Holmgren et al., 1974). On binding, only part of the monosialogangliotetraose, the carbohydrate moiety of $G_{Gtet}1$, is involved, i.e., $Gal(\beta1{\rightarrow}3)$-$GalNAc(\beta1{\rightarrow}4)Gal(3{\leftarrow}2\alpha)NeuAc$ (Stärk et al., 1974; Sattler et al., 1977, 1978). Binding to ganglioside $G_{Gtet}1$ or monosialogangliotetraose induces a conformational change in the toxin protein shown by a blue shift of fluorescence spectra (Mullin et al., 1976b; Moss et al., 1977b; Fishman et al., 1978b).

When ganglioside $G_{Gtet}1$–cholera toxin interaction occurs, it is assumed that ceramide provides an anchorage at the cell membrane and allows for multivalent interactions with membrane-bound ganglioside or other structures such as micelles (Sattler et al., 1977; Schwarzmann et al., 1978). Indeed, cholera toxin induces perturbations of ganglioside-containing liposome membranes with release of entrapped glucose (Moss et al., 1976b, 1977c; Ohsawa et al., 1977). Whereas Tosteson and Tosteson (1978) observed that cholera toxin could create ion permeable channels in bilayers of lecithin ganglioside $G_{Gtet}1$, Ochoa and Bangham (1976) could see no increase in ion permeability in a similar system.

At the cell surface membrane, cholera toxin induces a redistribution of membrane constituents that are believed to be linked to receptor ganglioside. Intramembrane proteins connected with the cytoskeletal system may be involved in patching and capping of the receptor–toxin complexes (Craig and Cuatrecasas, 1975; Revesz and Greaves, 1975; Sedlacek et al., 1976).

Although inhibition of cholera toxin in an in vivo system by gastric mucin was reported by Strombeck and Harrold (1974), at present it is widely accepted that ganglioside $G_{Gtet}1$ is the sole cell receptor for this toxin. Indeed, the responsiveness of cells to the toxin varies in parallel to the ganglioside composition (Hollenberg et al., 1974; Holmgren et al., 1974, 1975; Fishman et al., 1976b, 1977). NCTC2071 Cells chemically transformed mouse fibroblasts that contain no detectable $G_{Gtet}1$ are not responsive to cholera toxin. In this case exogenous $G_{Gtet}1$ could be functionally incorporated and serve as receptor for the toxin (Moss *et al.*, 1976*a*; Fishman *et al.*, 1977, 1978*a,b*). Endogenous and exogenous $G_{Gtet}1$ is protected by cholera toxin from the action of galactose oxidase (Moss *et al.*, 1977*a*).

Cholera toxin and the heat-labile exotoxin of *Escherichia coli* have many characteristics in common and may be similar (Dallas and Falkow, 1979). Thus, the steroidogenic effect of both toxins in adrenal tumor cells is inhibited by $G_{Gtet}1$ (Donta and Viner, 1975). Cholera toxin also interferes with the antiviral action of human interferon (Kohn *et al.*, 1976; Degré, 1978). A possible role for membrane ganglioside as receptor for interferon was first suggested by Besancon and Ankel (1974). Interferon was neutralized after preincubation with ganglioside and could be removed effectively from solution by ganglioside–Sepharose (Vengries *et al.*, 1976; Besancon *et al.*, 1976). The specificity of binding to interferon is not restricted to one ganglioside but decreases in effectiveness in the following order: $G_{Gtri}1 \gg G_{Gtet}3 > G_{Gtet}1 \gg G_{Gtet}2a > G_{Lac}1$. Binding of ganglioside to interferon can be reversed to a great extent by sialyllactose, indicating the involvement of this structural unit in the interaction (Besancon *et al.*, 1976).

The existence of two cell receptors for interferon was suggested by Chany *et al.* (1977). One receptor of the cell membrane-bound system is believed to be a "nonspecific" ganglioside, and the other is probably generated by a trypsin-sensitive glycoprotein that forms a species-specific activator site responsible for the amplification of the cellular response towards interferon. Ankel *et al.* (1980) showed two types of interferons from mouse fibroblasts, of which only one binds to ganglioside.

4.2. Interaction with Neurotropic Agents

Since the original observation by Woolley and Gommi (1964, 1965) that the serotonin sensitivity of a neuraminidase-treated fungus preparation can be restored by adding gangliosides, particularly $G_{Lac}2$, the question has not been answered unequivocally as to whether these sialoglycolipids constitute serotonin tissue receptors; for review, see W. E. van Heyningen (1974*b*). Ochoa and Bangham (1976) believe that the receptor site determinant is the sialic acid residue because other sialoglycoconjugates, such as fetuin, also bind serotonin. These authors could show that serotonin is fixed by liposomes containing various gangliosides with an affinity of only 10^2 1/mol, without affecting the ion permeability of their membrane. On the other hand, Maggio *et al.* (1977) reported the release of entrapped glucose from ganglioside-containing liposomes induced by serotonin and other biogenic amines. The involvement of bound sialic acid in the serotonin transport system was demonstrated by Dette and Weseman (1978). Pretreatment with neuraminidase noncompetitively inhibited the high affinity uptake of serotonin into rat brain synaptosomes. A specific and strong interaction between serotonin and ganglioside was also suggested from NMR studies which showed pronounced broadening of the aromatic resonance of the amine at 60MHz (Krishnan and Balaram, 1976). Chlorpromazine has an antiserotonin effect, and similarly binds to ganglioside (Krishnan and Balaram, 1976). Binding of d-tubocurarine to ganglioside was discovered by Rösner et al. (1979).

Colchiceine binds to ganglioside in a Ca^{2+}-dependent way. However, the specificity of this interaction is not very pronounced. The relative binding capacities of the ganglioside $G_{Gtet}3b$, $G_{Gtet}2a$, and $G_{Gtet}1$ for colchiceine (7:4:1) are not linearly related to their respective sialic acid contents (Rösner and Schönharting, 1977).

4.3. Interaction with Fibronectin (LETS Protein)

The observation made by Lingwood et al. (1978) that antiganglioside, as well as antifibronectin antibodies, had similar effects on the growth of transformed cells was already suggestive of some connection between ganglioside and fibronectin at the cell surface membrane (see Section 3.4). Indeed, Kleinman et al. (1979) discovered that fibronectin-mediated cell adhesion to collagen was inhibited by addition of gangliosides. Cell adhesion was also inhibited by the corresponding sialo-oligosaccharides that represent the carbohydrate portion of the respective gangliosides. Various gangliosides differed in their capacity to prevent cell attachment in the following order: $G_{Gtet}3b \gg G_{Gtet}2a > G_{Gtet}2b > G_{Gtet}1 > G_{Gtri}1$. $G_{Lac}1$ was found to be noninhibitory. Kleinman et al. (1979) also showed that the inhibition caused by gangliosides was not due to interference with the binding of fibronectin to collagen, but rather to an inability of the cell to attach to the fibronectin–collagen complex.

5. CONCLUDING REMARKS

The period of rapid expansion of our knowledge of the chemical constitution of the classical gangliosides appears to be coming to a close. As a consequence, research in this field is moving in the direction of clarification of their biological implications. It already appears evident that the physical, chemical, and metabolic properties of the gangliosides are well-balanced and may have great relevance in an understanding of their role. From their amphiphilic nature, we can assume that gangliosides are probably positioned with the ceramide moiety inserted within the lipid phase of the membrane. Beyond this one can say little, since we are still ignorant of basic facts. We do not yet know how the ganglioside molecule is distributed within the biomembrane, either statically or dynamically; nor is it understood which functional properties are imparted to biomembranes through the presence of gangliosides. In this respect, the association of gangliosides with other structures within the bio-membrane, particularly proteins, either as enzymes or as elements of information-mediating systems of the membrane, is an obvious possibility. We know little about the regulation of ganglioside metabolism that might predict which species should influence a cell's responsiveness to external stimuli. More refined experimental methods at the cellular level will undoubtedly be used to gain a further understanding of their biological importance.

6. REFERENCES

Abrahamson, M. B., Yu, R. K., and Zaby, V., 1972, Ionic properties of beef brain gangliosides, *Biochim. Biophys. Acta* **280**:365–372.

Aloj, S. M., Kohn, L. D., Lee, G., and Meldolesi, M. F., 1977, The binding of thyrotropin to liposomes containing gangliosides, *Biochem. Biophys. Res. Commun.* **74**:1053–1059.

Anderson, R., and Dales, S., 1978, Biogenesis of Pox viruses: Glycolipid metabolism in vaccinia-infected cells, *Virology* **84**:108–17.

Ando, S., and Yu, R. K., 1977*a*, Isolation and characterization of human and chicken brain tetrasialoganglioside, *Proc. Int. Soc. Neurochem.* **6**:535.

Ando, S., and Yu, R. K., 1977*b*, Isolation and characterization of a novel trisialo-ganglioside, G_{T1a}, from human brain, *J. Biol. Chem.* **252**:6247–6250.

Ando, S., Isobe, M., and Nagai, Y., 1976, High performance preparative column chromatography of lipids using a new porous silica, iatrobeads: separation of molecular species of sphingoglycolipids, *Biochim. Biophys. Acta,* **424**:98–105.

Ando, S., Kan, K., Nagai, Y., and Mureta, T., 1977, Chemical ionization and electron impact mass spectra of oligosaccharides derived from sphingolipids, *J. Biochem.* **82**:1623–1631.

Ando, S., Chang, N.-Ch., and Yu, R. K., 1978, High performance thin layer chromatography and densitometric determination of brain ganglioside compositions of several species, *Anal. Biochem.* **89**:437–450.

Ankel, H., Krishnamurti, Ch. Besancon, F., Stefanos, S., and Falcoff, E. (1980) Mouse fibroblast (type I) and immune (type II) interferons: Pronounced differences in affinity for gangliosides and in antiviral and antigrowth effects on mouse leukemia L-1210R cells, *Proc. Natl. Acad. Sci.* **77**:2528–2532.

Arce, A., Maccioni, H. J., and Caputto, R., 1971, The biosynthesis of gangliosides. The incorporation of galactose, *N*-acetylgalactosamine and *N*-acetylneuraminic acid into endogenous acceptors of subcellular particles from rat brain *in vitro, Biochem. J.* **121**:483–493.

Avrova, N. F., 1971, Brain ganglioside patterns of vertebrates, *J. Neurochem.* **18**:667–674.

Avrova, N. F., and Zabelinsky, S. A., 1971, Fatty acids and long chain bases of vertebrate brain gangliosides, *J. Neurochem.* **18**:675–681.

Avrova, N. F., Chenkaeva, E. Yu., and Obukhova, E. L., 1973, Ganglioside composition and content of rat brain subcellular fractions, *J. Neurochem.* **20**:997–1004.

Bach, G., Cohen, M. M., and Kohn, G., 1975 Abnormal ganglioside accumulation in cultured fibroblasts from patients with mucolipidosis IV, *Biochem. Biophys. Res. Commun.* **66**: 1483–1490.

Baecque, C., Johnson, A. B., Naiki, M., Schwarting, G., and Marcus, D. M., 1976, Ganglioside localisation in cerebellar cortex: an immunoperoxidase study with antibody to G_{M1} ganglioside, *Brain Res.* **114**:117–122.

Baker, H. J., Mole, J. A., Lindsey, J. R., and Creel, R. M., 1976, Animal models of human ganglioside storage diseases, *Fed. Proc. Fed. Am. Soc. Exp. Biol.* **35**:1193–1201.

Barkai, A., and DiCesare, J. L., 1975, Influence of sialic acid groups on the retention of glycosphingolipids in blood plasma, *Biochim. Biophys. Acta* **398**:287–293.

Basu, S., Kaufmann, B., and Roseman, S., 1973, Enzymatic synthesis of glucocerebroside by glucosyltransferase from embryonic chicken brain, *J. Biochem. Chem.* **248**:1388–1394.

Behr, J. P., and Lehn, J. M., 1973, The binding of divalent cations by purified gangliosides, *FEBS Lett.* **31**:297–300.

Bennett, V., Craig, S., Hollenberg, M. D., O'Keefe, E., Sahyoun, N., and Cuatrecasas, P., 1976, Structure and function of cholera toxin and hormone receptors, *J. Supramol. Struct.* **4**:99–210.

Bernacki, R. J., and Kim, N., 1977, Concomittant elevations in serum sialytransferase activity and sialic acid content in rats with metastasizing mammary tumor, *Science* **195**:577–580.

Besancon, F., and Ankel, H., 1974, Binding of interferon to ganglioside, *Nature London* **252**:478–480.

Besancon, F., Ankel, H., and Basu, Sh., 1976, Specificity and reversibility of interferon ganglioside interaction, *Nature London* **259**:576–578.

Bjorndahl, H., Hellerquist, C. G., Lindberg, G., and Svenson, S., 1970, Gas-Flüssigkeits-Chromatographie Massenspektrometrie bei der Methylierungsanalyse von Polysacchariden, *Angew. Chem.* **82**:643–674.

Blomberg, J., 1978, Acetylation analysis of saccharides. 2. Microanalysis of neutral glycosphingolipids by means of acetylation with radioactive acetic anhydride, *Anal. Biochem.* **88**:302–313.

Bosman, H. B., 1971, Platelet adhesiveness and aggregation: The collagen: glycosyl, polypeptide: *N*-acetylgalactosaminyl and glycoprotein: galactosyl transferases of human platelets, *Biochem. Biophys. Res. Commun.* **43**:118–1124.

Bosman, H. B., 1972, Cell surface glycosyl transferases and acceptors in normal and RNA- and DNA-virus transformed fibroblasts, *Biochem. Biophys. Res. Commun.* **48**:523–529.

Bosman, H. B., and Hemsworth, B. A., 1970, Intraneural mitochondria. Incorporation of amino acids and monosaccharides into macromolecules by isolated synaptosomes and synaptosomal mitochondria, *J. Biol. Chem.* **245**:363–371.

Brady, R. O., 1978, Sphingolipidoses, *Annu. Rev. Biochem.* **47**:687–713.

Brady, R. O., and Fishman, P. H., 1974, Biosynthesis of glycolipids in virus transformed cells, *Biochim. Biophys. Acta* **355**:121–148.

Brady, R. O., Borek, C., and Bradly, R. M., 1969, Composition and synthesis of gangliosides in rat hepatocyte and hepatoma cell lines, *J. Biol. Chem.* **244**:6552–6554.

Breckenridge, W. C., Gombos, G., and Morgan, J. G., 1972, The lipid composition of adult rat brain synaptosomal plasma membranes, *Biochim. Biophys. Acta* **266**:695–707.

Breckenridge, W. C., Gombos, G., and Morgan, J. G., 1973, The lipid composition of adult brain synaptosomal plasma membranes, *Biochim. Biophys. Acta* **320**:681–686.

Breer, H., 1975, Ganglioside pattern and thermal tolerance of fish species, *Life Sci.* **16**:1459–1464.

Breer, H., and Rahmann, H., 1976, Involvement of brain gangliosides in temperature adoption of fish, *J. Thermal. Biol.* **1**:233–235.

Breer, H. and Rahmann, H., 1977, Cholinesteraseaktivität und Hirnganglioside während der Fischentwicklung, *Wilhelm Roux Arch. Develop. Biol.* **181**:65–72.

Callies, R., Schwarzmann, G., Radsak, K., Siegert, R., and Wiegandt, H., 1977, Characterization of cellular binding of exogenous gangliosides, *Eur. J. Biochem.* **80**:425–432.

Cantz, M., and Messer, H., 1979, Oligosaccharide and ganglioside neuramindase activities of mucolipidosis I (sialidosis) and mucolipidosis II (I-cell disease) fibroblasts. *Eur. J. Biochem.* **97**:113–118.

Cantz, M., Gehler, K., and Spranger, J., 1977, Mucolipidosis I: increased sialic acid content and deficiency of an α-N-acetylneuraminidase in cultured fibroblasts, *Biochem. Biophys. Res. Commun.* **74**:732–738.

Caputto, R., Maccioni, A. H. R., and Caputto, B. L., 1977, Activation of deoxycholate adenosine triphosphatase by ganglioside and asialoganglioside preparations, *Biochem. Biophys. Res. Commun.* **74**:1046–1052.

Carter, H. E., and Gaver, R. C., 1967, Improved reagent for trimethylsilylation of sphingolipid bases, *J. Lipid Res.* **8**:391–395.

Carubelli, R., and Griffin, M. J., 1968, On the presence of N-glycolylneuraminic acid in HeLa cells, *Biochim. Biophys. Acta* **170**:446–448.

Cassidy, J. T., Jouridian, G. W., and Rosemann, S., 1965, The sialic acids. VI. Purification and properties of sialidase from clostridium perfringens. *J. Biol. Chem.* **240**:3501–3506.

Ceccarelli, B., Aporti, F., and Friesco, M., 1976, Effects of brain gangliosides on functional recovery experimental regeneration and reinnervation, *Adv. Exp. Med. Biol.* **71**:275–293.

Chany, C., Pauloin, A., and Chany-Fournier, F., 1977, Role of the membrane-bound receptor system in the biological activity of interferon. *Tex. Rep. Biol. Med.* **35**.

Chatterjee, S., and Sweeley, C. C., 1973, The effect of thrombin induced aggregation on human platelet glycosphingilipids *Biochem. Biophys. Res. Commun.* **53**:1310–1316.

Chatterjee, S., Sweeley, C. C., and Velicer, L. F., 1973, Biosynthesis of proteins, nucleic acids and glycosphingolipids by synchronized KB cells, *Biochem. Biophys. Res. Commun.* **54**:585–592.

Chatterjee, S., Sweeley, C. C., and Velicer, L. F., 1975a, Glycosphingolipids on human KB cells grown in monolayer, suspension, and synchronized cultures, *J. Biol. Chem.* **250**:61–66.

Chatterjee, S., Velicer, L. F., and Sweeley, C. C., 1975b, Glycosphingolipid glycosyl hydrolases and glycosidases of synchronized human KB cells, *J. Biol. Chem.* **250**:4972–4979.

Chem. Phys. Lipids, 1974, **13**:261–265.

Cheema, P., Yogeeswaran, G., Morris, H. P., and Murray, R. K., 1970, Ganglioside patterns of three Morris minimal deviation hepatomas, *FEBS Lett.* **11**:181.

Clarke, J. T. R., 1975, Gangliosides of the bovine neurohypophysis, *J. Neurochem.* **24**:533–538.

Coleman, P. L., Fishman, P. H., Brady, R. O., and Todaro, G. J., 1975, Altered ganglioside biosynthesis in mouse cell cultures following transformation with chemical carcinogens and X-irradiation, *J. Biol. Chem.* **250**:55–60.

Constanino-Ceccarini, E., and Suzuki, K., 1978, Isolation and partial characterization of an endogenous inhibitor of ceramide glycosyltransferases from rat brain, *J. Biol. Chem.* **253**:340–342.

Conzelmann, E., and Sandhoff, K., 1978, A B-variant of infantile G_{M2}-gangliosidosis deficiency of a factor necessary for stimulation of hexosaminidase A-catalyzed degradation of ganglioside G_{M2} and glycolipid G_{A2}, *Proc. Natl. Acad. Sci.* **75**:3979–3983.

Cork, C. G., Munnell, J. F., Lorenz, M. D., Murphy, J. V., Baker, H. J., and Rattazi, 1977, G_{M2} ganglioside lysosomal storage disease in cats with B-hexosaminidase deficiency, *Science* **196**:1014–1017.

Craig, S. W., and Cuatrecasas, P., 1975, Mobility of cholera toxin receptors on rat lymphocyte membranes, *Proc. Natl. Acad. Sci.* **72**:3844–3848.

Critchley, D. R., Graham, J. M., and MacPherson, 1973, Subcellular distribution of glycolipids in a hamster cell line, *FEBS Lett.* **32**:37–40.

Crone, H. D., 1976, On the inactivation by ganglioside of the haemolytic protein toxin from the sea wasp (chironex Fleckeri), *Toxicology* **14**:494–498.

Cumar, F. A., and Caputto, R., 1976, Split chromatographic spot produced by supposedly single gangliosides treated with trichloroacetic acid-phosphotungstic acid reagent *J. Neurochem.* **26**:227–228.

Cumar, F. A., Brady, R. O., Kolodny, E. H., McFarland, V. W., and Mora, P. T., 1970, Enzymatic block in synthesis of gangliosides in DNA virus-transformed tumorigenic mouse cell lines, *Proc. Natl. Acad. Sci.* **67**:757–764.

Cumar, F. A., Fishman, P. H., and Brady, R. O., 1971, Analogous reactions for the biosynthesis of monosialo- and disialo-gangliosides in brain, *J. Biol. Chem.* **246**:5075–5084.

Cumar, F. A., Tallmann, J. F., and Brady, R. O., 1972, The biosynthesis of monosialo- and disialo-ganglioside by galactosyltransferase from rat brain tissue, *J. Biol. Chem.* **247**:2322–2327.

Cumar, F. A., Maggio, B., and Caputto, R., 1978, Dopamine release from nerve endings induced by polysialogangliosides, *Biochem. Biophys. Res. Commun.* **84**:65–69.

Curatolo, W., Donald, M., Small, D. M., and Shipley, G. G., 1977, Phase behaviour and structural characteristics of hydrated bovine brain ganglioside, *Biochim. Biophys. Acta* **468**:11–20.

Czarniecki, M. F., and Thornton, E. R., 1977*a*, A carbon-13 nuclear magnetic resonance spin-lattice relaxation in the *N*-acylneuraminic acids. Probes for internal dynamics and conformation analysis, *J. Am. Chem. Soc.* **99**:8273–8278.

Czarniecki, M. F., and Thornton, E. R., 1977*b*, Carbon-13-nuclear magnetic resonance of ganglioside sugars. Spin-lattice relaxation probes for structure and microdynamics of cell surface carbohydrates, *J. Am. Chem. Soc.* **99**:8279–8282.

Czarniecki, M. F., and Thornton, E. R., 1977*c*, ^{13}C-NMR chemical shift titration of metal ion-carbohydrate complexes. An unexpected dichotomy for Ca^{2+} binding between anomeric derivatives of *N*-acetyl-neuraminic acid, *Biochem. Biophys. Res. Commun.* **74**:553–558.

Dallas, W. S., and Falkow, St., 1979, The molecular nature of heat-labile enterotoxin (LT) of Escherichia coli, *Nature London* **277**:406–407.

Dawson, G., 1979, Regulation of glycosphingolipid metabolism in mouse neuroblastoma and glial cell lines, *J. Biol. Chem.* **254**:155–162.

Dawson, G. and Stoolmiller, A. C., 1976, Comparison of the ganglioside composition of established mouse neuroblastoma cell strains grown in vivo and in tissue culture, *J. Neurochem.* **26**:225–226.

Dawson, G. and Sweeley, C. C., 1970, In vivo studies on glycosphingolipid metabolism in porcine blood, *J. Biol. Chem.* **245**:410–416.

Dawson, G., and Sweeley, Ch. C., 1971, Mass spectrometry of neutral, mono-, and disialoglycosphingolipids, *J. Lipid Res.* **12**:56–64.

Dawson, G., Kemp, S. F., Stoolmiller, A. C., and Dorfman, A., 1971, Biosynthesis of glycosphingolipids by mouse neuroblastoma (NB41A), rat glia (RGC-6) and human glia (CHB-4) in cell culture, *Biochem. Biophys. Res. Commun.* **44**:687–694.

Dawson, G., McLawhon, R., and Miller, R. J., 1979, Opiates and enkephalins inhibit synthesis of gangliosides and membrane glycoproteins in mouse neuroblastoma cell line N4TG 1 *Proc. Natl. Acad. Sci.* **76**:605–609.

de Cicco, D. and Greaves, M. F., 1978, Independent mobility of cholera toxin binding sites and Thy-1 alloantigen on mouse thymocytes *Immunology* **35**,183–188.

Degré, M., 1978, Cholera toxin inhibits antiviral and growth inhibitory activities of human interferon (40032), *Proc. Soc. Exp. Biol. Med.* **157**:253–255.

Den, H., and Kaufman, B., 1968, Ganglioside and glycoprotein glycosyltransferase in synaptosomes, *Fed. Proc. Fed. Am. Soc. Exp. Biol.* **27**:346.

Deppert, W., and Walter, G., 1978, Cell surface glycosyltransferases—Do they exist? *J. Supramol. Struct.* **8**:19–37.

Dette, G. A., and Weseman, W., 1978, On the significance of sialic acid in high affinity 5-hydroxytryptamine uptake by synaptosomes, *Hoppe Seylers z. Physiol. Chem.* **359**:399–405.

DeVries, G. H., and Norton, W. T., 1974, The lipid composition of axons from bovine brain, *J. Neurochem.* **22**:259–264.

DiCesare, J. L., and Dain, J. A., 1971, The enzymic synthesis of gangliosides. IV. UDP-N-acetylgalactosamine: (N-acetylneuraminyl)-galactosylglucosyl-ceramide N-acetylgalactosaminyl transferase in rat brain, *Biochem. Biophys. Acta* **231**:385–393.

DiCesare, J. L., and Rapport, M. M., 1973, Availability to neuraminidase of gangliosides and sialoglycoproteins in neuronal membranes, *J. Neurochem.* **20**:1781–1783.

DiCesare, J. L., and Rapport, M. M., 1974, Preparation of some labelled glycosphingolipids by catalytic addition of tritium, *Chem. Phys. Lipid.* **13**:447–452.

Dnistrian, A. M., Skipski, V. P., Barclay, M., Essner, E. S., and Stock, C. C., 1975, Gangliosides of plasma membranes from normal rat liver and Morris hepatoma, *Biochem. Biophys. Res. Commun.* **64**:367–375.

Donta, S. T., and Viner, J. P., 1975, Inhibition of the steroidogenic effects of cholera toxin and heat labile Escherichia coli enterotoxins by G_{M1} ganglioside: evidence for a similar receptor site for the two toxins, *Infect. Immun.* **11**:982–985.

Dreyfus, H., Urban, P. F., Bosch, P., Edel-Harth, S., Rebel, G., and Mandel, P., 1974, Effect of light on gangliosides from calf retina and photoreceptors, *J. Neurochem.* **22**:1073–1078.

Dreyfus, H., Aunis, D., Harth, S., and Mandel, P., 1977, Gangliosides and phospholipids of the membranes from bovine adrenal medullary chromaffine granules, *Biochim. Biophys. Acta* **489**:89–97.

Drzeniek, R., 1967, Differences in splitting capacity of virus and V. cholerae neuraminidases on sialic acid type, *Biochem Biophys. Res. Commun.* **26**:631–638.

Drzeniek, R., and Gauhe, A., 1970, Differences in substrate specificity of myxovirus neuraminidases, *Biochem. Biophys. Res. Commun.* **38**:651–656.

Drzeniek, R., Seto, J. T., and Rott, R., 1966, Characterization of neuraminidases from myxoviruses, *Biochem. Biophys. Acta* **128**:547–558

Duffard, R. O., and Caputto, R., 1972, A natural inhibitor of sialyl transferase and its possible influence on this enzyme activity during brain development, *Biochemistry* **11**:1396–1400.

Dutton, G. R., and Barondes, S. H., 1972, Macromolecular behaviour of gangliosides on electrophoresis in sodium dodecylsulphate, *J. Neurochem.* **19**:559–562.

Dyatlovitskaya, E. V., Novikov, A. M., and Bergelson, L. D., 1974, Gangliosides, liver, and hepatoma of rats *Biokhimiya* **39**:552–556.

Edel-Harth, S., Dreyfus, H., Bosch, P., Rebel, G., Urban, P. F., and Mandel, P., 1973, Gangliosides of whole retina and rod outer segments, *FEBS Lett.* **35**:284–288.

Egge, H., 1978, The application of mass spectrometry in the structural elucidation of glycosphingolipids, *Chem. Phys. Lipid.* **21**:349–360.

Esselman, W. J., and Miller, H. C., 1974*a*, The ganglioside nature of θ-antigen, *Fed. Proc. Fed. Am. Soc. Exp. Biol.* **33**:771.

Esselman, W. J., and Miller, H. C., 1974*b*, Brain and thymus lipid inhibition of antibrain associated θ-cytotoxicity, *J. Exp. Med.* **139**:445–450.

Evans, J. E., and McCluer, R. H., 1969, The structure of brain dihexosylceramide in globoid cell leukodystrophy, *J. Neurochem.* **16**:1393–1399.

Festoff, B. W., Appel, S. M., and Day, E., 1971, Incorporation of ^{14}C-glucosamine into synaptosomes *in vitro*, *J. Neurochem.* **18**:1871–1876.

Filipovic, J., Schwarzmann, G., Mraz, W., Wiegandt, H., and Buddecke, E., 1978, Sialic acid content of low density liproprotein controls their binding and uptake by cultured cells, *Eur. J. Biochem.* **93**:51–59.

Fishman, P. H., 1974, Normal and abnormal biosynthesis of gangliosides, *Chem. Phys. Lipid.* **13**:305–326.

Fishman, P. H., and Brady, R. O., 1976, Biosynthesis and function of gangliosides, *Science* **194**:906–915.

Fishman, P. H., MacFarland, V. W., Morat, P. T., and Brady, R. O., 1972, Ganglioside biosynthesis in mouse cells: Glycosyltransferase activities in normal and virally transformed cells, *Biochem. Biophys. Res. Commun.* **48**:48–57.

Fishman, P. H., Brady, R. O., Bradley, R. M., Aaronson, St. A., and Todaro, G. J., 1974*a*, Absence of a specific ganglioside galactosyltransferase in mouse cells transformed by murine sarcoma virus, *Proc. Natl. Acad. Sci.* **71**:298–301.

Fishman, P. H., Simmons, J. L., Brady, R. O., and Freeze, E., 1974*b*, Induction of glycolipid biosynthesis by sodium butyrate in HeLa cells. *Biochem. Biophys. Res. Commun.* **59**:292–299.

Fishman, P. H., Max, S. R., Tallman, J. E., Brady, R. O., MacLaren, N. K., and Cornblath, M., 1975, Deficient ganglioside biosynthesis: A novel human sphingolipidosis, *Science* **187**:68–70.

Fishman, P. H., Moss, J., and Vaughan, M., 1976*a*, Uptake and metabolism of gangliosides in transformed mouse fibroblasts, *J. Biol. Chem.* **251**:4490–4494.

Fishman, P. H., Bradley, R. M., and Henneberry, R. C., 1976*b*, Butyrate-induced glycolipid biosynthesis in HeLa Cells: Properties of the induced sialyltransferase, *Arch. Biochem. Biophys.* **172**:618–626.

Fishman, P. H., Moss, J., and Manganiello, V. C., 1977, Synthesis and uptake of gangliosides by choleragen-responsive human fibroblasts, *Biochemistry* **16**:1871–1875.

Fishman, P. H., Bradley, R. M., Moss, J., and Manganiello, V. C., 1978*a*, Effect of serum on ganglioside uptake and choleragen responsiveness of transformed mouse fibroblasts, *J. Lipid. Res.* **19**:77–81.

Fishman, P. H., Moss, J., and Osborne, J., 1978*b*, Interaction of choleragen with the oligosaccharide of ganglioside G_{M1}: evidence for multiple oligosaccharide binding sites, *Biochemistry* **17**:711–716.

Folch, J., Lees, M. and Sloane Stanley, G. H., 1957, A simple method for the isolation and purification of total lipids from animal tissues, *J. Biol. Chem.,* **226**:497–509.

Fong, J. W., Ledeen, R. W., Kundu, S. K., and Brostoff, S. W., 1976, Gangliosides of peripheral nerve myelin, *J. Neurochem.* **26**:157–162.

Formisano, S., Johnson, M. L., Lee, G., Aloj, S. M., and Edelhoch, H, 1979, Critical mcell concentrations of gangliosides, *Biochemistry* **18**:1119–1124.

Fredman, P., Mansson, J. E., Svennerholm, L., Karlsson, K. A., Pascher, I., and Samuelson, B. E., 1980*a*, The structure of the tetrasialoganglioside from human brain, *FEBS Lett.* **110**:80–84.

Fredman, P., Nilsson, O., Tayot, J.-L., and Svennerholm, L., 1980*b*, Separation of gangliosides on a new type of anion-exchange resin, *Biochim. Biophys. Acta* **618**:42–52.

Fukuda, M. N., Watanabe, K., and Hakomori, S.-J., 1978, Release of oligosaccharides from various glycosphingolipids by endo-β-galactosidase, *J. Biol. Chem.* **253**:6814–6819.

Gahmberg, C. G., and Hakomori, S. J., 1974, Organisation of glycolipids and glycoprotein in surface membranes: Dependency on cell cycle and on transformation, *Biochem. Biophys. Res. Commun.* **59**:283–291.

Gammack, D. B., 1963, Physicochemical properties of ox-brain gangliosides, *Biochem. J.* **88**:373–383.

Gaver, R. C., and Sweeley, C. C., 1965, Methods for methanolysis of sphingolipids and direct determination of long chain bases by gas chromatography, *J. Am. Oil Chem. Soc.* **42**:294–298.

Geiger, B., and Arnon, R., 1976, Chemical characterization and subunit structure of human *N*-acetylhexosaminidases A and B, *Biochemistry* **15**:3484–3492.

Geiger, B., Arnon, R., and Sandhoff, K., 1977, Immunochemical and biochemical investigation of hexosaminidase S, *Am. J. Hum. Genet.* **29**:508–522.

Ghidoni, R., Tettamanti, G., and Zambotti, V., 1974, An improved procedure for the *in vitro* labeling of ganglioside, *J. Biochem.* **23**:320–328.

Ghidoni, R., Sonnino, S., Tettamanti, G., Wiegandt, H., and Zambotti, V., 1976, On the structure of two new gangliosides from beef brain, *J. Neurochem.* **27**:511–515.

Ghidoni, R., Sonnino, S. Tettamanti, G., Baumann, N. Reuter, G., and Schauer, R., 1979, On the structure of a new, 9-0-Ac-NeuAc-containing ganglioside from mouse brain, *Glycoconjugates, Proceedings of the 5th International Symposium*, pp. 51–52, Kiel Thieme, Stuttgart.

Gill, D. M., 1977, The mechanism of action of cholera toxin, *Adv. Cyclic Nucleotide Res.* **8**:85–118.

Habermann, E., 1976, Affinity chromatography of tetanus toxin, tetanus toxoid, and botulinum A toxin on synaptosomes, and differentiation of their acceptors, *Naunyn Schmiedebergs Arch. Pharmacol.* **293**:1–9.

Habig, W. H., Grollmann, E. R., Ledley, F. D., Meldolesi, M. F., Aloj, S. M., Hardegree, M. C., and Kohn, L. D., 1978, Tetanus interactions with the thyroid: decreased toxin binding to membranes from a thyroid tumor with a thyrotropin receptor defect and in vivo stimulation of thyroid function, *Endocrinology* **102**:844–851.

Hajra, A. K., Bowen, D. M., Kishimoto, Y., and Radin, N. S., 1966, Cerebroside galactosidase of brain, *J. Lipid Res.* **7**:379–386.

Hakomori, S-I., 1964, Rapid permethylation of glycolipid and polysaccharide catalyzed by methylsulfinylcarbanion in dimethyl sulfoxide, *J. Biochem.* **55**:205–211.

Hakomori, S-I., 1970, Cell density dependent changes of glycolipid concentration in fibroblasts, and and loss of this respons in virus-transformed cells, *Proc. Natl. Acad. Sci.* **67**:1741–1747.

Hakomori, S-I., 1972, Preparation of antisera against glycolipids, *Methods Enzymol.* **28**:232–236.

Hakomori, S-I., 1973, Glycolipids of tumor cell membrane, *Adv. Cancer Res.* **18**:268–313.

Hakomori, S-I., and Siddiqui, B., 1972, Release of oligosaccharide from glycolipids, *Methods Enzymol.* **28**:156–159.

Hakomori, S-I., Saito, T., and Vogt, P., 1971, Transformation by rous sacroma virus: effects on cellular glycolipids, *Virology* **44**:609–621.

Hakomori, S-I., Watanabe, K., and Laine, R. A., 1977, Glycosphingolipids with blood group A, H, and I activity and their changes associated with ontogenesis and oncogenesis, *Pure Appl. Chem.* **49**:1215–1227.

Hamberger, A., and Svennerholm, L., 1971, Composition of gangliosides and phospholipids of neuronal and glial cell enriched fractions. *J. Neurochem.* **18**:1821–1829.

Hamanaka, S., Handa, S., and Yamakawa, T., 1979, Ganglioside composition of erythrocytes from various strains of inbred mice, *J. Biochem. Tokyo* **86**:1623–1626.

Handa, S., and Burton, R. M., 1969, Lipids of retina. I. Analysis of gangliosides in beef retina by thin layer chromatography, *Lipids* **4**:205–208.

Handa, S., and Yamakawa, T., 1971, Biochemical studies in cat and human gangliosidosis, *J. Neurochem.* **18**:1275–1280.

Hansson, H. A., Holmgren, J., and Svennerholm, L., 1977, Ultrastructural localization of cell membrane G_{M1} ganglioside by cholera toxin, *Proc. Nat. Acad. Sci.* **74**:3782–3786.

Harris, P. L., and Thornton, E. R., 1978, Carbon-13 and proton nuclear magnetic resonance studies of gangliosides, *J. Am. Chem. Soc.* **100**:6738–6745.

Harth, S. Dreyfus, H., Urban, P. F., and Mandel, P., 1978, Direct thin-layer chromatography of gangliosides of a total lipid extract, *Anal. Biochem.* **86**:543–551.

Haverkamp, J., Kamerling, J. P., Vliegenthart, J. G. F., Veh, R. W., and Schauer, R., 1977*a*, Methylation analysis determination of acylneuraminic acid residue type 2→8 glycosidic linkage, application to G_{Tlb} ganglioside and colominic acid, *FEBS Lett.* **73**:215–219.

Haverkamp, J., J. G. F., Veh, R. W., Sander, M., Schauer, R., Kamerling, J. P., and Vliegenhart, J. G. F., 1977*b*, Demonstration of 9-*0*-acetyl-*N*-acetylneuraminic acid in brain gangliosides from various vertebrates including man, *Hoppe Seylers Z. Physiol. Chem.* **358**:1609–1612.

Hayashi, K., and Katagiri, A., 1974, Studies on the interaction between gangliosides, proteins and divalent cations, *Biochem. Biophys. Acta* **337**:107–117.

Haywood, A. M., 1974*a*, Characteristics of Sendai virus receptors in a model membrane, *J. Mol. Biol.* **87**:625–628.

Haywood, A. M., 1974*b*, Fusion of Sendai virus with model membranes, *J. Mol. Biol.* **87**:625–628.

Hechtmann, P. and LeBlanc, D., 1977, Purification and properties of the hexosaminidase A-activating protein from human liver, *Biochem. J.* **167**:693–701.

Heckers, H, and Stoffel, W., 1972, Sphingolipids in blood platelets of the pig, *Hoppe Seylers Z. Physiol. Chem.* **353**:407–418.

Helting, T. B., Zwisler, O., and Wiegandt, H., 1977, Structure of tetanus toxin. II. Toxin binding to ganglioside, *J. Biol. Chem.* **252**:194–198.

Henning, R., and Stoffel, W., 1973, Glycolipids in lysosomal membranes, *Hoppe Seylers Z. Physiol. Chem.* **354**:760–770.

Hess, H. H., Stoffyn, P., and Sprinkle, K., 1971, Gangliosides in frog photoreceptors, 3rd International Meeting of Neurochemistry, Budapest, p. 295.

Heuser, E., Lipp, K., and Wiegandt, H., 1974, Detection of sialic acid containing compounds and the behaviour of gangliosides in polyacrylamide disc electrophoresis, *Anal. Biochem.* **60**:382–388.

Higashi, H., and Naiki, M., 1977, Antigen of "serum sickness" type of heterophile antibodies in human sera: identification as gangliosides with *N*-glycolyl-neuraminic acid, *Biochem. Biophys. Res. Commun.* **79**:388–395.

Hill, M. W., and Lester, R., 1972, Mixtures of gangliosides and phosphatidylcholine in aqueous dispersions, *Biochim. Biophys. Acta* **282**:18–30.

Hirabayashi, Y., Taki, T., and Matsumoto, M., 1979, Tumor ganglioside—natural occurrence of GM_{1b}, *FEBS Lett.* **100**:253–257.

Hof, L. and Faillard, H., 1973, The serum dependence of the occurrence of *N*-glycolylneuraminic acid in Hela cells, *Biochim. Biophys. Acta* **297**,561–563.

Hollenberg, M., Fishman, P. H., Bennett, V., and Cuatrecasas, P., 1974, Cholera toxin and cell growth: role of membrane gangliosides, *Proc. Nat. Acad. Sci.* **71**:4224–4228.

Holm, M., and Mansson, J. E., 1974*a*, Differences in sphingosine and fatty acid patterns of the mayor gangliosides of bovine retina, *FEBS Lett.* **38**:261–262.

Holm, M., and Mansson, J. E., 1974*b*, Gangliosides of bovine optic nerve, *FEBS Lett.* **45**:159–161.

Holm, M., and Mansson, J. E., 1974*c*, Differences in incorporation of *N*-acetyl-^{3}H mannosamine into the sialic acid of the major retinal gangliosides, studies in vivo, *FEBS Lett.* **46**:200–202.

Holm, M., Mansson, J. E., Vanier, M. Th., and Svennerholm, L., 1972, Gangliosides of human, bovine and rabbit retina, *Biochim. Biophys. Acta* **280**:356–364.

Holmgren, M., Mansson, J. E., and Svennerholm, L., 1974, Tissue receptor for cholera exotoxin: structural requirements of G_{M1} ganglioside in toxin binding and inactivation, *Med. Biol.* **52**:229–233.

Holmgren, J., Lönnroth, J., Mansson, J. E., and Svennerholm, L., 1975, Interaction of cholera toxin and membrane with ganglioside of small intestine, *Proc.Nat. Acad. Sci.* **72**:2520–2524.

Holmgren, J., Svennerholm, L., Elwing, H., Fredman, P., and Strannegård, Ö, 1980, Sendai virus receptor: proposed recognition structure based on binding to plastic-adsorbed gangliosides, *Proc. Natl. Acad. Sci.* **77**:1947–1950.

Holmquist, L., and Ostman, B., 1975, The anomeric configuration of *N*-acetylneuraminic acid released by the action of vibrio cholerae neuraminidase, *FEBS Lett.* **60**:327–330.

Hoshi, M., and Nagai, Y., 1975, Biochemistry of lipids of sea urchin gametes and embryos. 5. Novel sialo-sphingolipids from spermatozoa of the sea urchin *Anthocidaris crassispina, Biochim. Biophys. Acta* **388**:152–162.

Howard, K. E., and Burton, R. M., 1964, Studies on the ganglioside micelle, *Biochim. Biophys. Acta* **84**:435–440.

Huang, R. T. C., 1973, Isolation and characterization of the gangliosides of butter milk, *Biochim. Biophys. Acta* **306**:82–84.

Huang, R. T. C., and Klenk, E., 1972 α-Ketosidic linkage of the neuraminidase-resistant neuraminic acid in brain gangliosides, *Hoppe Seylers Z. Physiol. Chem.* **353**:679–682.

Huang, R. T. C., and Orlich, M. 1972, Substrate specificities of neuraminidase of Newcastle disease and fowl plague viruses, *Hoppe Seylers Z. Physiol. Chem.* **353**:318–322.

Huterer, S., and Wherret, Y. R., 1974, Glycosphingolipids in secondary lysosomes prepared from rat liver, *Can. J. Biochem.* **52**:507–513.

Igarashi, M., Belchis, D., and Suzuki, K., 1976, Brain gangliosides in adenoleukodystrophy, *J. Neurochem.* **27**:327–328.

Inouye, Y., Handa, S., and Osawa, T., 1974, Conversion of glucose and galactose to lipids by normal and phytohemagglutium-stimulated lymphocytes, *J. Biochem.* **76**:791–799.

Irwin, L. N., and Samson, E., 1971, Content and turnover of gangliosides in rat brain following behavioural stimulation, *J. Neurochem.* **18**:203–211.

Irwin, L. N., Chen, H. H., and Barraco, R. A., 1976, Ganglioside, protein hexose and sialic acid changes in the trisected optic tectum of the chick embryo, *Dev. Biol.* **49**:29–39.

Ishizuka, J., and Wiegandt, H., 1972, An isomer of trisialoganglioside and the structure of tetra- and pentasialoganglioside from fish brain, *Biochim. Biophys. Acta* **260**:279–289.

Ishizuka, J., Kloppenburg, M., and Wiegandt, H., 1970, Characterization of gangliosides from fish brain, *Biochim. Biophys. Acta* **210**:299–305.

Itaya, K., and Hakomori, S-I., 1976, Gangliosides and galactoprotein A″ (LETS' -protein) of temperature-sensitive mutant of transformed 3T3 cells, *FEBS Lett.* **66**:65–69.

IUPAC-IUB, 1967, *Eur. J. Biochem.* **2**:127–131.

IUPAC-IUB, 1978, The nomenclature of lipids, *J. Lipid Res.* **19**:114–128.

Iwamori, M., and Nagai, Y., 1978a, Isolation and characterization of a novel ganglioside, monosialosyl pentahexaosyl ceramide from human brain, *J. Biochem.* **84**:1601–1608.

Iwamori, M., and Nagai, Y., 1978b, A new chromatographic approach to the resolution of individual gangliosides *Biochim. Biophys. Acta* **528**:257–267.

Iwamori, M., Moser, H. W., and Kishimoto, Y., 1975a, Specific tritium labeling of cerebrosides at the 3-position of erythro-sphingosine and threo-sphingosine, *J. Lipid Res.* **16**:332–335.

Iwamori, M., Moser, H. W., McCluer, R. N., and Kishimoto, Y., 1975b, 3-Ketosphingolipids: application to determination of ceramides, cerebrosides, sulfatide, and sphingomyelin, *Biochim. Biophys. Acta* **380**:308–319.

Jaques, L. W., Brown, E. B., Barret, J. M., Brey, W. S., and Welner, W., 1977, Sialic acid, a calcium-binding carbohydrate, *J. Biol. Chem.* **252**:4533–4538.

Kanda, S., Inoue, K., Nojima, S., Utsumi, K. and Wiegandt, H., 1979, The incorporation of gangliosides and their derivatives to liposomal and natural membranes, *Seikagaku* **51**:686.

Karlsson, K. A., 1970*a*, Sphingolipid long chain bases, *Lipids* **5**:878–891.

Karlsson, K. A., 1970*b*, On the chemistry and occurrence of sphingolipid long-chain bases, *Chem. Phys. Lipid.* **5**:6–43.

Karlsson, K. A., 1973, Carbohydrate composition and sequence analysis of cell surface components by mass spectrometry. Characterization of the major monosialoganglioside of brain. *FEBS Lett.* **32**:317–320.

Karlsson, K. A., 1974, Carbohydrate composition and sequence analysis of a derivative of brain disialoganglioside by mass spectrometry, with molecular weight ions of m/e 2245. Potential use in the specific microanalysis of cell surface components, *Biochemistry* **13**:3643–3647.

Karlsson, K. A., Pascher, J., Pimlott, W., and Samuelsson, B. E., 1974*a*, Use of mass spectrometry for the carbohydrate composition and sequence analysis of glycosphingolipids, *Biochem. Mass Spectrom.* **1**:49–56.

Karlsson, K. A., Pascher, J., and Samuelson, B. E., 1974*b*, Analysis of intact gangliosides by mass spectrometry. Comparison of different derivatives of a hematoside of a tumor and the major monosialoganglioside of brain, *Chem. Phys. Lipid.* **12**:971–981.

Karpiak, S. E., Graf, L., and Rapport, M. M., 1976*a*, Antiserum to brain gangliosides produced recurrent epileptiform activity *Science* **194**:735–737.

Karpiak, S. E., Graf, L., and Rapport, M. M., 1976*b*, EEG-changes induced by antisera to brain gangliosides, *Trans Am. Soc. Neurochem.* **7**:171.

Karpiak, S. E., Graf, L., and Rapport, M. M., 1976*c*, Passive avoidance learning is inhibited by antiserum to brain gangliosides, *Soc. Neurosci* **2**:443.

Karpiak, S. E., Mahadik, S. P., and Rapport, M. M., 1978, Ganglioside receptors and induction of epileptiform activity: cholera toxin and choleragenoid (B-subunits) *Exp. Neurol.* **62**:256–259.

Kato, J., and Naiki, M., 1976, Ganglioside and rabbit erythrocyte membrane receptor for staphylococcal alpha-toxin, *Infect. Immun.* **13**:289–291.

Kasai, M., Iwamori, M., Nagai, Y., Okumura, K., and Tada, T., 1980, A glycolipid on the surface of mouse natural killer cells, *Eur. J. Immunol.* **10**:175–180.

Kawamura, N., and Taketomi, T., 1977, A new procedure for the isolation of brain gangliosides, and determination for their long chain base composition, *J. Biochem.* **81**:1217–1225.

Keenan, T. W., 1974*a*, Membranes of mammary gland. IX. Concentration of glycosphingolipid galactosyl and sialyltransferases in Golgi apparatus from bovine mammary gland, *J. Dairy Sci.* **57**:187–192.

Keenan, T. W., 1974*b*, Composition and synthesis of gangliosides in mammary gland and milk of the bovine, *Biochim. Biophys. Acta* **337**:255–270.

Keenan, T. W., and Dodak, R. L., 1973, Enzymatic block in higher ganglioside biosynthesis in avian transplantable lymphoid tumor, *FEBS Lett.* **37**:124–228.

Keenan, T. W., and Morré, D. J., 1973, Mammary carcinoma: enzymatic block in disialoganglioside biosynthesis, *Science* **182**:935–937.

Keenan, T. W., and Morré, D. J., 1975, Glycotransferases: do they exist on the surface membrane of mammalian cells? *FEBS Lett.* **55**:8–13.

Keenan, T. W., Huang, C. M. and Morré, D. J., 1972*b*, Gangliosides: nonspecific localization in the surface membranes of bovine mammary gland and rat liver, *Biochem. Biophys. Res. Commun.* **47**:1277–1283.

Keenan, T. W., Morré, D. J., and Huang, C. M., 1972*a*, Distribution of gangliosides among subcellular fractions from rat liver and bovine mammary gland, *FEBS Lett.* **24**:204–208.

Keenan, T. W., Franke, W. W., and Wiegandt, H., 1974a, Ganglioside accumulation by transformed murine fibroblasts (3T3) cells and canine erythrocytes, *Hoppe Seylers Z. Physiol. Chem.* **355**:1543–1558.

Keenan, T. W., Morré, D. J., and Basu, S., 1974b, Concentration of glycosphingolipid glycosyltransferase in Golgi apparatus from rat liver, *J. Biol. Chem.* **249**:310–315.

Keenan, T. W., Schmid, E., Franke, W. W., and Wiegandt, H., 1975, Exogenous glycosphingolipids suppress growth rate of transformed and untransformed 3T3 mouse cells. *Exp. Cell. Res.* **92**:259–270.

Kemp, S. F., and Stoolmiller, A. C., 1976, Studies on the biosynthesis of glyosphingolipids in culture mouse neuroblastoma cells: characterization and acceptor specificities of N-acetylneuraminyl and N-acetylgalactosaminyltransferases, *J. Neurochem.* **27**:723–732.

Keranen, A., 1975, Gangliosides of the human gastrointestinal mucosa *Biochim. Biophys. Acta* **409**:320–328.

Keranen, A., 1976, Methylation analysis of the major gangliosides of the human alimentary mucosa, *Biochim. Biophys. Acta* **431**:96–104.

Kishimoto, Y., and Mitry, N. T., 1974, A new procedure for synthesis of 3-keto derivatives of sphingolipids and its application for study of fatty acid compositives of brain ceramides, *Arch. Biochem. Biophys.* **169**:426–434.

Klein, F., and Mandel, P., 1975, Gangliosides of the peripheral nervous system of the rat, *Life Sci.* **16**:751–758.

Kleinman, H. K., Martin, G. R., and Fishman, P., 1979, Ganglioside inhibition of fibronectin-mediated cell adhesion to collagen, *Proc. Natl. Acad. Sci.* **76**:3367–3371.

Klenk, E., and Georgias, L., 1967. Über zwei weitere Komponenten des Gemisches der Gehirnganglioside, *Hoppe Seylers Z. Physiol. Chem.* **348**:1261–1267.

Kloppel, T. M. Keenan, T. W., Freeman, M. J., and Morré, D. J., 1977, Glycolipid-bound sialic acid in serum: increased levels in mice and humans bearing mammary carcinomas, *Proc. Nat. Acad. Sci.* **74**:3011–3013.

Kobata, A., and Ginsberg, V., 1972, Oligosaccharide of human milk. IV. Isolation and characterization of a new hexasaccharide, lacto-N-neohexaose, *Arch. Biochim. Biophys.* **150**:273–281.

Kohn, L. D., Friedman, R. M., Holmes, J. M., and Lee, F., 1976, Use of thyrotropin and cholera toxin to probe the mechanism by which interferon initiates its antiviral activity, *Proc. Nat. Acad. Sci.* **73**:3695–3699.

Kolodny, E. H., Kanfer, H., Quirk, J. M. and Brady, R. O., 1971, Properties of a particle-bound enzyme from rat intestine that cleaves sialic acid from Tay Sachs ganglioside, *J. Biol. Chem.* **246**:1426–1431.

Koscielak, J., Maślinski, W., Zielinski, J., Zdebska, E., Brudzyński, T., Miller-Podraza, H., and Cedergren, B., 1978, Structures and fatty acid composition of neutral glycosphingolipids of human plasma, *Biochim. Biophys. Acta* **530**:385–393.

Krishnan, K. S., and Balaram, D., 1976, A nuclear magnetic resonance study of the interactions of serotonin with gangliosides, FEBS Lett. **63**:313–315.

Kronick, P. L., Campbell, G. L. and Joseph, K., 1979, Magnetic microspheres prepared by redox polymerisation used in a cell separation based on gangliosides, *Science* **200**:1074–1076.

Kuhn, R. and Wiegandt, H., 1963a, Die Konstitution der Gangliotetraose und des Gangliosids G_{I}, *Chem. Ber.* **96**:866–880.

Kuhn, R., and Wiegandt, H., 1963b, Die Konstitution der Ganglioside G_{II}, G_{III}, and G_{IV}, *Z. Naturforsch. Teil B* **18**:541–543.

Kuhn, R., and Wiegandt, H., 1964, Weitere Ganglioside aus Menschenhirn, *Z. Naturforsch Teil B.* **19**:256–257.

Kuhn, R., Wiegandt, H., and Egge, H., 1961, Zum Bauplan der Ganglioside, *Angew. Chem.* **73**:580–581.

Kundu, S. D., and Roy, S. K., 1978, A rapid and quantitative method for the isolation of gangliosides and neutral glycosphingolipids by DEAE-silica gel chromatography. *J. Lipid Res.* **19**:390–395.

Laine, R. A., Yogeeswaran, G., and Hakomori, S-I., 1974, Glycosphingolipids covalently linked to agarose gel or glass beads, *J. Biol. Chem.* **249**:4460–4466.

Lalley, P. A., Rattazi, M. C., and Shows, T. B., 1974, Human β-D- N-acetylhexosaminidases A and B: Expression and linkage-relationships in somatic cell hybrids, *Proc. Natl. Acad. Sci.* **71**:1569–1573.

Landa, C. A., Maccioni, H. J. F., and Caputto, R., 1979, The site of synthesis gangliosides in the chick optic system, *J. Neurochem.* **33**:825–838.

Langenbach, R., and Kennedy, S., 1978, Gangliosides and their cell density dependent changes in control and chemically transformed C3M/10T1/2 cells, *Exp. Cell Res.* **112**:361–372.

Leblond-Larouche, L., Marais, R., Nigam, V. N., and Karasaki, S., 1975, A comparative study of the carbohydrate content protein, glycoprotein and ganglioside patterns of cell membranes. Isolated from Novikoff ascites hepatoma and normal liver, *Arch. Biochem. Biophys.* **167**:1–12.

Ledeen, R. W., 1978, Ganglioside structures and distribution: are they localized at the nerve endings? *J. Supramol. Struct.* **8**:1–17.

Ledeen, R. W., Salsman, K., and Cabrera, M., 1968, Gangliosides of bovine adrenal medulla, *Biochemistry* **7**:2287–2295.

Ledeen, R. W., Yu, R. K., and Eng, L. F., 1973, Gangliosides of human myelin, sialosylgalactosylceramide (G_7) as a major component, *J. Neurochem.* **21**:829–839.

Ledley, F. D., Lee, G., Kohn, L. D., Habig, W. H., and Hardegree, M. C., 1977, Tetanus toxin interactions with thyroid plasma membrane, *J. Biol. Chem.* **252**:4049–4055.

Lee, G., Consiglio, E., Habig, W., Dyer, Sh., Hardegree, C., and Kohn, L. D., 1978, Structure: function studies of receptors for thyrotropin and tetanus toxin: lipid modulation of effects binding to the glycoprotein receptor component, *Biochem. Biophys. Res. Commun.* **83**:313–320.

Li, S.-Ch. and Li, Y.-T., 1976, An activator stimulating the enzymic hydrolysis of sphingolipids, *J. Biol. Chem.* **251**:1159–1163.

Li, S.-Ch., Wan, Ch.-Ch., Mazotte, M. Y., and Li, Y. T., 1974, Requirements of an activator for the hydrolysis of sphingoglycolipids by glycosidases of human liver, *Carbohydr. Res.* **34**:189–193.

Li, S.-Ch., Chien, J.-L., Wan, C. C., and Li, Y.-T., 1978, Occurence of glycosphingolipids in chicken egg yolk *Biochem. J.* **173**:697–699.

Li, S.-Ch., Nakumura, T., Ogamo, A., and Li, Y. T., 1979, Evidence for the presence of two separate protein activators for the enzymic hydrolysis of G_{M1} and G_{M2} gangliosides, *J. Biol. Chem.* **254**:592–595.

Li, Y.-T., and Li, S.-Ch., 1979, The activator proteins for enzymic degradation of G_{M1} and G_{M2} gangliosides, *Glycoconjugates, Proceedings of the 5th International Symposium,* pp. 380–381 Kiel Thieme, Stuttgart.

Li, Y. T., Mansson, J. E., Vanier, M. T., and Svennerholm, L., 1973a, Structure of the major glucosamine containing ganglioside of human tissues. *J. Biol. Chem.* **248**:2634–2636.

Li, Y.-T., Mazzota, M. Y., Wan, Ch-Ch, Orth, R., and Li, S.-Ch., 1973b, Hydrolysis of Tay-Sachs ganglioside by β-hexosaminidase A of human liver and urine, *J. Biol. Chem.* **248**:7512–7515.

Lingwood, C. A. Ng, A., and Hakomori, S-I., 1978, Monovalent antibodies directed to transformation-sensitive membrane component inhibit the process of viral transformation, *Proc. Natl. Acad. Sci* **75**:6049–6053.

Lipovac, V., Bigalli, G., and Rosenberg, A., 1971, Enzymatic action of sialidase of *Vibro chol-erae* on brain gangliosides above and below the critical micelle concentration, *J. Biol. Chem.* 246:7642–7648.

Löfgren, H., and Pascher, J., 1977, Molecular arrangements of sphingolipids; the monolayer behaviour of ceramides, *Chem. Phys. Lipid.* 20:273–284.

Maccioni, H. J. F., Arce, A., and Caputto, R., 1971a, The biosynthesis of gangliosides, labelling of rat brain gangliosides *in vivo*, *Biochem. J.* 125:1131–1137.

Maccioni, H. J. F., Gimenez, M. S., and Caputto, R., 1971b, The labelling of the gangliosidic fraction from brains of rats exposed to different levels of stimulation after injection of [6-^{3}H] glucosamine, *J. Neurochem.* 18:2363–2370.

Maccioni, H. J. F., Arce, A., Canda, C., and Caputto, R., 1974, Rat brain microsomal ganglio-sides, *Biochem. J.* 138:291–298.

Macher, B. A., Pacuszka, T., Mullin, R. B., Sweeley, C. C., Brady, R. O., and Fishman, P. H., 1979, Isolation and identification of a fucose-containing ganglioside from bovine thyroid gland, *Biochim. Biophys. Acta* 588:35–43.

Maggio, B., Mestrallet, M. G., Cumar, F. A., and Caputto, R., 1977, Glucose release from lipo-somes containing gangliosides or other membrane lipids induced by biogenic amines and myeline basic protein, *Biochem. Biophys. Res. Commun.* 77:1265–1272.

Maggio, B., Cumar, F. A., and Caputto, R., 1978a, Induction of membrane fusion by polysialo-gangliosides, *FEBS Lett.* 90:149–152.

Maggio, B., Cumar, F. A., and Caputto, R., 1978b, Surface behaviour of gangliosides and related glycosphingolipids, *Biochem. J.* 171:559–565.

Mahieu, P., and Winand, R. J., 1970, Chemical structure of tubular and glomerular basement membranes of human kidney, *Eur. J. Biochem.* 12:410–418.

Mansson, J. E., Vanier, M.-Th., and Svennerholm, L., 1978, Changes in fatty acid and sphin-gosine composition of the major gangliosides of human brain with age, *J. Neurochem.* 30:273–275.

Manuelidis, L., and Manuelidis, E. E., 1976a, Ultrastructural study of plasma membrane G_{MI} in neuroectrodermal cells using cholera-peroxidase, *J. Neurocytol.* 5:575–589.

Manuelidis, L., and Manuelidis, E. E., 1976b Cholera toxin peroxidase: Changes in surface labeling of glioblastoma cells with increased time in tissue culture, *Science* 193:588–590.

Marcus, D. M., 1976, Applications of immunological techniques to the study of glycosphingo-lipids, in: *Glycolipid Methodology* (L. A. Witting, ed.), pp. 233–245, American Oil Chem-ical Society.

Marcus, D. M., and Schwarting, G. A., 1976, Immunochemical properties of glycolipids and phospholipids, *Adv. Immunol.* 23:203–240.

Markey, S. P., and Wegner, D. A., 1974, Mass spectra of complex molecules. I. Chemical ioni-zation of sphingolipids, *Chem. Phys. Lipid.* 12:182–200.

Matsumoto, M., and Taki, T., 1976, Blood group H active glycolipid from rat ascites hepatoma AH 7974F, *Biochem. Biophys. Res. Commun.* 71:472–476.

Max, St. R., 1970, The effect of denervation on the ganglioside composition of skeletal muscle, *Fed. Proc. Fed. Am. Soc. Exp. Biol.* 29:903.

Max, St. R., MacLaren, N. K., Brady, R. O., Bradley, R. M., Rennels, M. B., Tanaka, J., Gar-cia, J. H., and Cornblath, M., 1974, G_{M3} (hematoside) sphingolipodystrophy, *New Engl. J. Med.* 291:929–931.

McCabe, P. J., and Green, C., 1977, The dispersion of cholesterol with phospholipids and gly-colipids, *Chem. Phys. Lipid.* 20:319–330.

Meldolesi, M. F., Fishman, P. H., Aloj, S. M., Kohn, L. D., and Brady, R. O., 1976, Relationship of gangliosides to the structure and function of thyrotropin receptors: their absence on plasma membranes of a thyroid tumor defective in thyrotropin receptor activity, *Proc. Natl. Acad. Sci.* 73:4060–4064.

Mellanby, J., and Whittaker, V. P., 1968, The fixation of tetanus toxin by synaptic membranes, *J. Neurochem.* **15**:205–208.

Merat, A., and Dickerson, J. W. T., 1973, The effect of development on the gangliosides of rat and pig brain, *J. Neurochem.* **20**:873–880.

Merritt, W. D., Richardson, C. L., Keenan, T. W., and Morré, D. J., 1978, Gangliosides of liver tumors induced by N-2-fluorenylacetamide, 1. Ganglioside alterations in liver tumorigenesis and normal development, *J. Natl. Cancer Inst.* **60**:1313–1328.

Mestrallet, M. G., Cumar, F. A. and Caputto, R., 1974, On the pathway of biosynthesis of tri-sialoganglioside, *Biochem. Biophys. Res. Commun.* **59**:1–7.

Micelli, G., Caltagirone, C., and Gainotti, G., 1977, Gangliosides in the treatment of mental deterioration, *Acta Psychiatr. Scand.* **55**:102–110.

Miller, H. C., and Esselman, W. J., 1975, Identification of O-bearing T-cells derived from bone marrow cells treated with thymic factor, *Ann. N. Y. Acad. Sci.* **249**:54–60.

Michalski, J. C., Strecker, G., Fournet, B., Cantz, M., and Spranger, J., 1977, Structures of sialyloligosaccharides excreted in the urine of a patient with mucopolidosis. I, *FEBS Lett.* **79**:101–104.

Momoi, T., Ando, S. and Nagai, Y., 1976, High resolution preparative column chromatographic system for gangliosides using DEAE-sephadex and a new porous silica iatrobeads, *Biochim. Biophys. Acta* **441**:488–497.

Momoi, T., Wiegandt, H., Arndt, R., and Thiele, H. G., 1980, Gangliotetraosylceramide, the rat T-lymphocyte-macrophage associated antigen, *J. Immunol.* **125**:2496–2500.

Mora, P. T., Cumar, F. R., and Brady, R. O., 1971, A common biochemical change in SV 40 and polyoma virus transformed mouse cells coupled to control of cell growth in culture, *Virology* **46**:60–72.

Morgan, J. G., Reith, M., Marinaru, U., Breckenridge, W. C., and Gombos, G., 1972, The isolation and characterization of synaptosomal plasma membranes, *Adv. Expt. Med. Biol.* **25**:209–228.

Morgan, J. G., Zanetta, J. P., Breckenridge, W. C., Vincendon, G., and Gombos, G., 1973, The chemical structure of synaptic membrane. *Brain Res.* **62**:405–411.

Morgan, J. G., Tettamanti, G., and Gombos, G., 1976, Biochemical evidence on the role of gangliosides in nerve endings, *Adv. Exp. Med. Biol.* **71**:137–150.

Morré, D. J., Kloppel, T. M., Merritt, W. D., and Keenan, T. W., 1978, Glycolipids as indicators of tumorigenesis, *J. Supramol. Struct.* **9**:157–177.

Moskal, J. R., Gardner, D. N., and Basu, S., 1974, Changes in glycolipid glycosyltransferases and glutamate decarboxylase and their relationship to differentiation in neuroblastoma cells, *Biochem. Biophys. Res. Commun.* **61**:751–758.

Moss, J., Fishman, P. H., Magniello, V. C., Vaughan, M., and Brady, R. O., 1976*a*, Functional incorporation of ganglioside into intact cells. Induction of choleragen responsiveness, *Proc. Natl. Acad. Sci.* **73**:1034–1037.

Moss, J., Fishman, P. H., Richards, R. L., Alving, C. R., Vaughan, M., and Brady, R. O., 1976*b*, Choleragen-mediated release of trapped glucose from liposomes containing ganglioside G_{M1}, *Proc. Natl. Acad. Sci.* **73**:3480–3483.

Moss, J., Manganiello, V. C., and Fishman, P. H., 1977*a*, Enzymatic and chemical oxidation of gangliosides in cultured cells: effects of choleragen, *Biochemistry* **16**:1876–1881.

Moss, J., Osborne, J. C., Fishman, P. H., Brewer, H. P., Vaughan, M., and Brady, R. O., 1977*b*, Effect of gangliosides and substrate analogues on the hydrolysis of nicotinamide adenine dinucleotide by choleragen, *Proc. Natl. Acad. Sci.* **74**:74–78.

Moss, J., Richards, R. L., Alving, C. R., and Fishman, H. P., 1977*c*, Effect of the A and B protomers of choleragen on release of trapped glucose liposomes containing or lacking ganglioside G_{M1}, *J. Biol. Chem.* **252**:797–798.

Mraz, M., Schwarzmann, G., Sattler, J., Seeman, B., Momoi, T., and Wiegandt, H., 1979,

Aggregate formation of gangliosides in water, *Glyconjugates, Proceedings of the 5th International Symposium,* pp. 112–113, Kiel Thieme, Stuttgart.

Mraz, M., Schwarzmann, G., Sattler, J., Momoi, T., Seemann, B., and Wiegandt, H., 1980, Aggregate formation of gangliosides at low concentrations in aqueous media, *Hoppe Seylers Z. Physiol. Chem.* **361**:177–185.

Mullin, B. R., Aloj, S. M., Fishman, P. H., Lee, G., Kohn, L. D., and Brady, R. O., 1976*a,* Cholera toxin interactions with thyrotropin receptors on thyroid plasma membranes, *Proc. Natl. Acad. Sci.* **73**:1679–1683.

Mullin, B. R., Fishman, P. H., Lee, G., Aloj, S. M., Ledley, F. D., Winand, R. J., Kohn, L. D., and Brady, R. O., 1976*b,* Thyrotropin ganglioside interactions and their relationship to the structure and function of thyrotropin receptors, *Proc. Natl. Acad. Sci.* **73**:842–846.

Murray, R. K., Chatterjee, S, and Yogeeswaran, G., 1973, Glycolipids, cultured cells and neoplastic transformation, *PAABS Pan. Am. Assoc. Biochem. Soc.* **2**:721–735.

Nagai, Y., and Hoshi, M., 1975, Sialosphingolipids of sea urchin eggs and spermatozoa showing a characteristic composition for species and gamete, *Biochim. Biophys. Acta* **388**:146–151.

Nagai, Y., and Ohsawa, T., 1974, Production of high titer antisera against sialosphingolipids and their characterization using sensitized liposomes, *Jpn. J. Exp. Med.* **44**:451–464.

Nagai, Y. Momoi, T., Saito, M., Mitsuzawa, E., and Ohtani, S., 1976, Ganglioside syndrome, a new autoimmune neurologic disorder, experimentally induced with brain gangliosides, *Neurosci. Lett.* **2**:107–111.

Nagai, Y., Uchida, T., Takeda, Sh., and Ikuta, F., 1978, Restoration of activity for induction of experimental allergic peripheral neuritis by a combination of mylin basic protein P_2 and gangliosides from peripheral nerve, *Neurosci. Lett.* **8**:247–254.

Naiki, M., Marcus, D. M., and Ledeen, R., 1974, Properties of antisera to ganglioside G_{M1} and asialo G_{M1}, *J. Immunol.* **113**:84–93.

Narasimhan, R., and Murray, R. K., 1978, Comparative study of the glycosphingolipids of chicken Bursa of Fabricius and of chicken, rat and human thymus, *Biochem. J.* **173**:475–482.

Narasimhan, R., Murray, R. K., and Maclennan, D. H., 1974, Presence of glycosphingolipids in the sacroplasmic reticulum fraction of rabbit skeletal muscle, *FEBS Lett.* **43**:23–26.

Narasimhan, R., Hay, J. B., Greaves, M. F., and Murray, R. K., 1976, studies on the glycolipids of sheep thymus and of normal and concanavalin A-stimulated sheep peripheral lymphocytes, *Biochim. Biophys. Acta* **431**:578–591.

Nieman, H., Watanabe, K., and Hakomori, S-I., 1978, Blood group i and I activities of "lacto-*N*-norhexaosyl-ceramide" and its analogues: the structural requirements for i-specificities, *Biochem. Biophys. Res. Commun.* **81**:1286–1293.

Norden, A. G. W., and O'Brien, J. S., 1975, An electrophoretic variant of β-galactosidase with altered catalytic properties in a patient with GM_1 gangliosidosis, *Proc. Natl. Acad. Sci.* **72**:240–244.

Norton, W. T., and Poduslo, S. E., 1971, Neuronal perikarya and astroglia of rat brain chemical composition during myelination, *J. Lipid Res.* **12**:84–90.

O'Brien, J. S., Okada, S., Ho, M. W., Fillerup, D. L., Veath, M. L., and Adams, K., 1971, Ganglioside storage diseases, *Fed. Proc. Fed. Am. Soc, Exp. Biol.* **30**:956–969.

Ochoa, E. L. M., and Bangham, A. D., 1976 *N*-acetylneuraminic acid molecules as possible serotonin binding sites, *J. Neurochem.* **26**:1193–1198.

Ohman, R., 1970, Metabolism of gangliosides, Elanders Bockdrychkeri Actiebolag, Göteborg Doctor chem. Medicinska Fakultete, University, Göteborg, Sweden.

Ohashi, M., 1979*a,* Structure of ∝-galactosyl unit-containing gangliosides from frog fat body, *Glycoconjugates, Proceedings of the 5th International Symposium,* pp. 53–54. Kiel Thieme, Stuttgart.

Ohashi, M., 1979b, A comparison of the ganglioside distributions of fat tissues in various animals by two-dimensional thin layer chromatoraphy, *Lipids* **14**:52–57.

Ohashi, M., and Yamakawa, T., 1977, Isolation and characterization of glycosphingolipids in pig adipose tissue, *J. Biochem.* **81**:1675–1690.

Ohsawa, T., and Nagai, Y., 1975, Immunological evidence for the localization of sialoglyco-sphingolipids at the cell surface of sea urchin spermatozoa, *Biochim. Biophys. Acta.* **389**:69–83.

Ohsawa, T., Nagai, Y., and Wiegandt, H., 1977, Functional incorporation of gangliosides into liposomes, *Jpn. J. Exp. Med.* **47**:221–222.

Paglini, S., and Zapata, M. T., 1975, Swiss albino mouse brain gangliosides:biophysical studies, *Acta Physiol. Lat. Am.* **25**:188–196.

Pascher, J., 1976, Molecular arrangements in sphingolipids; conformation and hydrogen bonding of ceramide and their implication on membrane stability and permeability, *Biochim. Biophys. Acta* **455**:433–451.

Patt, L. M., and Grimes, W. J., 1974, Cell surface glycolipid and glycoprotein by glycosyltrans-ferases of normal and transformed cells, *J. Biol. Chem.* **249**:4157–4265.

Patt, L. M., Itaya, K, and Hakomori, S.-I., 1978, Retinol induces density-dependent growth inhibition and changes in glycolipids and LETS, *Nature London* **273**:379–381.

Peterson, J., Lospalluto, R., and Finkelstein, R., 1972, Localization of cholera toxin *in vivo, J. Infect. Dis.* **126**:617–628.

Poduslo, S. E., and Norton, W. T., 1973, The lipid composition of isolated brain cells and axons, 4th Meeting of the International Society of Neurochemistry, Tokyo, p. 46.

Portoukalian, J., Zwingelstein, G., Abdul-Malak, N., and Doré, J.-F., 1978, Alteration of gan-gliosides in plasma and red cells of human bearing melanoma tumors, *Biochim. Biophys. Res. Commun.* **85**:916–920.

Poss, A., Dellers, M., and Ruysschaert, J. M., 1978, Evidence for a specific interaction between G_{T1} ganglioside incorporated into bilayer membranes and thyrotropin, *FEBS Lett.* **86**:160–162.

Price, H., Kundu, S., and Ledeen, R., 1975, Structures of gangliosides from bovine adrenal medulla, *Biochemistry* **14**:1512–1518.

Pricer, W. E., and Ashwell, G., 1971, The binding of desialylated glycoproteins by plasma mem-branes of rat liver, *J. Biol. Chem.* **246**:4825–4833.

Radin, N. S., Hof, L., Bradley, R. M., and Brady, R. O., 1969, Lactosyl-ceramide galactosidase: comparison with other sphingolipid hydrolases in developing rat brain, *Brain Res.* **14**:497–505.

Radsak, K., Schwarzmann, G., Slenczka, W. and Wiegandt, H., 1979, Studies on the uptake of exogenous glycolipid by synchronized cells *Glycoconjugates, Proceedings of the 5th Inter-national Symposium,* pp. 448–449 Kiel Thieme, Stuttgart.

Rahmann, H., 1978, Gangliosides and thermal adaptation in vertebrates, *Jpn. J. Exp. Med.* **48**:85–96.

Rapport, M. M., and Graf, L., 1969, Immunochemical reactions of lipids, *Prog. Allergy* **13**:272–331.

Rapport, M. M., and Karpiak, S. E., 1976, Descrimative effects of antiserum to brain constitu-ents on behaviour and EEG activity in the rat, *Res. Comm. Psychol. Psychiatr. Behav.* **1**:115–124.

Rauvala, H., 1976a, Gangliosides of human kidney, *J. Biol. Chem.* **251**:7517–7520.

Rauvala, H., 1976b, Action of Cl. perfr. neuraminidase on gangliosides above and below the CMC of the substrate, *FEBS Lett.* **65**:229–233.

Rauvala, H., 1976c, Isolation and partial characterization of human kidney gangliosides, *Biochim. Biophys. Acta* **424**:284–295.

Ray, E. K., and Bough, H. A., 1978, The effect of herpes virus infection and 2-deoxy-D-glucose on glycosphingolipids in BHK-21 cells, *Virology* **88**:118–127.

Renkonen, O., Gahmberg, C. G., Simons, K., and Käriäinen, L., 1970, Enrichment of gangliosides in plasma membranes of hamster kidney fibroblasts, *Acta Chem. Scand.* **24**:733–735.

Revesz, T., and Greaves, M., 1975, Ligand-induced redistribution of lymphocyte membrane ganglioside G_{M1}, *Nature London* **257**:103–106.

Richardson, C. L., Baker, S. R., Morré, D. J., and Keenan, T. W., 1975, Glycosphingolipid synthesis and tumorigenesis, a role for the golgi apparatus in the origin of specific receptor molecules of the mammalian cell surface, *Biochim. Biophys. Acta* **417**:175–187.

Rickert, S. J., and Sweeley, C. C., 1978, Quantitative analysis of carbohydrate residues of glycoproteins and glycolipids by gas liquid chromatography; an appraisal of experimental details, *J. Chromatogr.* **147**:317–326.

Robert, J., Freysz, L., Sensenbrenner, M., Mandel, P., and Rebel, G., 1975, Gangliosides of glial cells: a comparative study of normal astroblasts in tissue culture and glial cells isolated on sucrose-ficol gradients, *FEBS Lett.* **50**:144–146.

Robbins, P. W., and MacPherson, J. C., 1971, Control of glycolipid synthesis in a cultured hamster cell line, *Nature London* **229**:569–570.

Rösner, H., 1977, Gangliosides, Sialoglycoprotein and acetylcholinesterase in the developing mouse brain, *Wilhelm Roux Arch. Develop. Biol.* **183**:325–335.

Rösner, H., and Schönharting, M., 1977, Bindung von Colchicein an isolierte Ganglioside und gangliosidhaltige Membranen, *Hoppe Seylers Z. Physiol. Chem.* **358**:915–919.

Rösner, H., Wiegandt, H., and Rahman, H., 1973, Sialic acid incorporation into gangliosides and glycoproteins of the fish brain, *J. Neurochem.* **21**:655–665.

Rösner, H., Merz, G., and Rahmann, H., 1979, Binding of *d*-tubocurarine by gangliosides, *Hoppe Seylers Z. Physiol. Chem.* **360**:413–420.

Roseman, S., 1970, The synthesis of complex carbohydrates by multiglycosyltransferase systems and their potential function in intercellular adhesion, *Chem. Phys. Lipid* **5**:270–297.

Rosenberg, A., and Schengrund, C., 1976, *Biological Roles of Sialic Acid*, Plenum Press, New York.

Rosenfelder, G., Young, W. W., and Hakomori, S. J., 1977, Association of the glycolipid pattern with antigenic alteration in the mouse fibroblasts transformed by murine sarcoma virus, *Cancer R.* **37**:1333–1339.

Rosenfelder, G., van Eijk, R. V. W., Monnes, D. A., and Mühlradt, P. F., 1978, glycolipids in mouse thymocytes stimulated by concanavalin A, *Eur. J. Biochem.* **83**:571–580.

Rosenfelder, G., van Eijk, R. V. W., and Muhlradt, P. F., 1979, Carbohydrate labeling of glycolipids from mouse splenocytes- mitogen stimulated B-cell and T-cell show different labeling patterns, *Eur. J. Biochem.* **97**:229–237.

Roth, S., and White, D., 1971, Intercellular contact and cell-surface galactosyl transferase activity, *Proc. Natl. Acad. Sci.* **48**:523–529.

Ruhlig, M. A., and Person, S., 1977, Alterations of neutral glycolipids in cells infected with syncytium producing mutants of herpes simplex virus type 1, *J. Virol.* **24**:602–608.

Rupprecht, E., Hans, Ch., Leonard, G., and Decker, K., 1976, Impaired ganglioside synthesis in rat liver after D-galactosamine administration in vivo, *Biochim. Biophys. Acta* **450**:45–56.

Saida, T., Saida, K., Dorfman, S., Silberberg, D. H., Sumner, A. J., Manning, M. C., Lisak, R. P., and Brown, M. J., 1979, Experimental allergic neuritis induced by sensitization with galactocerebroside *Science* **204**:1103–1106.

Saito, T., and Hakomori, S-I., 1971, Quantitative isolation of total glycosphingolipids from animal cells, *J. Lipid Res.* **12**:257–259.

Saito, M., Sugano, K., and Nagai, Y., 1979, Action of Arthobacter ureafaciens sialidase on sialoglycolipid substrates, *J. Biol. Chem.* **254**:7845–7851.

Sakiyama, H., Gross, S. K., and Robbins, Ph. W., 1972, Glycolipid synthesis in normal and virus-transformed hamster cell lines, *Proc. Natl. Acad. Sci.* **69**:872–876.

Samuelsson, K., and Samuelsson, B., 1970, Gas chromatographic and mass spectrometric studies of synthetic and naturally occurring ceramides, *Chem. Phys. Lipid.* **5**:44–79.

Sandford, P. A., and Conrad, H. E., 1966, The structure of the aerobacter aerogenes A3 (S1) polysaccharide. I. A reexamination using improved procedures for methylation analysis, *Biochemistry* **5**:1508–1516.

Sandhoff, K., 1977, Biochemie der Sphingolipidspeicherkrankheiten, *Angew. Chem.* **89**:283–295.

Sandhoff, K., Conzelmann, E, and Nehrkorn, H., 1977, Specificity of human liver hexosaminidases A and B against glycosphingolipids G_{M2} and G_{A2}, *Hoppe Seylers Z. Physiol. Chem.* **358**:779–787.

Sato, G., (ed.), 1973, *Tissue Culture of the Nervous System,* Plenum Press, New York.

Sattler, J., Wiegandt, H., Stärk, J., Kranz, Th., Ronnenberger, H.-J., Schmidtberger, R., and Zilg, H., 1975, Studies of the subunit structure of cholera toxin, *Eur. J. Biochem.* **57**:309–316.

Sattler, J., Schwarzmann, G., Stärk, J., Ziegler, W., and Wiegandt, H., 1977, Studies of the ligand binding to cholera toxin. II. The hydrophilic moiety of sialoglycolipids, *Hoppe Selyers Z. Physiol. Chem.* **358**:159–163.

Sattler, J., Schwarzmann, G., Knack, J., Röhm, K.-H., and Wiegandt, H., 1978, Studies of the ligand binding to cholera toxin. III. Cooperativity of oligosaccharide binding, *Hoppe Seylers Z. Physiol. Chem.* **359**:719–723.

Schauer, R., 1978, Isolation and characterization of sialic acids, *Methods Enzymol.* **50**:64–89.

Schauer, R., and Faillard, H., 1968, Das Verhalten isomerer NO-Diacetyl-neuraminsäureglykoside im Submaxillarismucin von Pferd und Rind bei Einwirkung bakterieller Neuraminidase, *Hoppe Seylers Z. Physiol. Chem.* **349**:961–968.

Schauer, R., Sander, M., Veh, R. W., and Wember, M., 1979, Resistance of 4-*O*-acetyl-*N*-acyl-neuraminic acids towards the action of fowl plague and Newcastle disease virus neuraminidases, *Glycoconugates, Proceedings of the 5th International Symposium,* pp. 360–361, Kiel Thieme, Stuttgart.

Schauer, R., Veh, R. W., Sander, M., Corfield, A. P., and Wiegandt, H., 1980, "Neuroaminidase-resistant" sialic acid residues of gangliosides, *Adv. Exptl. Med. Biol.* **125**:283–294.

Schengrund, C.-L., and Garrigan, O. W., 1969, A comparative study of gangliosides from the brain of various species, *Lipids* **4**:488–495.

Schengrund, C.-L., and Rosenberg, A., 1970, Intracellular location and properties of bovine brain sialidase, *J. Biol. Chem.* **245**:6196–6200.

Schengrund, C.-L., and Rosenberg, A., 1971, Gangliosides, glycosidases, and sialidase in the brain and eyes of developing chickens, *Biochemistry* **10**:2424–2428.

Schengrund, C.-L., Lausch, R. N. and Rosenberg, A., 1973, Sialidase activity in transformed cells, *J. Biol. Chem.* **248**:4424–4428.

Schwarting, G. A., and Summers, A., 1980, Gangliotetraosylceramide is a T-cell differentiation antigen associated with natural cell-mediated cytotoxicity, *J. Immunol.* **124**:1691–1694.

Schwarzmann, G., 1978, A simple and novel method for tritium labelling of gangliosides and other sphingolipids, *Biochim. Biophys. Acta* **529**:106–114.

Schwarzmann, G., Mraz, W., Sattler, J., Schindler, R. and Wiegandt, H., 1978, Comparison of the interaction of mono- and oligovalent ligands with cholera toxin: demonstration of aggregate formation at low ligand concentration, *Hoppe Seylers Z. Physiol. Chem.* **359**:1277–1286.

Sedlacek, H. H., Stärk, J., Seiler, F. R., Ziegler, W., and Wiegandt, H., 1976, Cholera toxin induced redistribution of sialoglycolipid receptor at the lymphocyte membrane, *FEBS Lett.* **61**:272–276.

Seiler, F. R., Sedlacek, H. H., Lüben, G., and Wiegandt, H., 1976, Alteration of the lymphocyte surface by vibrio cholerase neuraminidase, gangliosides and lysolecithins, *Behring Inst. Mitt.* **59**:22–29.

Sela, B.-A., 1980, Splenocytes incorporated with exogenous gangliosides induce a mixed lymphocyte reaction in autologous lymphocytes *Cell. Immunol.* **49**:196–201.

Sela, B.-A., Raz, A., and Geiger, B., 1978, Antibodies to ganglioside G_{M1} induce mitogenic stimulation and cap formation in rat thymocytes, *Eur. J. Immunol.* **8**:268–274.

Seyama, Y., and Yamakawa, T., 1974, Chemical structure of glycolipid of guinea pig red blood cell membrane, *J. Biochem.* **75**:837–842.

Seyama, Y., Yamakawa, T., Komai, T., 1968, Application of isotope dilution method to microanalytical determination of five classes of sphingolipids in tissues, *J. Biochem.* **64**:487–493.

Shapiro, D., and Rachaman, S., 1964, Total synthesis of cytolipin H, *Nature London* **201**:878–879.

Shapiro, D, Segal, H. and Flowers, H. W., 1957, The total synthesis of sphingosine, *J. Am. Chem. Soc.* **80**:1194–1197.

Shapiro, D., Acker, A. J., and Robinsohn, Y., 1973, Studies in the ganglioside series. VIII. Total synthesis of Tay-Sachs' globoside, *Chem. Phys. Lipid.* **10**:28–36.

Sharom, F. J., and Grant, C. W. M., 1978, A model for ganglioside behaviour in cell membranes, *Biochim. Biophys. Acta* **507**:280–293.

Sheahan, B. J., Roche, E., and Donelly, W. Y. C., 1977, Studies on cultured skin fibroblasts from calves with G_{M1}-gangliosidosis, *J. Comp. Pathol.* **87**:205–211.

Shoyama, Y., Okabe, H., Kishimoto, Y., and Costello, C., 1978, Total synthesis of stereospecific sphingosine and ceramide, *J. Lipid Res.* **19**:250–259.

Siddiqui, B, and Hakomori, S-I., 1970, Change of glycolipid pattern in Morris hepatomas 5123 and 7800, *Cancer Res.* **30**:2930–2936.

Siddiqui, B., and McCluer, R. H., 1968, Lipidcomponents of sialosylgalactosylceramide of human brain, *J. Lipid Res.* **9**:366–370.

Sillerud, L. O., Prestegard, J. M., Yu, R. K., Schafer, D. E., and Konigsberg, W. H., 1978, Assignment of the ^{13}C nuclear magnetic resonance spectrum of aqueous ganglioside G_{M1} micelles, *Biochemistry* **17**:2619–2628.

Simmons, J. L., Fishman, P. H., Freese, E., and Brady, R. O., 1975, Morphological alterations and ganglioside sialyltransferase activity induced by small fatty acids in Hela cells, *J. Cell Biol.* **66**:414–425.

Simpson, L. L., and Rapport, M. M., 1971, Ganglioside interaction with botulinum toxin, *J. Neurochem.* **18**:1341–1343.

Skipski, V. P., Katopodis, N., Prendergast, J. S. and Stock, C. C., 1975, Gangliosides in blood serum of normal rat and Morris hepatoma 5123tc-bearing rats, *Biochem. Biophys. Res. Commun.* **67**:1122–1127.

Smid, F., and Reinisova, J., 1973, A densitometric method for the determination of gangliosides after their separation by thin layer chromatography and detection with resorcinol reagent, *J. Chromatogr.* **86**:200–204.

Sonnino, S., Ghidoni, R., Galli, G., and Tettamanti, G., 1978, On the structure of a new, fucose containing ganglioside from pig cerebellum, *J. Neurochem.* **31**:947–956.

Sonnino, S., Ghidoni, R., Marchesini, S., and Tettamanti, G., 1979, Cytosolic gangliosides: occurrence in calf brain as ganglioside-protein complexes, *J. Neurochem.* **33**:117–121.

Spranger, J., and Cantz, M., 1978, Mucolopidosis I, the cherry red-spot-myoclonus syndrome and neuraminidase deficiency, *Birth Defects* **14**:105–112.

Spranger, J., Gehler, J., and Cantz, M., 1977, Mucolipidosis I—a sialidosis, *Am. J. Med. Genet.* **1**:21–29.

Stärk, J., Ronneberger, H. J., Wiegandt, H., and Ziegler, W., 1974, Interaction of ganglioside $G_{Gtet}1$ and its derivatives with choleragen, *Eur. J. Biochem.* **48**:103–110.

Steigerwald, J. C., Basu, S., Kaufman, B., and Roseman, S., 1975, Enzymatic synthesis of Tay-Sachs ganglioside, *J. Biol. Chem.* **250**:6727–6734.

Stein-Douglas, K., Schwarting, G. A., Naiki, M., and Mareus, D. M., 1976, Gangliosides as markers for murine lymphocyte subpopulations, *J. Exp. Med.* **143**:822–832.

Stellner, K., Saito, H., and Hakomori, S-I., 1973, Determination of aminosugar linkages in glycolipids by methylation. Amino sugar linkages of ceramide pentasaccharides of rabbit erythrocytes and of Forssman antigen. *Arch. Biochem. Biophys.* **155**:464–472.

Stoeckel, K., Schwab, M., and Thoenen, H., 1975, Comparison between the retrogade axonal transport of nerve growth factor and tetanus toxin in motor, sensory and adrenergic neurons, *Brain Res.* **99**:1–16.

Stoeckel, K., Schwab, M., and Thoenen, H., 1977, Role of gangliosides in the uptake and retrograde axonal transport of cholera and tetanus toxin as compared to nerve growth factor and wheat germ agglutinin, *Brain Res.* **132**:273–285.

Stoffel, W., and Sorgo, W., 1976, Asymmetry of the lipid-bilayer of sindbis virus, *Chem. Phys. Lipid.* **17**:324–335.

Stoker, M., and MacPherson, J., 1961, Studies on transformation of hamster cells by polyoma virus *in vitro, Virology* **14**:359–370.

Stoolmiller, A. C., Dawson, G., and Kemp, St. F., 1974, Regulation of ganglioside synthesis in mouse neuroblastoma cells (INB 41A and NE2a) in tissue culture, *Fed. Proc. Fed. Am. Soc. Exp. Biol.* **33**:1212.

Stoolmiller, A. C., Dawson, G., and Schachner, M., 1975, Comparison of glycosphingolipid metabolism in mouse glial tumors and cultured cell strains of neural origin, *Fed. Proc. Fed. Am. Soc. Exp. Biol.* **34**:634.

Strombeck, D. R., and Harrold, D., 1974, Binding of cholera toxin to mucins and inhibition by gastric mucin, *Infect. Immun.* **10**:1266–1272.

Sugano, K., Saito, M. and Nagai, Y., 1978, Susceptibility of ganglioside GM_1 to a new bacterial neuraminidase, *FEBS Lett.* **89**:321–325.

Sugita, M., 1979*a*, Studies on the glucosphingolipids of the starfish *Asterina pectinifera*, 2. Isolation and characterization of a novel ganglioside with an internal sialic acid residue, *J. Biochem.* **86**:289–300.

Sugita, M., 1979*b*, Studies on the glycosphingolipids of the starfish, *Asterina pectinifera*, 3. Isolation and structural studies of two novel gangliosides containing internal sialic acid residues, *J. Biochem.* **86**:765–772.

Sugita, M. and Hori, T., 1976, New types of gangliosides in star fish with sialic acid residues in the inner part of their carbohydrate chains, *J. Biochem.* **80**:637–640.

Suttajit, M. and Winzler, R. J., 1971, Effect of modification of *N*-acetylneuraminic acid on the binding of glycoproteins to influenza virus and on suspectibility to cleavage by neuraminidase, *J. Biol. Chem.* **246**:3398–3404.

Suzuki, A., Ishizuka, I., and Yamakawa, T., 1975, Isolation and characterization of a ganglioside containing fucose from boar testis, *J. Biochem.* **78**:947–954.

Suzuki, K., 1965, The pattern of mammalian brain gangliosides—II Evaluation of the extraction procedures, postmortem changes and the effect of formalin preservation, *J. Neurochem.* **12**:629–638.

Suzuki, Y., and Suzuki, K., 1972, Specific radioactive labeling of terminal *N*-acetylgalactosa-mine of glycosphingolipids by the galactose oxidase—sodium borohydride method, *J. Lipid Res.* 13:687–690.

Svennerholm, L., 1974, Sphingolipid changes during development, pre- and postnatal development of the human brain, *Mod. Probl. Paediatr.* 13:104–115.

Svennerholm, L., 1976, Interaction of cholera toxin and ganglioside G_{M1}, *Adv. Exp. Med. Biol.* 71:191–204.

Svennerhom, L., Bruce, A., Mansson, J. E., Raynsmark, B. M., and Vanier, M. T., 1972, Sphin-golipids of human skeletal muscle Biochim. *Biochim. Biophys. Acta* 280:626–636.

Svennerholm, L., Mansson, J. E., and Li, Y.-T., 1973, Isolation and structural determination of a novel ganglioside, a disialosylpenta-hexaosylceramide from human brain, *J. Biol. Chem.* 248:740–742.

Sweeley, C. C., and Dawson, G., 1969, Determination of glycosphingolipid structures by mass spectrometry, *Biochem. Biophys. Res. Commun.* 37:6–14.

Takeda, J., Takeda, T., Honda, T., and Miwatani, T., 1976, Inactivation of the biological activ-ities of the thermostable direct hemolysin of *Vibrio parahaemolyticus* by ganglioside G_{T1}, *Infect. Immun.* 14:1–5.

Taketomi, T., and Kawamura, N., 1970, Preparation of lysohematoside (neuraminyl-galactosyl-glycosyl-sphingosin) from hematoside of equine erythrocyte and its chemical and hemolytic properties, *J. Biochem. Tokyo* 68:475–485.

Taketomi, T., Hara, A., and Uemura, K., 1975, Immunochemical studies of lipids, IV. Chemical modification of Forssman globoside and immunological activities, *Jpn. J. Exp. Med.* 45:293–298.

Tallman, J. F., and Brady, R. O., 1972, The catabolism of Tay-Sachs ganglioside in rat bain lysosomes, *J. Biochem. Chem.* 247:7570–7575.

Tallman, J. F., and Brady, R. O., 1973, The purification and properties of a mammalian neur-aminidase (sialidase), *Biochim. Biophys. Acta* 293:434–443.

Tamai, Y., Araki, S. M., Katsuto, K., and Satake, M., 1974, Molecular composition of the sub-microsomal membranes lipid of rat brain, *J. Cell Biol.* 63:749–758.

Tettamanti, G., Bertona, L., Berra, B., and Zambotti, V., 1965, Glycolyl-neuraminic acid in ox brain gangliosides, *Nature London* 206:192.

Tettamanti, G., Morgan, J. G., Gombos, G., Vincendon, G., and Mandel, P., 1972, Sub-synap-tosomal localisation of brain particulate neuraminidase, *Brain Res.* 47:515–518.

Tettamanti, G., Bonali, F., Marchesini, S. and Zambotti, V., 1973, A new procedure for the extraction, purification and fractionation of brain gangliosides, *Biochim. Biophys. Acta* 296:160–170.

Tiffany, J. M., 1973, Artificial lipoprotein membranes as models for virus-cell surface interac-tions, *Membr. Mediat. Inform.* 2:103–146.

Tosteson, M. T., and Tosteson, D. C., 1978, Bilayers containing gangliosides develop channels when exposed to cholera toxin, *Nature London* 275:142–144.

Triggle, D. J., 1971 *Neurotransmitter-Receptor Interactions,* Academic Press, New York.

Uemura, K., Yuzawa, M., and Taketomi, T., 1978, characterization of major glycolipids in bovine erythrocyte membrane, *J. Biochem.* 83:463–471.

Ueno, K., Ishizuka, I., and Yamakawa, T., 1975, Glycolipids of fish testis, *J. Biochem.* 77:1223–1232.

Ueno, K., Ando, S., and Yu, R. K., 1978, Gangliosides of human, cat, and rabbit spinal cords and cord myelin, *J. Lipid Res.* 19:863–871.

Utchida, Y., Tsukada, Y., and Sugimor, T., 1976, Abstract, 5th Fermentology Symposium, p. 267.

Vakirtzi-Lemonias, C., and Evangelatos, G. P., 1978, Effect of puromycin and cycloheximid on glycosphingolipid biosynthesis in PHA-stimulated human lymphocytes. *Biochem. Biophys. Res. Commun.* **85**:1488–1495.

van Heyningen, S., 1974, Cholera toxin: interaction of subunits with ganglioside G_{M1}, *Science* **183**:656–657.

van Heyningen, S., 1976, Binding of ganglioside by the chains of tetanus toxin, *FEBS Lett.* **68**:5–7.

van Heyningen, W. E., 1959*a*, The fixation of tetanus toxin by nervous tissue, *J. Gen. Microbiol.* **20**:291–300.

van Heyningen, W. E., 1959*b*, Chemical assay of the tetanus toxin receptor in nervous tissue, *J. Gen. Microbiol.* **20**:301–309.

van Heyningen, W. E., 1959*c*, Tentative identification of the tetanus toxin receptor in nervous tissue, *J. Gen. Microbiol.* **20**:310–320.

van Heyningen, W. E., 1963, The fixation of tetanus toxin, strychnine, serotonin and other substances by gangliosides, *J. Gen. Microbiol.* **31**:375–387.

van Heyningen, W. E., 1974, Gangliosides as membrane receptors for tetanus toxin, cholera toxin and serotonin, *Nature London* **249**:415–417.

van Heyningen, W. E., and Mellanby, J., 1968, The effect of cerebroside and other lipids on the fixation of tetanus toxin by gangliosides, *J. Gen. Microbiol.* **52**:447–454.

van Heyningen, W. E., Carpenter, C. J., Pierce, N., Frank and Greenough, W. B., 1971, Desactivation of cholera toxin by ganglioside, *J. Infect. Dis.* **124**:415–418.

van Hoof, F., 1973, in: *Lysosomes and Storage Diseases,* (H. G. Hers and F. van Hoof, eds), p. 5305 Academic Press, New York.

Veh, R. W., Corfield, A. P., Sander, M., and Schauer, R., 1977, Neuraminic acid-specific modification and tritium labelling of gangliosides, *Biochim. Biophys. Acta* **486**:145–160.

Vengries, V. E., Reynolds, F. H., Hollenberg, M. D., and Pitha, P. M., 1976, Interferon action; role of membrane gangliosides, *Virology* **72**:486–493.

Visser, A. and Emmelot, P., 1973, Studies on plasma membranes. XX. Sialidase in hepatic plasma membranes, *J. Membrane Biol.* **14**:73–84.

Wang, T. J. Freimuth, W. W., Müller, H. C., and Esselman, W. J., 1978, Thy-1 antigenicity is associated with glycolipid of brain and thymocytes, *J. Immunol.* **121**:1361–1365.

Warren, L., Critchley, D., and MacPherson, I., 1972, Surface glycoproteins and glycolipids of chicken embryo cells transformed by a temperature-sensitive mutant of rous sarcoma virus *Nature London* **235**:275–277.

Wassermann, A., and Takaki, T., 1898, Über tetanus antitoxische Eigenschaften des normalen Centralnervensystems, *Ber. Klin. Wschr.* **35**:5–6.

Watanabe, K., and Hakomori, S.-I., 1979, Ganglioside of human erythrocytes. A novel ganglioside with a unique *N*-Acetyneuraminosyl-(2→3)- *N*-acetylgalactosamine structure, *Biochemistry* **18**:5502–5504.

Watanabe, K., Stellner, K., Yogeeswaran, G., and Hakomori, S. I., 1974, A branchend, long chain neutral glycolipid and gangliosides of human erythrocytes membranes. *Fed. Proc. Fed. Proc. Am. Soc. Exp. Biol.* **33**:1225.

Watanabe, K., Laine, R. A., and Hakomori, S-I., 1975, On neutral fucoglycolipids having long, branched carbohydrate chains: H-active and I-active glycosphingolipids of human erythrocytes membranes, *Biochemistry* **14**:2725–2733.

Watanabe, K., Powell, M., and Hakomori, S-I., 1978, Isolation and characterization of a novel fucoganglioside of human erythrocyte membranes, *J. Biol. Chem.* **253**:8962–8967.

Watanabe, K., Powell, M., and Hakomori, S-I., 1979*b*, Isolation and characterization of gangliosides with a new sialosyl linkage and core structures from human erythrocyte membranes. *Glycoconjugates. Proceedings of the 5th International Symposium*, p. 48, Kiel Thieme, Stuttgart.

Watanabe, K., Powell, M. E., and Hakomori, S.-I., 1979*b*, Isolation and characterisation of gangliosides with a new sialosyl linkage and core structure, *J. Biol. Chem.* 254:8223–8229.

Weinstein, D. B., Marsh, J. B., Glick, M. C., and Warren, L., 1970, Membranes of animal cells VI. The glycolipids of the L cell and its surface membrane, *J. Biol. Chem.* 245:3928–3937.

Wenger, D. A. and Wardell, S., 1973*a*, Action of neuraminidase from Cl. perfr. on Tay-Sachs ganglioside, *Physiol. Chem. Phys.* 4:224–230.

Wenger, D. A., Wardell, S., 1973*b*, Action of neuraminidase (EC 3.2.1.18) clostridium perfringens on brain gangliosides in the presence of bile salts, *J. Neurochem.* 20:607–616.

Werries, E., and Buddecke, E., 1973, Detection of α-glycosidic bands in the ganglioside G_{M1} by stereospecific enzymatic degradation, *Eur. J. Biochem.* 37:535–540.

Wherrett, J. R., 1973, Characterization of the major ganglioside in human red cells and of a related tetrahexosyl ceramide in white cells, *Biochim. Biophys. Acta* 326:63–73.

Wiegandt, H., 1967, The subcellular localization of gangliosides, *J. Neurochem.* 14:671–674.

Wiegandt, H., 1968, Structure and function of gangliosides, *Angew. Chem.* 80:89–98.

Wiegandt, H., 1971, Glycosphingolipids, *Adv. Lipid Res.* 9:249–289.

Wiegandt, H., 1973, Gangliosides of extraneural organs, *Z. Physiol. Chem.* 354:1049–1056.

Wiegandt, H., 1974, Monosialo-lactoisohexaosyl-ceramide: a ganglioside from human spleen, *Eur. J. Biochem.* 45:367–369.

Wiegandt, H., 1979, Toxin interactions with glycoconjugates, *Adv. Cytopharm.* 3:17–25.

Wiegandt, H., and Bücking, H. W., 1970, Carbohydrate components of extraneural gangliosides from bovine and human spleen, and bovine kidney, *Eur. J. Biochem.* 15:287–292.

Wiegandt, H., and Egge, H., 1970, Oligosaccharide der Frauenmilch, *Fortschr. Chem. Organ. Naturst.* 28:404–428.

Wiegandt, H., and Schulze, B., 1969, Spleen gangliosides: the structure of ganglioside $G_{Lntet}1$, *Z. Naturforsch. Teil B* 24:945–946.

Wiegandt, H., and Ziegler, W., 1974, Synthetic glycolipids containing glycosphingolipid-derived oligosaccharides *Hoppe Seylers Z. Physiol. Chem.* 355:11–18.

Wiegandt, H., Ziegler, W., Stärk, J., Kranz, Th, Ronnenberger, H. J., Zilg, H., Karlson, K.-A., and Samuelson, B. E., 1976, Studies of the ligand binding to cholera toxin I. The lipophilic moiety of sialoglycolipids, *Hoppe Seylers Z. Physiol. Chem.* 357:1637–1646.

Windeler, A., and Feldman, G. L., 1969, Silver acetate for stabilizing methyl galactosides after methanolysis of glycolipids, *Lipids* 4:167–168.

Windeler, A., and Feldman, G. L., 1970, The isolation and partial structural characterization of some ocular gangliosides, *Biochem. Biophys. Acta* 202:361–366.

Winterbourn, C. C., 1971, Separation of brain gangliosides by chromatography on DEAE-Cellulose, *J. Neurochem.* 18:1153–1155.

Williams, A. F., Barclay, A. N., Letarte-Muirhead, M., and Morris, A. J., 1977, Rat Thy-1 antigens from thymus and brain: their tissue distribution, purification and chemical composition. *Cold Spring Harbor Symp. Quant. Biol.* 41:51–61.

Wolfe, B. A., and Robbins, P. W., 1974, Cell mitotic cycle synthesis of NIL hamster glycolipids including the Forssman antigen, *J. Cell Biol.* 61:676–687.

Wooley, D. W., and Gommi, B. W., 1964, Serotonin receptors: V, selective destruction by neuramindase and reactivation with tissue lipids, *Nature London* 202:1074.

Woolley, D. W., and Gommi, B. W., 1965, Serotonin receptors, VII. Activities of various pure gangliosides as the receptor, *Proc. Natl. Acad. Sci.* 53:959–963.

Yamashita, K., Tachibana, Y., and Kobata, A., 1977, Oligosaccharides of human milk, *J. Biol. Chem.* 252:5408–5411.

Yates, A. J., and Thompson, D., 1977, An improved assay of gangliosides separated by thin-layer chromatography, *J. Lipid Res.* **18**:660–663.

Yates, A. J. and Wherrett, J. R., 1974, Changes in the sciatic nerve of the rabbit and its tissue constituents during development, *J. Neurochem.* **23**:993–1003.

Yeung, K. K., Moskal, J. R., Chien, J. L., Gardener, D. A., and Basu, S., 1974, Biosynthesis of globoside and Forssman-related glycosphingolipids in mouse adrenal Y-1 tumor cells, *Biochem. Biophys. Res. Commun.* **59**:252–260.

Yip, M. C., 1972, The enzymic synthesis of gangliosides: uridine diphosphate galactose: N-acetylgalactosaminyl-(N-acetylneuraminyl)-galactosyl-glucosyl ceramide galactosyltransfer-ase in rat tissues, *Biochim. Biophys. Acta* **273**:374–379.

Yip, M. C., and Dain, J. A., 1970, The enzymic synthesis of ganglioside. II. UDP-galactose: N-acetylgalactosaminyl-(N-acetylneuraminyl)-galactosyl-glucosyl ceramide galactosyltrans-ferase in rat brain, *Biochim. Biophys. Acta* **206**:252–260.

Yogeeswaran, G., and Hakomori, S-I., 1975, Cell contact-dependent ganglioside changes in mouse 3T3 fibroblasts and a suppressed sialidase activity on cells contact, *Biochemistry* **14**:2151–2156.

Yogeeswaran, G., and Murray, R. K., 1973, Glycosphingolipids of clonal lines of mouse neuro-blastoma and neuroblastoma X-L-cell hybrids, *J. Biol. Chem.* **248**:1231–1239.

Yogeeswaran, G., Sheinin, R., Wherrett, J. R., and Murray, R. K., 1972, Studies on the glyco-lipids of normal and virally transformed 3T3 mouse fibroblasts, *J. Biol. Chem.* **247**:5146–5158.

Yogeeswaran, G., Murray, R. K., Pearson, M. L., Sanwall, B. D., McMorris, F. A. and Ruddle, F. A., 1973, Glycosphingolipids of clonal lines of mouse neuroblastoma and neuroblastoma XL cell hybrids, *J. Biol. Chem.* **248**:1231–1239.

Yohe, H. C., and Rosenberg, A., 1972, Interaction of triiodide anion with gangliosides in aqueous iodine, *Chem. Phys. Lipid.* **9**:279–294.

Yohe, H. C. and Yu, R. K., 1980, *In vitro* biosynthesis of an isomer of brain trisialoganglioside, G_{T1a}, *J. Biol. Chem.* **255**, 608–613.

Yohe, H. C., Roark, D. E., and Rosenberg, A., 1976, C_{20} Sphingosine as a determining factor in aggregation of gangliosides, *J. Biol. Chem.* **251**:7083–7087.

Young, W. W. and Hakomori, S-I., 1981, Therapy of mouse lymphoma with monoclonal anti-bodies to glycolipid: selection of low antigenic varianta *in vivo, Science* **211**:487–789.

Young, W. W., Laine, R. A., and Hakomori, S-I., 1978, Covalent attachment of glycolipids to solid supporters and macromolecules, *Methods Enzymol.* **50**:137–140.

Young, W. W., Hakomori, S-I., Durdick, J. M., and Henney, C. S., 1980, Identification of gan-glio-N-tetraosylceramide as a new cell surface marker for murine natural killer (NK) cells, *J. Immunol.* **124**:199–201.

Yu, R. K., and Ando, S., 1977, Isolation and characterization of some new ganglioside from brain. Presented at the Seminar on "Structural and Functional Significance of Membrane Glycolipid", Honolulu, Hawaii, Oct. 5–7, 1977.

Yu, R. K., and Iqbal, K., 1979, Gangliosides of human myelin, oligodendroglia and neurons, 6th Meeting of the International Society of Neurochemistry, Copenhagen, p. 547.

Yu, R. K., and Ledeen, R. W., 1971, Gangliosides in bovine and human plasma, *Fed. Proc. Fed. Proc. Am. Soc. Exp. Biol.* **30**:1134.

Yu, R. K., and Ledeen, R. W., 1972, Gangliosides of human bovine and rabbit plasma, *J. Lipid Res.* **13**:680–686.

Yu, R. K., and Lee, S. H., 1976, *In vitro* biosynthesis of sialosylgalactosylceramide (G_7) by mouse brain microsomes, *J. Biol. Chem.* **251**:198–203.

Yu, R. K., Ledeen, R. W., and Eng, L. F., 1974, Ganglioside abnormalities in multiple sclerosis, *J. Neurochem.* **23**:169–174.

Yusuf, H. K. M., Merat, A., and Dickerson, J. W. T., 1977, Effect of development on the gangliosides of human brain, *J. Neurochem.* **28**:1299–1304.

Zhukova, J. G., and Smirnova, G. P., 1969, Occurence of glucofuranose residues in sialoglycolipids from *Echinodermata, Carbohydr. Res.* **9**:366–367.

Zimmerman, J. M., and Gifferetti, J.-Cl., 1977, Interaction of tetanus toxin and toxoid which cultured neuroblastoma cells, *Naunyn Schmiedebergs Arch. Pharmacol.* **296**:271–277.

INDEX